Narrative Discourse in Neurologically Impaired and Normal Aging Adults

Narrative Discourse in Neurologically Impaired and Normal Aging Adults

Edited by
Hiram H. Brownell
Boston College
Aphasia Research Center
Department of Neurology, Boston University School of Medicine
Boston Department of Veterans Affairs Medical Center

and
Yves Joanette
Laboratoire Th.-Alajouanine
Centre de recherche du C. H. Côte-des-Neiges
Ecole d'orthophonie et d'audiologie
Faculté de médicine, Université de Montréal

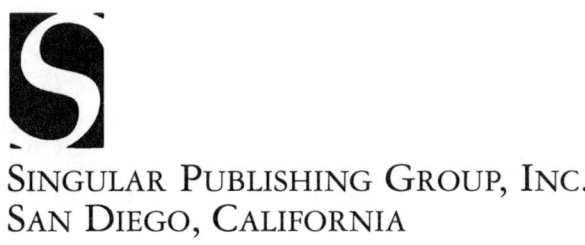

SINGULAR PUBLISHING GROUP, INC.
SAN DIEGO, CALIFORNIA

Singular Publishing Group, Inc.
4284 41st Street
San Diego, California 92105-1197

© 1993 by Singular Publishing Group, Inc.

All rights, including that of translation reserved. No part of this publication may be reproduced, stored in a retrieval system, or transmitted in any form or by any means, electronic, mechanical, recording, or otherwise, without the prior written permission of the publisher.

Typeset in 10/12 Palatino by So Cal Graphics
Printed in the United States of America by BookCrafters

Library of Congress Cataloging-in-Publication Data

Narrative discourse in neurologically impaired and normal aging adults / edited by Hiram H. Brownell and Yves Joanette.
    p. cm.
    Includes bibliographical references and index.
    ISBN 1-56593-083-5
    1. Language disorders in old age—Congresses. 2. Neuropsychiatry—Congresses. 3. Aphasia—Congresses. 4. Cognition disorders in old age—Congresses. 5. Verbal learning in old age—Congresses. I. Brownell, Hiram H. II. Joanette, Yves.
    [DNLM: 1. Verbal behavior—congresses. 2. Verbal behavior—in old age—congresses. 3. Aphasia—congresses. 4. Brain Damage, Chronic—congresses. WM 475 N234 1993]
RC429.N37 1993
618.97'6855—dc20
DNLM/DLC
for Library of Congress   93-15128
                                                                                CIP

Contents

Preface vii

Contributors xii

Addresses for Correspondence xiv

PART I THEORETICAL CONSIDERATIONS

1. Levels of Approach to Discourse 3
   Michel Fayol and Patrick Lemaire

2. Computational and Psychological Models of Discourse 23
   Peter C. Gordon

3. A Neurosemiotic Perspective on Text Processing 47
   Peter Grzybek

PART II NARRATIVE CAPACITIES OF HEALTHY ELDERLY SUBJECTS

4. Assessment of Intraindividual Change in Text Recall of Elderly Adults 77
   Roger A. Dixon, Christopher Hertzog, Ingrid C. Friesen, and David F. Hultsch

5. Qualitative Differences in Working Memory and Discourse Comprehension in Normal Aging 103
   Helen J. Kahn and Danielle Cordon

6. The Effect of Normal Aging on Discourse: A Sociolinguistic Approach 115
   William Labov and Julie Auger

7. Narrative Discourse Processing in Normal Aging: A Neuropsychological and Comparative Study 135
   Claudio L. N. Guimaraes dos Santos and Jean-Luc Nespoulous

PART III NARRATIVE CAPACITIES OF PATIENTS WITH FOCAL BRAIN DAMAGE

8. Comprehension of Narrative Discourse by Aphasic Listeners 151
   Robert H. Brookshire and Linda E. Nicholas

9.	Selected Aspects of Narratives in Polish-Speaking Aphasics as Illustrated by Aesop's Fables *Hanna K. Ulatowska, Maria Sadowska, Jan Kordys, and Danuta Kadzielawa*	171
10.	Discourse Production Patterns in Neurologically Impaired and Aged Populations *Guila Glosser*	191
11.	Contextual and Thematic Influences on Narrative Comprehension of Left and Right Hemisphere Brain-Damaged Patients *Monica Strauss Hough and Robert S. Pierce*	213
12.	Conceptual Processing of Discourse by a Right Hemisphere Brain-Damaged Patient *Carl H. Frederiksen and Brigitte Stemmer*	239
13.	Narrative Expressive Deficits Associated with Right Hemisphere Damage *Penelope S. Myers*	279

PART IV NARRATIVE CAPACITIES OF PATIENTS WITH DEMENTIA

14.	Narrative Schema in Dementia of the Alzheimer's Type *Bernadette Ska and Dominique Guénard*	299
15.	Narrative Discourse in Dementia *Dominique Cardebat, Jean-François Démonet, and Bernard Doyon*	317
Index		333

Preface

Language provides the primary means for people to interact with and understand their world. While language and its disorders are usually analyzed in terms of individual phonemes, words, or sentences, a moment's reflection shows that natural communication transcends isolated words or sentences. In fact, the basic unit of communication is the discourse, whether it be actualized as a series of sentences or even a single word (e.g., "Oh!"). The focus of this book is on one particular type of multisentential text, narrative discourse, which refers to the ways in which people link together the bits and pieces of language to create representations of events, objects, beliefs, personalities, and experiences. The key aspect of narrative discourse, which distinguishes it from simple lists of sentences, is the notion of structure—how the component parts of a "text" relate to one another to form a coherent whole. Thus, the primary goal of this field can be summarized as the characterization of the structure of discourse and the processes needed to create and communicate that structure.

Because narrative discourse involves so many aspects of human language and cognition, it has been the subject of investigation by researchers working in a number of different fields. In assembling the present studies, we have tried to provide a unique and balanced perspective, one that represents the range of approaches taken to studying narrative. Although there are already several edited books and even journals devoted to this general area of inquiry, most of the recent literature represents the mainstream in cognitive science and reports studies using what could be termed the "standard" subject population, that is, English-speaking college students. Certainly, this research tradition provides the basis for many of the studies discussed in the present collection, and some chapters report refinements and new applications of existing cognitive models. In addition, though, our book includes discussion of relevant work that is not routinely cited (e.g., studies in semiotics) and of new techniques (e.g., on-line analysis of brain activity during narrative processing) that represent important avenues for future investigation. Also, as complements to studies done with college student subjects, we offer reports of narrative ability in alternative populations including healthy elderly subjects, dementing patients, focally brain-injured patients, and speakers of languages other than English. Some of these chapters provide a clinically useful perspective on how different people's narrative abilities vary, and all of them represent means of testing current views of narrative which may have been developed in other disciplines. As a whole, then, this volume provides an up-to-date review that fairly represents the richness and diversity of work on narrative discourse, including research that has been done on the effects of brain damage on verbal communication abilities. We intend the book to be of interest to audiences in neuropsychology, speech-language pathology, cognitive psychology, linguistics, and, most generally, to researchers and students in any branch of cognitive science.

The chapters in this book are organized around four sections that focus on, in order, theoretical considerations, aspects of narrative ability in healthy elderly adults, the effects of focal damage to the right and left cerebral hemispheres, and the effects of diffuse brain damage such as associated with dementia of the Alzheimer's type. In addition to the citations of common background literature incorporated into the different chapters, readers will no doubt make their own connections while reading through the book. For example, a concept used or referred to in one of the empirical chapters will probably have been presented in the relevant historical and theoretical context in one of the chapters appearing in the first section. In addition, a theoretical framework developed in the introduction to one of the later, empirically oriented chapters should be useful in understanding the performances of other subject populations as well.

The first section contains three chapters which are, themselves, complementary. All three address theoretical aspects of narrative discourse theories. The first one by Michel Fayol and Patrick Lemaire is a general introduction to the different levels of approaches to discourse abilities illustrated by the most frequently studied topic, namely story comprehension. This chapter contains a pertinent review of the different models that can be used in such studies. It should certainly be read by all as a substantive introduction to the book. The two following chapters, one by Peter Gordon and the other by Peter Grzybek, are to some extent expansions on the themes presented in the first chapter. Gordon's chapter presents exciting new work based on a computational model of discourse comprehension. Grzybek's chapter reports extensively on other views of narrative discourse and text processing that incorporate more linguistically based approaches with a definite European flavor. This literature is relevant to current and future work in discourse but will be unfamiliar to many North American researchers. Grzybek also introduces the use of brain-damaged patients for studying narrative ability. All in all, it is hoped that these three chapters will not only benefit readers as they read the others chapters of this book, but will also influence new work in the field of cognitive neuropsychology of text-level impairments.

The second section of this book contains four chapters addressing the narrative capacities of healthy elderly subjects. Indeed, most studies in neuropsychology and aphasiology rely on subjects with stroke or dementia who, apart from their brain damage, are usually older than the typical subjects tested in narrative discourse studies. Because aging, by itself, can be a source of changes in narrative performance, it is of the utmost importance to become acquainted with these characteristics before trying to describe, and interpret, some of the narrative characteristics of brain-damaged patients. The section starts with Roger Dixon and colleagues' chapter discussing intraindividual changes in text recall. Helen Kahn and Danielle Cordon's chapter explores how a reduction in working memory capacity affects the strategies elderly listeners bring to a narrative task. William Labov and Julie Auger's chapter presents longitudinal data that suggest preserved and even increased linguistic sophistication associated with aging. Finally, this section ends with an innovative chapter by Claudio Guimaraes dos Santos and Jean-Luc Nespoulous that discusses some "on-line," neurobiological correlates of discourse processing in aging subjects. This chapter reports one of the very first SPECT studies to focus on narrative abilities in a normal population.

The third section of this book contains the largest number (six) of chapters. These chapters examine different aspects of the narrative abilities of patients who have suffered left- or right-hemisphere focal brain damage. In the case of left-sided damage, the patients are aphasic and typically impaired in many aspects of oral and/or written language. Although discourse and, more generally speaking, text-level abilities can frequently be affected in aphasic patients, these dimensions of communication impairment have not been included in the classical description of aphasia, simply because the necessary conceptual tools have not been available until recently. The situation is quite different for right brain damage, in which case language impairments lie more at the text level in the absence of an aphasia proper. These patients' communicative impairments have also been better described in recent years since the development of theories and associated empirical techniques for analyzing text-level processing. The first chapter in this section by Robert Brookshire and Linda Nicholas presents an accessible outline of major issues bearing on the comprehension abilities of aphasic patients and also summarizes a large body of empirical work. The contribution of Hanna Ulatowska and her colleagues similarly focuses on aphasic subjects, but who are speakers of Polish. Also, these authors have developed an original approach by virtue of using a distinctive type of narrative, that is, Aesop's fables, to evaluate subjects' narrative abilities. The next chapter by Guila Glosser illustrates a neuropsychological approach to distinguishing impairments at the narrative level from those at other levels of linguistic analysis. By testing for selective deficits in brain-injured patients, researchers can identify the component parts of discourse ability and how each component contributes to the creation of a narrative. Working within this tradition, Glosser reports comparisons of performances of normal elderly subjects, patients with focal, unilateral left and right brain damage, and patients with diffuse brain injury. The chapter by Monica Hough and Robert

Pierce represents a link between the previous chapters and the next ones. It reviews an extensive series of studies addressing specifically the contextual and thematic influences on narrative comprehension by both left- and right-brain-damaged patients and shows how narrative abilities can be dissociated by unilateral brain damage. The chapter by Penelope Myers is special because it discusses the expressive performance of right-brain-damaged patients and analyzes narrative performance in the context of their other cognitive abnormalities. Finally, the chapter by Carl Frederiksen and Brigitte Stemmer illustrates the case study approach. These authors use a fully elaborated model, such as described in the opening section of the book, as a basis for a theoretically detailed investigation of a single right-brain-damaged patient's narrative processing.

The chapters included in the last section review the narrative abilities of demented populations. Historically, diffusely brain-damaged patients have attracted the attention of aphasiologists and neuropsychologists interested in the effects of brain damage on text-level processes. Indeed, many of the early studies were performed using this population. The two chapters in this section represent state-of-the-art efforts. The first one is by Bernadette Ska and Dominique Guénard who use one of the theoretical frameworks presented in Fayol and Lemaire's chapter, namely narrative schemas, to analyze the performances of patients with dementia of the Alzheimer's type. The last chapter, by Dominique Cardebat, Jean-François Démonet, and Bernard Doyon, also reports on narrative abilities of patients with dementia but takes a broader theoretical approach to the problem.

Acknowledgments

This book is based in large part on a symposium entitled Narrative and Discourse Processes (organizers: H. Brownell and Y. Joanette) which was part of the second annual TENNET Conference (Theoretical and Experimental Neuropsychology/Neuropsychologie expérimentale et théoretique), held in Montréal, Québec, in May, 1991.

This book would not have been possible without the support of the following agencies and grants: Conseil des recherches médicales du Canada (PG-28) (Y. Joanette), le Fonds de la recherche en santé du Québec (Y. Joanette), NIH grants R01 NS27894 and 5P01 DC00081 (H. Brownell), and the Research Service of the Department of Veterans Affairs (H. Brownell).

We want to take this opportunity to thank Colette Cerny for her many contributions to the management of this enterprise.

Because this book was a completely collaborative project, our names are listed in alphabetical order.

Contributors

Julie Auger, B. A.
Linguistics Laboratory
University of Pennsylvania

Robert H. Brookshire, Ph. D.
Speech Pathology Service (127A)
Minneapolis V. A. Medical Center

Hiram H. Brownell, Ph. D.
Department of Psychology
Boston College

Dominique Cardebat, Ph. D.
Laboratoire d'imagerie, de neuropsychologie et de pharmacologie du vieillissement cérébral humain
INSERM U.230, C. H. U. Purpan

Danielle Cordon, M. S.
Department of Communication Science and Disorders
University of Vermont

Jean-François Démonet, M. D.
Laboratoire d'imagerie, de neuropsychologie et de pharmacologie du vieillissement cérébral humain
INSERM U.230, C. H. U. Purpan

Roger A. Dixon, Ph. D.
Department of Psychology
University of Victoria

Bernard Doyon, M. D.
Laboratoire d'imagerie, de neuropsychologie et de pharmacologie du vieillissement cérébral humain
INSERM U.230, C. H. U. Purpan

Michel Fayol, Ph. D.
Laboratoire d'Etude des Acquisitions et du Développement/CNRS
Université de Bourgogne

Carl H. Frederiksen, Ph. D.
Laboratory of Applied Cognitive Science
McGill University

Ingrid C. Friesen, M. A.
Department of Psychology
University of Victoria

Guila Glosser, Ph. D.
Department of Neurology
The Graduate Hospital

Peter C. Gordon, Ph. D.
Department of Psychology
Harvard University

Dominique Guénard, M. D.
Laboratoire Th. -Alajouanine
Centre de recherche du C. H. Côte-des-Neiges

Peter Grzybek, Ph. D.
Institut für Slawistik
Karl-Franzens-Universität Graz

Claudio L. N. Guimaraes dos Santos, M. D., Ph. D.
CNPq (Brazil) and
Laboratoire Jacques Lordat
Département des sciences du langage
Université de Toulouse-Le Mirail

Christopher Hertzog, Ph. D.
School of Psychology
Georgia Institute of Technology

Monica Strauss Hough, Ph. D.
Department of Speech-Language
 & Auditory Pathology
School of Allied Health Sciences
East Carolina University

David F. Hultsch, Ph. D.
Department of Psychology
University of Victoria

Yves Joanette, Ph. D.
Laboratoire Th.-Alajouanine
Centre de Recherche du
C. H. Côte-des-Neiges

Danuta Kadzielawa, Ph. D.
Faculty of Psychology
University of Warsaw

Helen J. Kahn, Ph. D.
Department of Communication
 Science and Disorders
University of Vermont

Jan Kordys, Ph. D.
Polish Academy of Sciences
Institute of Literary Studies

William Labov, Ph. D.
Linguistics Laboratory
University of Pennsylvania

Patrick Lemaire, Ph. D.
Laboratoire d'Etude des Acquisitions
et du Développement/CNRS
Université de Bourgogne

Penelope S. Myers, Ph. D.
Department of Neurology
Section of Speech Pathology
Mayo Clinic

Jean-Luc Nespoulous, Ph. D.
Laboratoire Jacques-Lordat
Département des sciences du langage
Université de Toulouse-Le Mirail

Linda E. Nicholas, M. A.
Speech Pathology Service (127A)
Minneapolis V. A. Medical Center

Robert S. Pierce, Ph. D.
School of Speech Pathology &
 Audiology
Kent State University

Maria Sadowska, Ph. D.
Polish Academy of Sciences

Bernadette Ska, Ph. D.
Laboratoire Th.-Alajouanine
Centre de recherche du C. H. Côte-
 des-Neiges

Brigitte Stemmer, M. D., Ph. D.
Laboratoire Th.-Alajouanine
Centre de recherche du C. H. Côte-
 des-Neiges

Hanna Ulatowska, Ph. D.
Callier Center for Communication
 Disorders
University of Texas at Dallas

Addresses for Correspondence

EDITORS

Hiram H. Brownell, Ph. D. *and*
Department of Psychology
Boston College
Chestnut Hill, MA 02167
U. S. A.

Yves Joanette, Ph. D.
Laboratoire Th. -Alajouanine
Centre de recherche du C. H. Côte-
   des-Neiges
4565, chemin de la Reine-Marie
Montréal (Québec) H3W 1W5
CANADA

AUTHORS

Chapter 1
Michel Fayol, Ph. D.
L.E.A.D./CNRS
Université de Bourgogne
6 B^d Gabriel
F - 21000 Dijon
FRANCE

Chapter 2
Peter C. Gordon, Ph. D.
Department of Psychology
University of North Carolina at
   Chapel Hill
CB #3270, Davie Hall
Chapel Hill, NC 27599
U. S. A.

Chapter 3
Peter Grzybek, Ph. D.
Institut für Slawistik
Karl-Franzens-Universität Graz
Heinrichstraβe 26
A-8010 GRAZ
AUSTRIA

Chapter 4
Roger A. Dixon, Ph. D.
Department of Psychology
University of Victoria
P.O. Box 3050
Victoria (B. C.) V8W 3P5
CANADA

Chapter 5
Helen J. Kahn, Ph. D.
Department of Communication Sci-
   ence and Disorders, Allen House
University of Vermont
Burlington, VT 05405
U. S. A.

Chapter 6
William Labov, Ph. D.
Linguistics Laboratory
1107 Blockley Hall
University of Pennsylvania
418 Guardian Drive
Philadelphia, PA 19104
U. S. A.

Chapter 7
Jean-Luc Nespoulous, Ph. D.
Laboratoire Jacques-Lordat
Département des sciences du langage
Université de Toulouse-Le Mirail
5, Allées Antonio Machado
F-31058 Toulouse Cedex
FRANCE

Chapter 8
Robert H. Brookshire, Ph. D.
Linda E. Nicholas, M. A.
Speech Pathology Service (127A)
V. A. Medical Center
1 Veterans Drive
Minneapolis, MN 55417
U. S. A.

Chapter 9
Hanna Ulatowska, Ph. D.
Callier Center for Communication Disorders
University of Texas at Dallas
1966 Inwood Road
Dallas, TX 75235
U. S. A.

Chapter 10
Guila Glosser, Ph. D.
Department of Neurology
The Graduate Hospital
1 Graduate Plaza
Philadelphia, PA 19146
U. S. A.

Chapter 11
Monica S. Hough, Ph. D.
Department of Speech-Language & Auditory Pathology
School of Allied Health Sciences
East Carolina University
Greenville, NC 27858
U. S. A.

Chapter 12
Carl H. Frederiksen, Ph. D.
Laboratory of Applied Cognitive Science
McGill University
3700 McTavish St., B199
Montreal (Quebec) H3A 1Y2
CANADA

or

Brigitte Stemmer, M. D., Ph. D.
Laboratoire Th. -Alajouanine
Centre de recherche du C. H. Côte-des-Neiges
4565, chemin de la Reine-Marie
Montréal (Québec) H3W 1W5
CANADA

Chapter 13
Penelope S. Myers, Ph. D.
Department of Neurology
Section of Speech Pathology
Mayo Clinic
Rochester, MN 55905
U. S. A.

Chapter 14
Bernadette Ska, Ph. D.
Laboratoire Th. -Alajouanine
Centre de recherche du C. H. Côte-des-Neiges
4565, chemin de la Reine-Marie
Montréal (Québec) H3W 1W5
CANADA

Chapter 15
Dominique Cardebat, Ph. D.
Laboratoire d'imagerie, de neuropsychologie et de pharmacologie du vieillissement cérébral humain
INSERM U.230, C. H. U. Purpan
F-31059 Toulouse Cedex
FRANCE

PART I

Theoretical Considerations

CHAPTER 1

Levels of Approach to Discourse

MICHEL FAYOL AND PATRICK LEMAIRE

The Chapter presents a critical review of the major trends in the cognitive psychology of discourse. The focus is put on the comprehension of narratives. Narrative is the type of discourse which has been extensively studied on the comprehension side and from different theoretical perspectives. Comparatively the research perspectives used on less-investigated types of discourse have been more limited. Reviewing the study of story comprehension may be the best way to provide an overview of the problems posed by the study of discourse in general as well as to present the theories and methods used in this research domain. Nevertheless, whenever possible, complementary information about other forms of discourse, such as description and argumentation will be introduced.

This chapter is divided into three parts—story grammars, causal networks, and procedural models—each corresponding to a different approach to story comprehension. For each of these different approaches we present the related research, the more significant results over the past 20 years, and the main criticism they have encountered.

STORY GRAMMARS

BASIC ASSUMPTIONS

Story grammars first appeared in 1975 (Mandler & Johnson, 1977; Rumelhart, 1975, 1977, 1980; Thorndyke, 1977). Two factors seem to have contributed to their appearance. First, the idea emerged that it was necessary to go beyond the level of sentences in order to study language and to look at larger units such as episodes, discourse, and so on. Second, there was the desire to use at the discourse level the formal linguistic framework provided by generative grammars. These influences led to the selection of the story form as the first unit larger than the sentence because the story is the most stereotypical type of discourse (and type of text) (cf. Barthes, 1986; Genette, 1966; for a review, see Fayol, 1985, Ch. 1; Fayol, 1991a).

Story grammars were devised to describe the structure of simple stories (problem-solving stories; Rumelhart, 1977). They consist of systems of rules defining the regularities actually found in narrative texts. Story grammars describe the abstract structure of stories as composed of a finite set of units (e.g., setting/goal/attempt/outcome/ending), connected to each other through a finite set of relations (e.g., cause/after/and). These grammars are both convenient notation systems and systems of rules that can be used to generate all narrative sequences, and only narrative sequences. Table 1–1 displays an example of an excerpt of rewrite rules used for simple stories.

Story grammars capture the regularities of conventional stories. However, they also provide a cognitive analysis of the story schema. The story schema is the set of all regularities that people have discovered through reading or hearing stories. This schema is therefore a general mental structure consisting of a set of expectations about the way stories unfold. The concept of story schema implies the existence of a mental organization specific to stories and independent of the contents evoked therein.

Stories are assumed to involve an invariable underlying structure despite differences in content. This structure (called the superstructure) has a mental counterpart, the story schema. The problem is to determine whether it is valid to assume that the existence of a story schema can account for the behavior of subjects when they comprehend, memorize, or produce stories (Mandler, 1987).

PSYCHOLOGICAL VALIDITY OF THE STORY SCHEMA

A great deal of research has been carried out on the story schema. The conclusions drawn from these studies are now widely accepted. In short, the notion of story schema has been used to explain many phenomena. Stories are organized into episodes, which constitute processing units. Episodes in turn are broken down into constituents, which are linked to each other via relations and presented in an optimal, so-called canonical, order. This organization is assumed to be independent of content and brought to bear during information intake (encoding), as well as during retrieval.

Table 1-1. Rewrite rules for the base structures of simple stories

STORY	→	Setting And EPISODE
EPISODE	→	{ BEGINNING Cause DEVELOPMENT Cause ENDING { { EPISODE (And EPISODE)^n 　　　　　　　(Then 　　　　　　)
BEGINNING	→	{ Beginning Event } { 　　　　　　　　　　} { EPISODE 　　　　　　}
DEVELOPMENT	→	{ COMPLEX REACTION Cause GOAL PATH 　　　} { Simple Reaction Cause Action 　　　　　　　　} { DEVELOPMENT (Cause DEVELOPMENT)^n 　　}
COMPLEX REACTION	→	Simple Reaction Cause Goal
GOAL PATH	→	Attempt Cause OUTCOME
OUTCOME	→	{ Outcome Event } { 　　　　　　　　　} { EPISODE 　　　　}
ENDIND	→	{ Ending Event } { 　　　　　　　　} { EPISODE 　　　}

Nonterminal nodes are written in upper case; nodes that are not rewritten except to States or Events are written in lower case.
Source: From Mandler, J. M. (1984). *Stories, scripts, and scenes. Aspects of schemata theory* (p. 24). Hillsdale, NJ: L.E.A. Publishing, reprinted by permission.

Encoding Processes

The effects of story schema on encoding processes have been investigated mainly with reading tasks. Two facts have been shown. First, a sentence is read more slowly on the average when the sentence appears at the beginning or ending of an episode than when the same sentence is presented alone or in a list of unrelated sentences (Haberlandt, Berian, & Sandson, 1980). This suggests that the episode, like the sentence, is a real-time processing unit that affects the information intake. Second, the reading and/or comprehension latencies are increased when the story constituents are presented into a non-standard order (Mandler & Goodman, 1982). This effect suggests that the order of information plays a critical role in understanding stories.

Memorization

A well-structured narrative text is known to involve several constituents: setting, goal, attempt, result, and so on. It has been shown that comprehension and memorization of narrative texts are better when the story contains all the necessary constituents, and when these constituents are in the standard or canonical order, that is: setting/beginning/reaction/goal/attempt/outcome/ending (Yussen et al., 1991). However, some of the constituents (setting, beginning, and outcome) are systematically better remembered than others. This effect has been found with elementary school children and with adult subjects from diverse cultures (Mandler, Scribner, Cole, & DeForest, 1980). Such performance stability on both immediate and delayed recall tasks has raised the problem of whether the effect of the story schema is due to encoding processes. Nevertheless, some researchers assume that the story schema has an effect only during information retrieval from memory (Alba & Hasher, 1983; Bloom, 1988; Kardash, Royer, & Greene, 1988; Yekovich & Thorndyke, 1981).

CRITICAL ANALYSIS

Story grammars have received substantial criticism. The following three types of problems have been evoked.

1. Some researchers consider story grammars to be insufficiently detailed or not quite adequate. For example, Garnham (1983) noticed that stories could not be broken down into constituents, as sentences can, because there is no parsed, finite lexicon of story elements. Mandler (1984) addressed this criticism by responding that story grammars are simply convenient means of notation: They are not used to parse narratives in constituents.

2. Other researchers have questioned some empirical findings. For example, the slower reading speed found at the beginning and ending of episodes has not always been replicated (Frochot, Zagar, & Fayol, 1987). In addition, no investigation has reported a text-type x constituent interaction effect on reading latencies. That is, no empirical research investigated the possibility that the slower reading rate effect at the beginning and/or the ending of episodes was specific to stories. It may as well occur for paragraphs in general.

3. Other researchers have found that some subjects use story schemata that do not always correspond exactly to the canonical schema. Accordingly, Mosenthal (1979) showed that readers and listeners perform better on recall of texts that were structured according to their

expectancies, even when this textual organization is different from the canonical narrative organization.

In sum, despite criticisms, the canonical narrative structure is still thought to be a relevant factor in processing stories, even though individual differences do pose a few problems.

EXTENSION TO OTHER TYPES OF TEXTS

Some researchers have attempted to extend at least some of the results collected in the study of stories to other types of texts or discourse. The question is always the same: Do text structures (conceived as independent of content) have an effect on subjects' performances? Can it be shown that (at least) some subjects efficiently use text structures (i.e., superstructures) that are independent of content when processing texts? A series of findings allows us to give a positive answer to this question (see Fayol, 1991a for a review).

Meyer and Freedle (1984) reported that when content remained constant, the most organized type of discourse (i.e., comparison and causation) promoted the most efficient processing of text (see also Meyer, Brandt, & Bluth, 1980). However, such facilitation occurred only if the reader or listener activated and used the text's top level structure.

Cook and Mayer (1988) showed that it was both possible and effective to teach the top level structures of scientific texts to students who had not been using them previously. Recall and comprehension performance was shown to improve after such training.

In conclusion, when content is controlled, the most organized and/or most conventional type of discourse (or text) induces the most efficient processing. It can be thought that this is so because the strongly organized texts provide a structure with highly specific relationships between components. This structure may in fact be used during encoding. But it is most often resorted to during retrieval, provided that the subjects have acquired the corresponding text type schemata. The use of text-type schemata can be compared to the use of categorical organizations in word-list recall. Recall is always better for words presented in an organized list than for words presented in random order. However, as noted by Mandler (1984) performance is even better with the canonical narrative structure than with any other ordered organization.

Nevertheless, some researchers contend that it was not necessary to refer to text superstructures to explain subjects' performance (Schank, 1975; Trabasso & Sperry, 1985). In particular, some researchers consider that the mental representation that follows the comprehension of a text depends essentially, and perhaps exclusively, on its content. From that perspective, text superstructures would be a kind of by-product of content-based organizations.

THE ROLE OF CONTENT: FROM SCRIPTS TO CAUSAL NETWORKS

SCRIPTS AND SCENE SCHEMATA

Understanding a text requires more than the simple activation of a superstructure. For example, if a narrative episode is represented simply as the hero's subgoal, an attempt to reach that subgoal, and a result, there is no way to distinguish between success and failure, or other possibilities (Reiser, Black, & Lehnert, 1985).

As early as 1975, several researchers began to elaborate alternative theories about story comprehension (Rumelhart, 1975; Schank, 1975), relying solely on the subject's knowledge of the situations involved. Schank and Abelson (1977) introduced the notion of script, that is, knowledge structure that subjects possess about common situations or routines (e.g., going to a restaurant, taking a plane, etc.; see Fayol & Monteil, 1988; Schallert, 1982). This type of knowledge structure is more concrete than the story schema, because it always pertains to specific content. Each script includes a title (or script header) and is divided into scenes (e.g., for "taking a plane," we have: going to the airport, checking in your luggage, waiting in the sitting room, getting into the plane, etc.). Each scene in the script is then divided into a variable number of actions. Certain typical roles (e.g., airline flight attendant, pilot, etc.) are then assigned to each action. Scripts are fuzzy concepts: They have fewer features than story schemata, and unlike story schemata, scripts do not necessarily include a fixed superstructure. The same remarks hold for scene schemata, which are representations of locational and spatial knowledge.

Scripts and scene schemata have been shown to affect text processing. They improve comprehension and recall, in particular by facilitating inferences, in addition to guiding information intake. However, they can induce the false recognition of typical actions. That is, if a reader or listener knows a script and is presented with a portion of this script, he or she will "spontaneously" activate the whole knowledge network associated with this script. As a consequence, when the subject is asked later to judge whether he or she has read or listened to some statements related to this script, the subject may falsely recognize some of the activated portions of the network. Because of the high level of activation some statements are cognitively available as if they actually had been previously presented.

Scripts and scene schemata comprise a sort of "backdrop" against which unexpected events or states occur. The comprehension of these unexpected events is possible via the construction of causal networks.

CAUSAL NETWORKS

Schank and Abelson (1977) began stressing how important causal relations were to narrative schemata. The causal relations in stories can be divided into two categories:

1. plan structures, which deal with action sequences carried out in view of reaching a goal (or subgoal; see Lichtenstein & Brewer, 1980; Rumelhart, 1977), and
2. state or event sequences, which form a chronological-causal chain.

Some researchers have used these two categories of relations as their basis for representing narrative schemata in causal network form (see Trabasso, Secco, & van den Broek, 1984; Trabasso & Sperry, 1985; Trabasso & van den Broek, 1985). It was hypothesized that understanding an event is to discover its causes and effects (via a naive theory of causality). The causal structure of the schemata is thus what determines comprehension, judgments of importance, and recall.

The causal structure associated with a text can be obtained by (a) dividing the narrative schema into states, and (b) establishing the relationships between those states on the basis of a criterion of "necessity in the circumstances" (e.g., A is said to have caused B if B would not have occurred in the circumstances presented in the text if A had not occurred). According to this criterion, enablement, motivation, psychological causality, and physical causation are all considered to be causal relations.

The states and events in a text are represented in such a causal network. The causal chain is opened by statements describing the setting. Then a series of events occurs; the events can be explained by the causality, and expectations are created. Two of the properties of causal networks are highly relevant:

1. Certain events, called causal chain events, are located along the causal chain, whereas others lead to dead ends;
2. A given event can be causally related to several other events via higher or lower connections.

An example of a narrative text and its associative causal network is displayed in Figure 1–1. These two properties enable one to explain the following effects:

- States or events that are part of the causal chain (connecting the text's opening to its final outcome) are better recalled and judged as

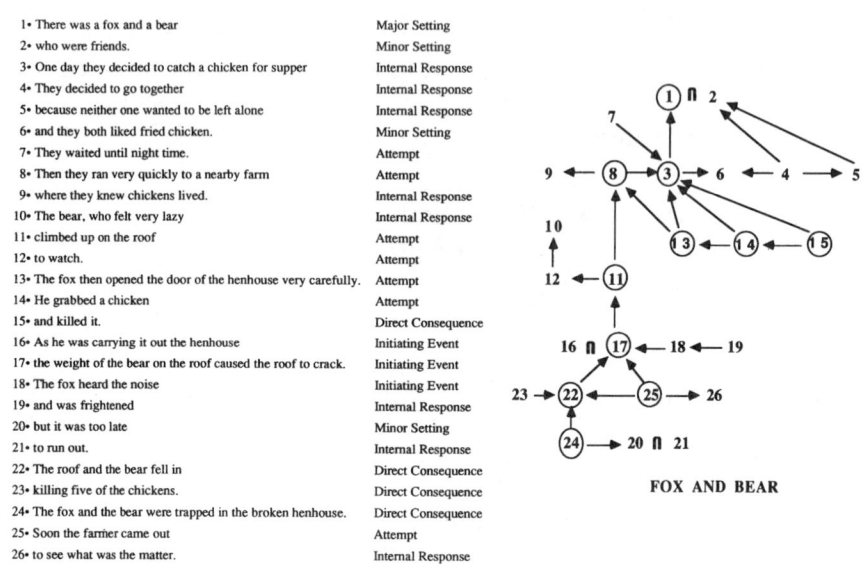

1• There was a fox and a bear	Major Setting
2• who were friends.	Minor Setting
3• One day they decided to catch a chicken for supper	Internal Response
4• They decided to go together	Internal Response
5• because neither one wanted to be left alone	Internal Response
6• and they both liked fried chicken.	Minor Setting
7• They waited until night time.	Attempt
8• Then they ran very quickly to a nearby farm	Attempt
9• where they knew chickens lived.	Internal Response
10• The bear, who felt very lazy	Internal Response
11• climbed up on the roof	Attempt
12• to watch.	Attempt
13• The fox then opened the door of the henhouse very carefully.	Attempt
14• He grabbed a chicken	Attempt
15• and killed it.	Direct Consequence
16• As he was carrying it out the henhouse	Initiating Event
17• the weight of the bear on the roof caused the roof to crack.	Initiating Event
18• The fox heard the noise	Initiating Event
19• and was frightened	Internal Response
20• but it was too late	Minor Setting
21• to run out.	Internal Response
22• The roof and the bear fell in	Direct Consequence
23• killing five of the chickens.	Direct Consequence
24• The fox and the bear were trapped in the broken henhouse.	Direct Consequence
25• Soon the farmer came out	Attempt
26• to see what was the matter.	Internal Response

Figure 1–1. Excerpt of a text ("Bumperstickers and the cops") and of the corresponding proposition list and coherence graph. From Kintsch, W., & van Dijk, 1978. Toward a model of text comprehension and text production. *Psychological Review, 85,* 363–394. Copyright (1978) by the American Psychological Association. Adapted by permission.

more important than states or events that are not on the causal chain (Trabasso, Secco, & van den Broek, 1984; Trabasso & Sperry, 1985);

- An event or state in the text is better recalled, judged more important (Black & Bern, 1981; O'Brien & Myers, 1987; Trabasso & van den Broek, 1985; van den Broek & Trabasso, 1986), and more often included in a summary (van den Broek, 1989; van den Broek & Trabasso, 1986) when it has more causal connections (forward or backward) to other events or states in the text.

CRITICAL ANALYSIS

The above analysis of causal networks pertains less to stories as a whole than to the event schemata described therein. In other words, causal networks represent the way in which events are strung together in the mental model describing the situation. Indeed:

- Causal networks apply both to narrative texts and to filmed action sequences (Lichtenstein & Brewer, 1980);
- Comprehending causal networks seems to depend on subjects' causal understanding capacity (Freeland & Scholnick, 1987).

Taking into account the causal organization of the described events appears to be essential. This provides a partial explanation of the "level" effect, whereby certain facts are judged more important than others, are better recalled than others, and are more often included in summaries (see however Bower, 1982—things are not always that simple). However, it has been noted that only a moderate amount of the variance can be explained by the causal organization of the events (approximately 30%). Therefore, other factors must be taken into account.

Two difficulties appear with causal networks.

1. They only apply to texts that describe sequences of events or states for which causal links exist, such as stories, recipes, user's manuals, and so on (Smith & Goodman, 1984). Very few studies concern expository text or argumentative texts. In argumentation and exposition, inductive and deductive relations, as well as relations of categorical membership, certainly play a major role in cohesion. Little is known, however, about their corresponding mental models.
2. Causal networks do not take into account linguistic and textual constraints. Comprehension is considered to be problem solving: The subject must discover the causal structure of the events. However, it has not been explained how this construction comes about through the processing of linguistic cues and prior knowledge. This gap in our understanding has been partially filled by procedural models.

FROM TEXT TO MENTAL MODEL: APPROACHES INVOLVING PROCESSES

KINTSCH AND VAN DIJK'S MODEL

Kintsch and van Dijk's approach (1978) assumes that comprehension is a real-time process. This process starts with a text. The text contains linguistic cues that are organized according to language-specific rules (i.e., morphology, syntax). The reader or listener processes those linguistic cues and relates them to prior conceptual knowledge. However, one of the constraints of this linguistic processing and of concept relating is the limited capacity of short-term memory (STM).

The limited capacity of STM constrains text comprehension by forcing cyclical processing. Therefore, the strategy used to select propositions to include in short-term memory is a critical component of this cyclical processing (Fletcher, 1981).

According to Kintsch and van Dijk's model, the meaning of a text can be specified at two levels (Miller & Kintsch, 1980):

1. **The microstructure:** A list of micropropositions representing the individual ideas in the text. This level is established by means of microprocessing.
2. **The macrostructure:** Main ideas are represented in a global structure (the gist). The macrostructure is extracted through macroprocesses.

Microprocessing

Kintsch and van Dijk (1977) assume that the meaning of a text is represented in memory as a network of propositions called a textbase (where each proposition is comprised of a predicate and one or more arguments). Two propositions are related to each other if their arguments overlap and if they co-occur in working memory during the comprehension process. Because of limited memory capacity, texts are processed in cycles: one clause or one sentence at a time. During each cycle, the working memory holds all the propositions from the current clause (or sentence) and a small number of propositions from prior portions of text. Every important proposition remains in working memory for several cycles. The longer it stays in working memory, the more likely it is to be recalled.

Propositions in working memory are assumed to be organized in a hierarchical network with a topical proposition as the superordinate node. All propositions sharing an argument with this superordinate proposition form the second level of the network. Thematic propositions are assigned the highest level. Propositions sharing an argument with the thematic propositions are assigned the next highest level, and so on (Vipond, 1980). It is assumed that the reader attempts to represent a text by a single hierarchically organized network. However, the reader can only form an integrated network if all arguments overlap. If a single network cannot be formed, the reader must initiate a search through long-term memory. If a proposition in long-term memory is found that shares an argument with the input set, this proposition is reinstated in working memory. If such a proposition cannot be connected due to a lack of argument overlap, a proposition may be inferred to establish a relationship. If it is not possible to "link" a proposition to the network, a new network is constructed. Figure 1–2 gives an example of a short text and of the corresponding proposition list and coherence graph.

A series of violent, bloody encounters between police and Black Panther Party members punctuated the early summer days of 1969. Soon after, a group of black students I teach at California State College, Los Angeles, who were members of the Black Panther Party, began to complain of continuous harassment by law officers.

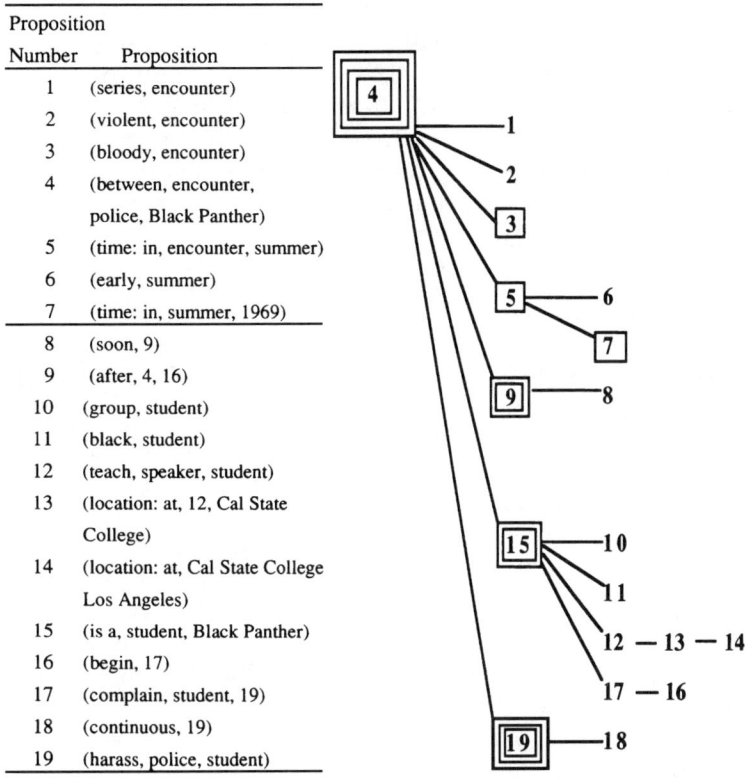

Proposition Number	Proposition
1	(series, encounter)
2	(violent, encounter)
3	(bloody, encounter)
4	(between, encounter, police, Black Panther)
5	(time: in, encounter, summer)
6	(early, summer)
7	(time: in, summer, 1969)
8	(soon, 9)
9	(after, 4, 16)
10	(group, student)
11	(black, student)
12	(teach, speaker, student)
13	(location: at, 12, Cal State College)
14	(location: at, Cal State College Los Angeles)
15	(is a, student, Black Panther)
16	(begin, 17)
17	(complain, student, 19)
18	(continuous, 19)
19	(harass, police, student)

Figure 1–2. The "Fox and Bear" story and its causal network representation. From Trabasso, T., Secco, T., & van den Broek, P., 1984. *Causal cohesion and story coherence.* Copyright (1984) by Lawrence Erlbaum Publisher.

Consequently, the difficulty of text comprehension can be indexed by:

- the number of levels in the network;
- the number of reinstatements; and
- the number of inferences and reorganizations.

These remarks concern the microstructure. However, in addition to comprehending the detailed microstructure, readers or listeners elaborate the gist of a passage. The gist is constructed via the execution of macroprocesses.

Macroprocessing

Macroprocesses are similar to microprocesses but apply to units that are larger than the sentence (e.g., paragraphs). Macropropositions are built out of micropropositions controlled by a schema. Micropropositions are assessed as relevant or irrelevant, depending on that schema. Relevant macropropositions are either retained, generalized, or constructed. Micropropositions that are not relevant to the schema are eliminated. The next step is the elaboration of the gist of the text, which is an ordered, connected list of macropropositions.

CRITICAL ANALYSIS

Several studies have provided empirical evidence supporting Kintsch and van Dijk's (1977) thesis, particularly the results concerning the repetition of references (i.e., argument overlap).

- Subjects remember texts with more repetitions of the same reference between sentences better than those with fewer referential connections (Kintsch, Kosminsky, Streby, McKoon, & Keenan, 1975);
- Subjects take longer to read a sentence when they have to make an inference to establish its referential connection with the previous sentence than when they do not (Cirilo, 1981; Cirilo & Foss, 1980; Haviland & Clark, 1974);
- Subjects read texts faster when they do not have to search in long-term memory for the referents (Miller & Kintsch, 1980);
- It is possible, at least to a certain extent, to organize the microstructure of texts to make microprocesses and/or macroprocesses easier to apply (Kieras, 1978).

However, even if empirical data have often been consistent with predictions based on Kintsch and van Dijk's model, some issues are not addressed, and a number of difficulties remain unresolved. For example, the mere repetition of an argument does not guarantee reference to the same entity: An entity may have the same referent but not the same name (as with synonyms), or it may have the same name but not the same referent (Garnham, Oakhill, & Johnson-Laird, 1982).

More generally, the criticism points out three shortcomings of Kintsch and van Dijk's model:

1. It seems unrealistic to consider coherence only through argument overlap. Other types of relations can affect coherence, notably those pertaining to world knowledge (Kintsch, 1979);
2. The fact that the reader or listener constructs the text's micro- and macrostructure does not guarantee comprehension. To illustrate this point, take Perrig and Kintsch's (1985) study on comprehension and recall of texts describing a walk through a town. The subjects were able to recall the texts quite well. But their performance indicated a poor ability to use the informations that they had acquired to make inferences about spatial relations in the town if those relations had not been explicitly stated in the text.
3. Kintsch and van Dijk's model uses semantic propositions obtained through an analysis "done by hand." The text had to be entirely rewritten. Therefore, what is processed is not the text's surface itself, but rather a more or less intuitive interpretation of the text's surface. Some current research has tried to address these issues.

RELATIONS BETWEEN LINGUISTIC AND COGNITIVE ASPECTS

Kintsch and van Dijk's (1987) breakdown into propositions was rather intuitive. Their choice of the superordinate proposition that renders the text as a whole coherent was also intuitive. Since that time, improvements have been made. These improvements were added to account for how a reader or listener who does not have any information about what follows in a text can gradually organize and build its macrostructure and "situation model" in real time (or mental model; see Johnson-Laird, 1983, and, more recently, Bower & Morrow, 1990).

A few examples of these improvements are given here, for instance Gernsbacher and Hargreaves (1988) showed that the first participant mentioned in a sentence is always more accessible than the others. That is, subjects recognize the name of the first participant more quickly than the name of any other participant when they are asked whether they have already seen this name. Moreover, when there are two participants in a text, if only one is introduced by a proper name, he or she will be taken as the thematic subject (Garrod & Sanford, 1988). Later in the text, the thematic subject is preferred as antecedent for referential pronouns (Garrod & Sanford, 1985).

In short, the first-mentioned participant tends to be considered as the thematic subject, especially if he or she is called by a proper name. In addition, the thematic subject has a special referential status.

The character who fills the role of thematic subject is the most prominent character in the reader or listener's mind. He or she is a preferred candidate for any device that signals reference, such as a pronoun. As stories pass from one episode to the next, secondary characters (i.e., scenario-dependent ones) cease to be focused or draw attention, while the main character(s) continue to be the center of focus.

Thus, first-mentioned participants or characters designated by proper names are more accessible because they form the foundation for the online building of a coherent representation (Gernsbacher, 1989). Subsequent information is then related to that foundation. Such a foundation gives the story a consistent point of view from which the entire narrative schema is constructed (Black, Turner, & Bower, 1979). Part of the problem posed by the intuitive determination of the thematic proposition is thus resolved, because the criteria that lead to the selection of the thematic subject are known.

The real-time construction of a situation model also requires that the reader or listener represents the movements of the characters and situates them in space. Morrow (1985) showed that prepositions and verb aspects help to guide narrative comprehension by indicating which are the most prominent parts of motion events. They do so by specifying the mover's location, which in turn determines what is most relevant to the mover's experience (see also Bower & Morrow, 1990; Morrow, Greenspan, & Bower, 1987).

Thus, proper names, first-mentioned participants, prepositions, verb aspects, and no doubt many other linguistic cues, enable the reader or listener to determine what are the important events for understanding the text's event structure, and thus for constructing a mental model of the situation being described. These linguistic cues seem to act as indicators of the cognitive operations to be carried out, that is, to focus one's attention on one particular aspect or another, to stop focusing one's attention on that aspect, and so on (Fayol, 1991b).

CONCLUDING REMARKS: A FOUR-LEVEL APPROACH

A review of research on story comprehension—in other words, an overview of the most widely studied activity as it operates on the best-known type of text—brings to light the existence of different levels of text processing. Indeed, four levels can be distinguished.

THE CONCEPTUAL LEVEL

For the narrative schema, this level can be represented as consisting of states and events linked via chronological-causal connections. The corresponding "mental model" depends on the subject's world knowledge and upon his or her ability to engage in "naive" causal reasoning. This level is definitely independent of the linguistic level. The problem is that it is currently difficult to determine which elements and relations are applicable to the conceptual organizations underlying other types of text, such as argumentation and explanation.

THE SUPERSTRUCTURAL LEVEL

The superstructural level pertains to the global organization of certain types of text. It can be seen as a fruitful "framework" which facilitates information monitoring, perhaps right from encoding, and most certainly during retrieval. It no doubt plays the same role as categorization in word list learning, that is it facilitates the on-line categorization of information and the establishment of superordinate relations between categories.

It seems irrelevant and even impossible to reduce this superstructural level to the conceptual level. There is no reason to assume, for example, that the setting of a story will necessarily be placed at the beginning. The usual placement of the setting does not stem from conceptual structuring into causal networks. Rather, it is most likely due to the cognitive constraints that have contributed to making Setting + Initial event + Reaction the conventional superstructure.

THE MICROSTRUCTURAL AND MACROSTRUCTURAL LEVELS

Until recently, little was known about the microstructural level. Kintsch and van Dijk (1977) did not really deal with the microstructure because they rewrote that level entirely in the form of propositions (predicates and arguments). Within the past few years, some researchers have shown that the way in which a reader or listener monitors his or her cognitive activity depends upon some linguistic cues: for example, position in the sentence, proper names, verb aspect, and pronouns. Some of these cues serve to draw attention. They facilitate the construction of a coherent representation of the described situation, a representation that is organized around a given point of view.

The greater our understanding of the role of the microstructure and its corresponding microprocesses, the more the role of the macrostructure presents a problem. Although recent work (Fletcher & Chrysler, 1990) has shown that it is relevant to make the distinction between surface forms, textbase, and situation model for recognition tasks, the status of the macrostructure is not clear. Indeed, as another study has shown (Fletcher & Bloom, 1988), the performance of Kintsch and van Dijk's

(1977) model can be improved by introducing a new strategy. This new strategy consists of retaining a proposition if it cannot be integrated into the causal network (rather than limiting the model to argument overlap).

It is conceivable that microprocesses are brought to bear within the confines of a limited capacity working memory and that the causal network organization suffices to account for the observed phenomena, thereby eliminating the need for a separate macrostructure level.

CONCLUSION

The aim of this chapter was to provide an integrated overview of the main trends in the study of discourse processing. Focusing on story understanding enabled us to show that several levels of processing could be involved in the understanding processes. Indeed, we were led to distinguish four potential levels: conceptual, superstructural, macrostructural, and microstructural. It can be suggested from the present analysis that dissociations between these levels should be found in the neuropsychology area. We hope that such a perspective will induce further empirical research.

REFERENCES

Alba, J. M., & Hasher, L. (1983). Is memory schematic? *Psychological Bulletin, 93*, 203–231.
Barthes, R. (1986). Introduction à l'analyse structurale des récits. *Communication, 8*, 1–27.
Black, J. B., & Bern, H. (1981). Causal coherence and memory for events in narratives. *Journal of Verbal Learning and Verbal Behavior, 20*, 267–275.
Black, J. B., Turner, J. T., & Bower, G. W. (1979). Point of view in narrative comprehension, memory, and production. *Journal of Verbal Learning and Verbal Behavior, 18*, 187–198.
Bloom, C. P. (1988). The role of schemata in memory for text. *Discourse Processes, 11*, 305–318.
Bower, G. H. (1982). Plans and goals in understanding episodes. In A. Flammer & W. Kintsch (Eds.), *Discourse processing* (pp. 2–15). Amsterdam: North-Holland.
Bower, G. H., & Morrow, D. G. (1990). Mental models in narrative comprehension. *Science, 247*, 44–48.
Cirilo, R. K. (1981). Referential coherence and text structure in story comprehension. *Journal of Verbal Learning and Verbal Behavior, 20*, 358–367.
Cirilo, R. K., & Foss, D. J. (1980). Text structure and reading time for sentences. *Journal of Verbal Learning and Verbal Behavior, 19*, 96–109.
Cook, L. K., & Mayer, R. E. (1988). Teaching readers about the structure of scientific texts. *Journal of Educational Psychology, 80*, 448–456.
Fayol, M. (1985). *Le récit et sa construction*. Neuchâtel, Paris: Delachaux & Niestlé.
Fayol, M. (1991a). Text typologies: A cognitive approach. In G. Denhière & J. P. Rossi (Eds.), *Text and text processing*. Amsterdam: North Holland.

Fayol, M. (1991b). Stories. A psycholinguistic and ontogenetic approach to the acquisition of narrative abilities. In Pieraut-Le-Bonniec & M. Dolitsky (Eds.), *From basic language to discourse basis*. Amsterdam: Benjamin.

Fayol, M., & Monteil, J. M. (1988). The notion of script. From general to developmental and social psychology. *C.P.C./European Bulletin of Cognitive Psychology, 8*, 335–361.

Flechter, C. R. (1981). Short-term memory processes in text comprehension. *Journal of Verbal Learning and Verbal Behavior, 20*, 564–574.

Flechter, C. R., & Bloom, C. P. (1988). Causal reasoning in the comprehension of simple narratives texts. *Journal of Memory and Language, 27*, 235–244.

Flechter, C. R., & Chrysler, S. T. (1990). Surface forms, textbases, and situational models: Recognition memory for three types of textual information. *Discourse Processes, 13*, 175–190.

Freeland, C. A. B., & Scholnick, E. K. (1987). The role of causality in young children's memory for stories. *International Journal of Behavioral Development, 10*, 71–98.

Frochot, M., Zagar, D., & Fayol, M. (1987). Effets de l'organisation narrative sur la lecture de récits. *L'Année Psychologique, 87*, 237–252.

Garnham, A. (1983). What's wrong with story grammars. *Cognition, 15*, 145–154.

Garnham, A. Oakhill, J., & Johnson-Laird, P. N. (1982). Referential continuity and the coherence of discourse. *Cognition, 11*, 29–46.

Garrod, S., & Sanford, A. J. (1985). On the real-time character of interpretation during reading. *Language and Cognitive Processes, 1*, 43–59.

Garrod, S., & Sanford, A. J. (1988). Thematic subjecthood and cognitive constraints on discourse structure. *Journal of Pragmatics, 12*, 357–372.

Genette, G. (1966). Frontières du récit. *Communications, 8*, 152–163.

Gernsbacher, M. A. (1989). Mechanisms that improve referential access. *Cognition, 32*, 99–156.

Gernsbacher, M. A., & Hargreaves, A. J. (1988). Accessing sentence participants: The advantage of first mention. *Journal of Memory and Language, 27*, 699–717.

Haberland, K., Berian, C., & Sandson, J. (1980). The episode schema in story processing. *Journal of Verbal Learning and Verbal Behavior, 19*, 635–650.

Haviland, S. E., & Clark, H. H. (1974). What's new? Acquiring new information as a process in comprehension. *Journal of Verbal Learning and Verbal Behavior, 13*, 512–521.

Johnson-Laird, P. N. (1983). *Mental models*. Cambridge, MA: Cambridge University Press.

Kardash, C. A. M., Royer, J. M., & Greene, B. A. (1988). Effects of schemata on both encoding and retrieval of information from prose. *Journal of Educational Psychology, 80*, 326–329.

Kieras, D. E. (1978). Good and bad structure in simple paragraphs: Effect on apparent theme, reading time, and recall. *Journal of Verbal Learning and Verbal Behavior, 17*, 13–28.

Kintsch, W. (1979). On modeling comprehension. *Educational Psychologist, 14*, 3–14.

Kintsch, W., & van Dijk, T. A. (1978). Toward a model of text comprehension and text production. *Psychological Review, 85*, 363–394.

Kintsch, W., Kozminsky, E., Streby, W. J., McKoon, G., & Keenan, J. M. (1975) Comprehension and recall of text as a function of content variables. *Journal of Verbal Learning and Verbal Behavior, 14*, 196–214.

Lichtenstein, E. H., & Brewer, W. F. (1980). Memory for goal-directed events. *Cognitive Psychology, 12*, 412–455.

Mandler, J. M. (1984). *Stories, scripts, and scenes. Aspects of schemata theory*. Hillsdale, NJ: L.E.A. Publishers.

Mandler, J. M. (1987). On the psychological reality of story structure. *Discourse Processes, 10*, 1–29.

Mandler, J. M., & Goodman, M. S. (1982). On the psychological validity of story structure. *Journal of Verbal Learning and Verbal Behavior, 21*, 507–523.

Mandler, J. M., & Johnson, N. S. (1977). Remembrance of things parsed: Story structure and recall. *Cognitive Psychology, 9*, 111–151.

Mandler, J. M., Scribner, S., Cole, M., & DeForest, M. (1980). Cross-cultural invariance in story recall. *Child Development, 51*, 19–26.

Meyer, B. J. F., Brandt, D. J., & Bluth, G. J. (1980). Use of top-level structure in text: Key for reading-comprehension on ninth grade students. *Reading Research Quarterly, 16*, 73–103.

Meyer, B. J. F., & Freedle, R. O. (1984). Effects of discourse type on recall. *American Educational Research Journal, 21*, 121–143.

Miller, J. R., & Kintsch, W. (1980). Readability and recall of short prose passage: A theoretical analysis. *Journal of Experimental Psychology: Human Learning and Memory, 6*, 334–354.

Morrow, D. G. (1985). Prepositions and verb-aspect in narrative understanding. *Journal of Memory and Language, 24*, 390–404.

Morrow, D. G., Greenspan, S. L., & Bower, G. H. (1987). Accessibility and situation models in narrative comprehension. *Journal of Memory and Language, 16*, 165–187.

Mosenthal, P. (1979). Three types of schemata in children's recall of cohesive and non-cohesive texts. *Journal of Experimental Child Psychology, 27*, 129–142.

O'Brien, E. J., & Myers, J. L. (1987). The role of causal connections in the retrieval of text. *Memory and Cognition, 15*, 419–427.

Perrig, W., & Kintsch, W. (1985). Propositional and situational representations of texts. *Journal of Memory and Language, 24*, 503–518.

Reiser, B. J., Black, J. B., & Lehnert, W. G. (1985). Thematic knowledge structure in the understanding and generation of narratives. *Discourse Processes, 8*, 357–389.

Rumelhart, D. E. (1975). Notes on a schema for stories. In D. G. Bobrow & A. Collins (Eds.), *Representation and understanding* (pp. 237–272). New York: Academic Press.

Rumelhart, D. E. (1977). Understanding and summarizing brief stories. In D. Laberge & S. J. Samuels (Eds.), *Basic processes in reading: Perception and comprehension*. Hillsdale, NJ: L.E.A. Publishers.

Rumelhart, D. E. (1980). Schema: The building block of cognition. In R. J. Spiro, B. C. Bruce, & W. F. Brewer (Eds.), *Theoretical issues in reading comprehension*. Hillsdale, NJ: L.E.A. Publishers.

Schank, R. C., & Abelson, R. P. (1977). *Scripts, goals, plans, and understanding*. Hillsdale, NJ: L.E.A. Publishers.

Smith, E. E., & Goodman, L. (1984). Understanding written instructions; The role of an explanatory schema. *Cognition and Instruction, 1*, 359–396.

Schallert, D. L. (1982). The significance of knowledge: A synthesis of research related to schema theory. In O. Wayne & S. White (Eds.), *Reading expository material* (pp. 13–48). New York: Academic Press.

Thorndyke, P. W. (1977). Cognitive structures in comprehension and memory of narrative discourse. *Cognitive Psychology, 9*, 77–110.

Trabasso, T., Secco, T., & van den Broek, P. (1984). Causal cohesion and story coherence. In H. Mandl, N. Stein, & T. Trabasso (Eds.), *Learning and comprehension of text* (pp. 83–111). Hillsdale, NJ: L.E.A. Publishers.

Trabasso, T., & Sperry, L. L. (1985). Causal relatedness and importance of story events. *Journal of Memory and Language, 24,* 595–611.

Trabasso, T., & van den Broek, P. (1985). Causal thinking and the representation of narrative events. *Journal of Memory and Language, 24,* 612–630.

van den Broek, P. (1989). Causal reasoning and inference making in judging the importance of story statements. *Child Development, 60,* 286–298.

van den Broek, P., & Trabasso, T. (1986). Causal networks versus goal hierarchies in summarizing text. *Discourse Processes, 9,* 1–15.

Vipond, D. (1990). Micro and macroprocesses in text comprehension. *Journal of Verbal Learning and Verbal Behavior, 19,* 276–296.

Yekovich, F. R., & Thorndyke, P. W. (1981). An evaluation of alternative functional models of narrative schemata. *Journal of Verbal Learning and Verbal Behavior, 20,* 454–469.

Yussen, S. R., Stright, A. D., Glysch, R. L., Bonk, C. E., Lu, I., & Al-Sabaty, I. (1991). Learning and forgetting of narratives following good and poor text organization. *Contemporary Educational Psychology, 16,* 346–374.

CHAPTER 2

Computational and Psychological Models of Discourse

PETER C. GORDON

Discourse has proven to be an attractive yet problematic topic for language researchers. It is attractive because intuitively we know that there has to be something more to language than just sentences; that something is discourse, which integrates sentences into coherent communication. It is problematic because the structure of discourse is considerably less salient than that of other levels of language, such as the syntactic structure of sentences or the phonological and morphological structure of words. In some ways, the structure of discourse is analogous to the structure of intonation. We *know* that intonation plays a vital role in spoken language, yet its characteristics are far more resistant to analysis than the segmental aspects of speech. Similarly, we *know* that discourse structure is important, yet it is elusive. Indeed, an argument can be made that discourse has no independent structure of its own beyond the structure given by world knowledge and domain-specific knowledge about the topic of communication. The goal of this chapter is to review theories and evidence that challenge such a position, and suggest that meaning is not the only structure present in discourse. With the goal stated that way, the reader might be tempted to infer that the argument to be challenged is something of a straw man. For some levels of discourse analysis this may be the case, but for other levels it is a challenge to show that discourse has a structure beyond the meanings it communicates.

The question of whether discourse has its own structure is fundamental to the question of whether the study of discourse addresses a computationally coherent problem or whether it simply examines a facet of some more general computational problem such as knowledge representation or reasoning. The valid expression of the computational level of a problem, in the sense developed by Marr (1982), requires a complete description of the mapping of different representations of information. For discourse, this mapping is between the text (or spoken narrative) and the structure of discourse. If discourse has no independent structure, then no such mapping can be formulated. An argument that discourse does have its own structure does not entail a denial that meaning and content interact with structure in the use of discourse; plainly, that would be false. Rather, the claim is that the analysis of discourse structure can be considered as a coherent problem on its own. In addition to this abstract computational level of analysis, theoretical understanding of discourse requires specification of processes that can generate discourse structure during language production and can recognize it during comprehension. Work at this algorithmic level of analysis is validated through the development of working natural language processing systems and through experimental tests of the psychology of discourse processing. Progress at this level allows us to develop an understanding of how and when different kinds of structure (and meaning) play a role in the production and comprehension of language. In addition to his computational and algorithmic levels of analysis, Marr (1982) also emphasized the importance of understanding the hardware that performed the computation. Because many of the other chapters in this book address that level, this chapter focuses on the computational and algorithmic levels.

This chapter is organized around the commonly acknowledged distinction between global and local discourse structure. It provides relatively brief reviews of discourse models that have been discussed elsewhere in the psychological literature and more extensive reviews of some research from computational linguistics that have not received such discussion.

GLOBAL STRUCTURE OF DISCOURSE

Global discourse structure is generally viewed as serving the functions of organizing and highlighting the important meanings of a discourse. These roles place it close to the structure of events described by a discourse, and the challenge becomes finding ways of characterizing discourse structure independently of the content of the meanings it organizes. Ideally, the hypothesized discourse structures should be general across discourses of different types and about different topics yet still be rich enough to provide useful information about the packaging of meaning in communication.

Some scholars clearly do not believe that this can be done. Research on some kinds of knowledge structures and on mental models takes the view that the structure of a discourse (at least at the global level) exists only through the structure of the concepts and events that are described. This research is not the topic of this chapter, but a few highlights are worth noting. Schank and Abelson (1977) developed a kind of knowledge structure, or schema, called a script, which describes some common sequence of events, the typical example being the activities that transpire on going to a restaurant. The possession of such scripts allows a language understanding system to make appropriate inferences about information that is merely implicit in a text. The standard criticisms of this, and other schema approaches, are that there is no good account of how the schemas are acquired, it is difficult to specify how only the appropriate schemas are activated and only the relevant inferences drawn, and it is clearly the case that we can understand the description of novel events for which we do not have schemas. The *mental models* approach developed by Johnson-Laird (1983) attempts to circumvent some of these problems by positing that discourse comprehension involves construction of a model based on the events that are described, rather than simply activating prestored packages of meaning. This approach has inspired some interesting research (e.g., Anderson, Garrod, & Sanford, 1983; Glenberg, Meyer, & Lindem; 1987), but is incomplete with regard to *how* the mental models for discourse are constructed. The *causal network* approach of Trabasso and his colleagues (e.g., Trabasso & van den Broek, 1985) uses patterns of causality in the events depicted by a narrative to predict which events in a story are considered important and are likely to be recalled. The causal patterns are determined by a procedure that relies on general philosophical tests for causality, such as counterfactual reasoning. This work is important in its attempt to formulate general, explicit tools for characterizing the structure of events, but the independence of those tools from the theorists' interpretation of the story has yet to be rigorously demonstrated.

STORY GRAMMARS, SCHEMAS, AND MACROSTRUCTURES

Story grammars provide an early instance of a theory that does postulate that discourse has its own structure at the global level. They achieved prominence in cognitive science in the mid 1970s through the work of several authors (notably Mandler & Johnson, 1977; Rumelhart, 1975; 1977; Thorndyke, 1977), who built on earlier linguistic studies of folk tales. As the name implies, story grammars were in part meant to extend the theoretical role of traditional grammars to a larger domain by providing rules specifying the well-formedness of stories ("observational adequacy") and their constituent structure ("descriptive adequacy").

For example, the grammar presented by Rumelhart (1975) attempted to account for a "wide range of simple stories" with rewrite rules such as:

Story → Setting + Episode
Setting → (State, State, State, . . .)
Episode → Event + Reaction

Formally, these rules are directly analogous to the rewrite rules used to describe sentence structure, such as:

Sentence → Noun Phrase + Verb Phrase

A semantic interpretation rule accompanies each syntactic rule in the story grammar, and together they provide a hierarchical structure that links the components of the story. Describing Rumelhart's (1975) grammar in detail would be lengthy business, but essentially the grammar expressed the idea that many stories concern some sort of problem solving; something happens to a protagonist resulting in a goal which the protagonist pursues to some result. Rumelhart (1975) showed how a rule system formalizing these principles could illuminate the structure of some stories. Other researchers (Mandler & Johnson, 1977; Thorndyke, 1977) formulated similar story grammars and showed that they captured the structure of other stories and narratives.

Empirical investigation of story grammars was undertaken in a number of ways. Rumelhart (1977) showed that his story grammars could be used to generate summaries that were comparable to those produced by people. Research on memory showed that story grammars could predict interesting aspects of story recall such as which events in a story were recalled and the effects of reordering or omitting constituents of a story (Mandler & Goodman, 1982; Mandler & Johnson, 1977; Thorndyke, 1977). Investigation of the role of story grammars in on-line comprehension showed that sentences at the boundaries of story constituents were read more slowly than those in the middle of constituents (Haberlandt, Berian, & Sandson, 1980; Mandler & Goodman, 1982).

To derive predictions from story grammars about various kinds of performance, it was necessary to elaborate purely structural models, such as the one illustrated above, into more complete processing models that specified the ways in which structure is abstracted from an input story and then used to generate a summary. Rumelhart (1977) proposed such a processing model, which at the time he could aptly characterize as the "modal model" of comprehension, one built around the notion of a schema. Schemas are knowledge representations for generic concepts. They specify the relations between the parts of a concept, which may themselves be considered as schemas, meaning that schemas can be embedded to give a hierarchical structure to concepts. The process of understanding involves fitting input (e.g., a text) into the schema. This occurs in both a bottom-up, data-driven way, and in a top-down, expectation-driven way. The schema may provide default values for some of its variables that are not determined by the input. Although schemas have been considered potentially applicable to all kinds of knowledge (Rumelhart, 1977), their invocation as "story" schemas can be regarded as having particular relevance for comprehension. That is because the story schema specifies knowledge about the structure of a certain kind of text—a story—in the same way that syntax specifies knowledge about a certain kind of word string—a sentence. The story schema may then drive the comprehension of the story, or play a critical role in planning its narration. Of course, the story structure must fit the semantic content of the story, meaning that there must be interaction between the processes responsible for story structure and content.

Research on story grammars was laudable in its efforts to bring explicit formalisms to the somewhat nebulous arena of discourse structure. However, critics quickly pointed out limitations in the work. Garnham (1983) noted that proponents of story grammars had for the most part failed to consider plausible alternative theories of the phenomena they were considering and therefore had failed to show that their theories were uniquely able to account for the nature of stories. Black and Wilensky (1979) argued that story grammars did not achieve observational adequacy because they could not generate some stories and could generate some nonstories. Rumelhart (1980) and Mandler and Johnson (1980) correctly noted that Black and Wilensky's examples of this sort were not part of the domain of stories they had studied. However, this response concedes that the domain of the story grammars was fairly limited and that they cannot be considered as general theories of the structure of narrative discourse. Additional criticism focused on the formalization of story grammars as rewrite rules (Black & Wilensky, 1979; Garnham, 1983). Though some of these criticisms were apparently mistaken (Black & Wilensky, 1979; cf. Frisch & Perlis, 1982; Mandler & Johnson, 1980; Rumelhart, 1980), Garnham (1983) noted that to be meaningful, rewrite rules must operate on a small set of nonterminal categories and a larger but still finite set of terminal elements that belong to those categories. The terminal elements for story grammars are semantic propositions which do not constitute a finite set.

It may seem that arguments about the formal structure of story grammars were premature given the relatively small number of stories that were studied and the rather loose relation between the theory and the data that were used to support it. However, the simple and explicit nature of early story grammars was a major aspect of their appeal, and this derived in good measure from the formalism that was used. The development of story grammars into the less tractable formalism of story schemas (Rumelhart, 1977) allowed them to be understood in processing terms, but also made it more difficult to clearly discern the claims that were specifically being made about stories. Of course, schemas have played a role in the explanation of diverse psychological phenomena since Bartlett (1932), but many researchers (e.g., Alba & Hasher, 1983) have noted the gap between their appeal and their ability to yield specific and valid predictions about measurable psychological phenomena.

In an approach related to story grammars, Kintsch and van Dijk (1978) proposed a model of global discourse structure called *macrostructure*. This work is presented separately from the other work on story grammars because it is more general and because it is part of an explicit overall processing model for discourse. The macrostructure is constructed out of a detailed representation of a text referred to as a microstructure. The microstructure is a local discourse structure in which the propositions in a text are linked together through shared arguments. The macrostructure corresponds to the gist of the text and is abstracted through the application of macrorules which generalize redundant propositions, delete irrelevant propositions, and infer new propositions where necessary. Application of the macrorules is under control of a schema which specifies which propositions are important. Kintsch and van Dijk (1978) discuss two possible types of schemas: The first type depends on the narrative type of the text and includes schemas for stories and scientific reports. This aspect of the model essentially generalizes the idea of story grammars to other kinds of texts by providing different "grammars" for different narrative styles. The value of this generalization depends on the richness of valid schemas for different kinds of text and the ease with which the appropriate schema type can be evoked. Unfortunately, little evidence was presented that allow this to be assessed. The second type of schema depends on the goals of the reader, for example a story can be read for enjoyment of its plot or to provide evidence about social conditions at the time it was written. The structure provided by this second type of schema is clearly not a discourse structure; rather, it is a structure based on language-independent meanings and goals. Accordingly, the Kintsch and van Dijk model should be regarded as a hybrid case which permits a global structure to be based on the text or on meaning and knowledge.

The Kintsch and van Dijk model has attracted a substantial amount of positive attention because it explicitly specifies the processing cycle whereby propositions are linked together into the microstructure and abstracted into the macrostructure. This specification has allowed comparatively precise and accurate predictions to be made about the probability that the propositions in a text will be recalled or included in a story summary. Later developments of the model (van Dijk & Kintsch, 1983) have considered a wider variety of macrostructures. This has given it greater range of application, though at some cost to its clarity. In addition, the model suffers many of the faults of the related work on story grammars and schemas; deriving a macrostructure for a narrative involves some component of ad hoc interpretation.

INTENTIONAL STRUCTURE

Grosz and Sidner (1986) propose a theory in which the global structure of discourse consists of the ways in which various discourse purposes (or intentions) are related. Though the theory is meant to apply to all types of discourses, its roots are in the study of task-oriented dialogues (Grosz, 1977). This type of discourse (a commonly used example is one person giving directions to another about how to fix an air compressor) makes particularly clear the fact that speakers use language to fulfill purposes—to *do* something. That idea has been central to philosophical analyses which tie the meaning of language to a speaker's intentions and a listener's recognition of those intentions (Austin, 1962; Grice, 1969; Searle, 1969). The work by Grosz and Sidner (1986) generalizes formalizations of speaker intentions for single utterances in conversation to discourses of different kinds made up of multiple utterances. Numerous authors (e.g., Levelt, 1989) have pointed out that conversation is developmentally primary and the most frequent form of language use. For these reasons, a unified theoretical analysis of conversation and other types of discourse is desirable.

Grosz and Sidner's (1986) intentional structure is built out of those intentions (or purposes) that the speaker or author intends to be recognized and the listener or reader must recognize for communication to be successful. (This is as distinct from some types of speaker purposes, such as to impress, that are not intended to be recognized.) According to the theory, every discourse has a single purpose that is primary. That purpose determines the choice of discourse as a form of action and the content of what is communicated. The primary *discourse purpose* (DP) is achieved through the contribution of subordinate purposes, each of which is conveyed by a separate discourse segment. The subordinate purposes are therefore called *discourse segment purposes* (DSPs). Grosz and Sidner (1986) specify two kinds of relationships between the DP and the various DSPs: dominance and satisfaction-precedence. When one DSP helps to satisfy another DSP, the first DSP is said to contribute to the second; conversely, the second dominates the first. The dominance relation therefore gives the intentions a hierarchical structure. The second relation, satisfaction-precedence, indicates that the order in which two DSPs are satisfied is important. Grosz and Sidner argue that the range of possible discourse purposes is open ended and that therefore a theory of discourse structure cannot be built around the content of individual intentions. Rather, the theory must be built around the relations that can exist between discourse purposes and the processes for planning and recognizing them.

The division of the utterances in a discourse into discourse segments is intimately bound to the recognition of discourse purposes and the relations between them. Grosz and Sidner (1986) point out that several previous researchers have argued that discourse naturally breaks down into segments, but that there have been no systematic psychological studies of the consistency with which this can be done. In their model, the fundamental decomposition of a discourse into segments derives from the presence of specific purposes (i.e., DSPs) that make important contributions to the overall purpose. While the segmentation of utterances is due to this intentional structure, utterances themselves may contain linguistic cues indicating segment boundaries. By doing so, these linguistic cues contribute to the recognition of discourse purposes and in some cases to the recognition of the relations between segment purposes. The most carefully studied of these linguistic cues are: the nature of referring expressions, intonation, and cue phrases.

Referring expressions provide evidence about discourse segmentation because their form tends to vary within and across the boundaries of discourse segments. Within a discourse segment, referring expressions tend to be reduced forms such as pronouns and ellipses (a good deal more will said about this in the section on local discourse structure). The form of referring expressions across discourse boundaries is more complicated. The use of an unreduced form (such as a name or definite description) can indicate the start of a new discourse segment. In addition, the use of a reduced form to refer to an entity that was not mentioned in the previous utterance can signal a return to a previous discourse segment. Referring expressions of this last type may be confusing if there are not additional cues to the selection of the correct referent.

Intonation, and prosody more generally, also provides cues about discourse segmentation. One such cue is that speech rate tends to be slower at the start of a discourse segment than at the end (Butterworth, 1975; Lehiste, 1979). Research on a second cue, pitch range, has shown that the variation in pitch that occurs over a sentence increases in sentences that begin a discourse segment (Lehiste, 1979; Silverman, 1987). Perceptual studies have shown that listeners exploit this as a cue to discourse structure (Hirschberg & Pierrehumbert, 1986; Silverman, 1987).

"Cue phrases" is the term used by Grosz and Sidner (1986) to refer to a class of expressions that they, and other investigators, have argued play an explicit role in indicating the segmental structure of discourse as well as its underlying intentional structure. Cue phrases include expressions such as "next," "anyway," "by the way," and "in any case." The purpose of such expressions is manifestly aimed at providing information about the intentional structure of the discourse (or its "attentional focus," see below). In some cases, specific cue phrases provide information about the relation between discourse purposes. Phrases such as "for example" and "to wit" indicate a dominance relation. Phrases such as "first" and "finally" provide information about satisfaction-precedence. It is important to note that these expressions can serve roles in addition to conveying discourse structure. However, acoustic analyses (Hirschberg & Litman, 1987) have shown that the cue-phrase uses of the word "now" were distinguishable from the temporally deictic uses through phrasing and accent.

Grosz and Sidner (1986) apply their theory systematically to the analysis of two kinds of discourse phenomena: interruptions and cue phrases. They show that various kinds of interruptions (e.g., flashbacks and digressions), as well as cue phrases, must be performed in a way that respects the intentional structure of the discourse. Further development of Grosz and Sidner's (1986) theory requires specification of algorithms for turning intentions into plans for discourse acts and for recognizing intentions from discourse acts. In discussing such algorithms, Grosz & Sidner (1986, 1990) point to considerable research in computer science on these problems, not just in the domain of discourse, but also as they pertain to action more generally (e.g., robot control). This follows quite naturally from their view of discourse as a kind of natural activity.

SUMMARY

The various approaches discussed above (story grammars or schemas, macrostructures, and intentional structures) are similar in characterizing global discourse structure as hierarchical. This hierarchy is built out of a fixed set of goals in the story approach, and a more open set in the macrostructure approach. In the intentional approach, the structure is built out of an open set of intentions among which there is a fixed, small set of relations. The range of possible goals (or intentions) presents a clear trade-off: Is it better to work with a small set of goals in relatively fixed relations that gives a detailed account of a narrow domain of narratives? Or, is it better to work with an open set of goals or intentions that is potentially applicable to a broad range of narratives, but requires further development in order to provide a powerful account of discourse structure?

A basic difference between the approaches to global discourse structure is whether it is built out of goals or intentions. Exact definitions of these terms would require quite close attention to philosophical nuance, but at least some of the difference between them in the present context is easy to see. The goals in story grammars belong to the participants in the events described by the story, and a story by definition must be about events with the kind of goal structure described by a story grammar. In contrast, the intentional structure of Grosz and Sidner (1986) refers to the intentions of the speaker (or author) of the narrative. This distinction is consistent with how the different approaches see discourse in regard to other psychological phenomena. Story schemas (Rumelhart, 1977) treat discourse as a special case of knowledge representation, whereas the intentional approach (Grosz & Sidner, 1986) treats discourse as a special case of action. The relative merits of these different affiliations is again hard to assess and may depend on the type of discourse. Analysis of conversation clearly relies at least to some extent on recognizing the importance of the speaker's utterances as acts that are intended to influence the listener. It is less clear that such recognition is necessary for other kinds of narratives, such as a novel, where there is less engagement between discourse participants.

Independent of their differences, all of these approaches to global discourse confront the common challenge of developing more principled ways of describing the structures of narratives. As many critics have commented (e.g., Johnson-Laird, 1983; Rayner & Pollatsek, 1989), applying such models relies heavily on intuitive analyses of a text. The use of intuition per se is not the problem; most linguistic analyses of language structure rely on it extensively. However, structural analyses that use intuition as primary data are risky unless people's intuitions about the basic elements of the structure are clear and general. This has not been demonstrated for the global discourse structures that have been postulated.

INTERACTION OF GLOBAL AND LOCAL DISCOURSE STRUCTURE

Two of the models discussed above address the structure of discourse at both the global and local levels. According to the Kintsch and van Dijk (1978) model, discourse comprehension makes use of a limited-capacity short-term buffer that contains arguments of propositions that are readily available for linking with identical arguments of newly encountered propositions. This buffer contains arguments from recently processed text and also arguments that are schematically important. Thus, the buffer mixes elements of both the local discourse structure through recency and global discourse structure through schematic importance. When an input proposition cannot be linked to an argument in the short-term buffer, an exhaustive search is performed of long-term memory for the text. Psychological research on *reinstatement* of arguments from long-term memory has shown that it is a time-consuming process (e.g., Lesgold, Ross, & Curtis, 1979; O'Brien, 1987).

For Grosz and Sidner (1986), the corresponding structure is the *focus space stack*, which models the discourse participants attentional state. A focus space in the stack contains the entities mentioned (or strongly implied) in a discourse segment, as well as the discourse segment purpose. The stack contains a subset of the focus spaces previously operative in the discourse, with the current discourse segment at the top of the stack. The inclusion and ordering of focus spaces on the stack is determined by the dominance structure of the discourse segment purposes. If the purpose of a new discourse segment contributes to the purpose of the immediately preceding segment, then the focus space of the preceding segment is *pushed* on the stack; if it does not contribute, then the preceding focus space is *popped* off the stack.[1] Thus, the ordering of the focus space retains a reduced representation of the intentional structure of a discourse. This reduced representation determines the ease with which references can be made to entities that are not contained in the focus space of the current discourse segment.

Although there are clear differences between the two models, the short-term buffer of Kintsch and van Dijk (1978) and the focus space stack of Grosz and Sidner (1986) are similar in constraining the semantic information that is available for interpreting an utterance as locally coherent. In that context, it is interesting to note that psychologists generally view the capacity of short-term memory as limiting human cognitive ability. The motivation of computational linguists for postulating the analogous focus spaces is different; they constrain the amount of information that is relevant for interpretation and therefore make the computational task more tractable.

---

[1] In computer architecture, a "stack" is an easily accessible memory structure. Like a stack of papers, it is organized sequentially with the first unit of stored information on the top. Adding a new unit of information to the stack is called a "push" because the rest of the information is pushed further down. Removing a unit of information is called a "pop" because everything else moves up one step.

LOCAL DISCOURSE STRUCTURE

There is much broader agreement about the existence of discourse structure at the local level than at the global level. Further, there is substantial agreement that this structure depends critically on patterns of *co-reference* between sentences. For example, in Passage 1:

Passage 1
John ran all the way to the bustop.
He wanted to be sure to catch the 8:00 a.m. bus.

both "John" and "he" co-refer. The term co-reference (or sometimes co-specification or co-indexation) is used to make it clear that one linguistic expression (e.g., "he") does not refer to a second linguistic expression (i.e., "John"), but rather that both linguistic expressions refer to the same semantic object (i.e., "the person named John"). Various linguists (Halliday & Hassan, 1976), psychologists (Johnson-Laird, 1983; Kintsch & van Dijk, 1978), and computer scientists (Grosz, Joshi, & Weinstein, 1986; Hobbs, 1979) have argued that the extent and manner in which successive sentences make reference to common entities is related to the local coherence of discourse.

EXTENT OF CO-REFERENCE

The intuitive reason why co-reference is important to coherence is that it is hard to see how a series of sentences can go together without talking about the same things. More formal expressions of this reason are also available. As noted above, in the Kintsch and van Dijk (1978) model, comprehension involves an attempt to link propositions together if they have common arguments. The arguments of propositions are entities that are referred to in a narrative. Overlapping arguments provide a basis for linking if they are in short-term memory (STM) at the same time. As recency provides an important basis for a proposition's being in STM, references to the same entity in successive sentences will increase the likelihood that propositions can be linked easily. Experimental research on reading time and recall has shown that argument repetition does facilitate discourse comprehension (Kintsch, Kozminsky, Streby, McKoon & Keenan, 1975; Manelis & Yekovich, 1976).

BRIDGING INFERENCES

In some cases, definite references can be made in such a way that the reader (or listener) is led to believe that the entity being referred to has been previously introduced into the discourse, even when it has not. In such cases, the reader is invited to infer the relationship between the entity and other aspects of the discourse that have been previously introduced. Haviland and Clark (1974) studied such bridging inferences as part of the Given-New Strategy in language comprehension. According to this strategy, a felicitously uttered sentence will convey some given (or old) information that allows it to be linked to the preceding discourse, as well as some new information that modifies what was previously known. The first task of the reader is to match the given part of the sentence to the appropriate memory representation for the previously given information. If there is no direct match, then the reader must infer it. The classic example of such bridging inferences comes from comparison of the following two passages:

Passage 2
We got some beer out of the trunk.
The beer was warm.
Passage 3
We checked the picnic supplies.
The beer was warm.

In Passage 2, "beer" is explicitly mentioned in the first sentence, providing an easy match for its mention in the second sentence. In Passage 3, "beer" is not explicitly mentioned in the first sentence, and the reader must infer that it was included in the picnic supplies in order to provide a match for its mention in the second sentence. Haviland and Clark (1974) showed that comprehension times for sentences were longer when such inferences must be drawn. For present purposes, this result shows quite clearly that local discourse coherence is dependent on referential continuity. If this continuity is not present in the explicit text, then the necessary inferences are drawn during comprehension to allow sentences to be linked together.

MANNER OF REFERENCE

Referring expressions can be made in a variety of forms such as definite descriptions, names, pronouns, and ellipses. The choice of manner of reference depends in part on discourse structure. Both linguistic analyses (e.g., Chafe, 1976) and experimental research on language production (Fletcher, 1984; Marslen-Wilson, Levy, & Tyler, 1982) have shown that speakers use reduced forms (e.g., pronouns and ellipses) to refer to highly focused entities, whereas unreduced forms (e.g., definite descriptions) are used to refer to nonfocused entities. Intuitively, there are two reasons for this. First, the greater information present in the unreduced form may be necessary to determine the correct referent for a nonfocused entity. In contrast, a reduced form is sufficient to specify an entity that is highly focused. Second, the use of a marked form to refer to a highly focused entity conveys more information than is necessary, thereby violating Grice's (1969) maxim of quantity and inviting the implicature that the reference is intended to do more than provide a basis for referential coherence with the previous sentence.

INTERPRETATION OF AMBIGUOUS PRONOUNS

Although reference to common entities helps sentences cohere into discourse segments, the assumption that discourse segments are coherent can aid in determining the referents of syntactically ambiguous pronouns. Syntactic ambiguity arises when gender, number, animacy, and disjoint reference are not sufficient to specify the entity referred to by a pronoun, and there is evidence that it makes pronoun interpretation more difficult (e.g., Frederiksen, 1981). One structural factor that aids pronoun interpretation derives from a tendency for pronouns to refer to the grammatical subjects of previous sentences (Frederiksen, 1981). A second structural factor, which often subsumes the first, is called *parallel function* (Caramazza, Grober, & Garvey, 1977; Sheldon, 1974); a pronoun will be interpreted as being co-referential with an earlier noun phrase if the two play the same grammatical role in their respective sentences or clauses.

CENTERING: A THEORY OF LOCAL DISCOURSE COHERENCE

Centering theory, developed by Grosz, Joshi and Weinstein (1983, 1986) provides a specific formulation of how reference contributes to local discourse coherence. Within the more encompassing framework of Grosz and Sidner (1986), centering is meant to capture operations within a focus space on the focus stack. It aims to account for the characteristics of reference described above, as well as other phenomena associated with reference that have not been treated by other theorists. Centering is a revision of a theory of immediate focusing by Sidner (1979). It has been employed in the development of natural language processing systems (see Gordon, Grosz, & Gilliom, 1993 for references) and has been tested and refined as a psychological theory.

Discourse centers are semantic objects that provide coherence in a discourse segment; in many ways they are analogous to the propositional arguments of Kintsch and van Dijk (1978). However, centering makes a further distinction between backward-looking and forward-looking centers. Each utterance in a discourse segment is thought to have a single backward-looking center (the **Cb**) that provides a link back to the previous utterance. Each utterance also has an ordered set of forward-looking centers (the **Cf**) that provide potential links to the subsequent utterance. The centers in Passage 4 are partially identified.

Passage 4
1. Susan gave Betsy a pet hamster.
   Cf = {Susan, Betsy, hamster$_1$}
2. She reminded her that such hamsters were quite shy.
   Cb = {Susan} **Cf** = {Susan, Betsy, hamsters}
3. She asked Betsy whether she liked the gift.
   Cb = {Susan} **Cf** = {Susan, Betsy, hamster$_1$}

There is no **Cb** in the first utterance, because there is no preceding utterance for it to link back to. The **Cf** of this utterance includes Susan, Betsy, and some particular hamster—hamster$_1$. The second and third utterances have the same **Cb** (Susan), and their **Cf** lists are shown.[2]

The **Cb** of an utterance is the entity that provides the strongest semantic link back to the previous utterance; thus, it plays an essential role in coherence. As originally developed (Grosz et al., 1983, 1986), centering theory did not completely identify the factors that made an entity the **Cb** of an utterance; however, it was believed that factors such as realization as a pronoun, surface-initial position, grammatical status, and prominence in the previous utterance were all potentially important. Psycholinguistic research to be discussed below (Gordon et al., 1993) has shown that realization as the grammatical subject of an utterance, if that is possible, is the critical factor in making an entity the **Cb** of an utterance.

The **Cf** is the set of entities realized in an utterance, ordered in terms of prominence. The members of the **Cf** provide potential links to the next utterance; the ease of the link being determined by an entities ranking in the **Cf** set. As with the **Cb**, the factors determining this ranking were not completely specified in Grosz et al., (1983, 1986), but were thought to include realization as a pronoun, surface-initial position and grammatical status. Psycholinguistic research (Gordon et al., 1993) has demonstrated the importance of status as grammatical subject and of surface-initial position in the ranking of the **Cf**. Other likely determinants remain to be investigated.

Centering theory was developed to provide a formal account of two constraints on the coherence of discourse segments: the linguistic realization of discourse centers and the continuity of centers across utterances. With regard to the first of these, centering theory specified a rule that said in essence that no entity in an utterance could be realized by a

---

[2] These are only partial *Cf* lists. More complete lists might include semantic entities such as the one realized by the verb phrase "gave Betsy a pet hamster."

pronoun unless the **Cb** was also realized by a pronoun. This rule adds substantial precision to previous research that had noted a tendency to use reduced forms (such as pronouns) to refer to topics (see the discussion above). It was motivated by consideration of examples such as Passage 5, which repeats Passage 4 with an alternative final sentence.

Passage 5
1. Susan gave Betsy a pet hamster.
2. She reminded her that such hamsters were quite shy.
3. Susan asked her whether she liked the gift.

The only difference between the two passages is that in Passage 5, sentence 3 realizes Susan with a name, whereas in Passage 4, sentence 3 realized Susan with a pronoun. Intuitively, this difference makes the second version of the passage far less coherent than the first. Centering theory explains this incoherence as due to the **Cb** (Susan) being realized in Passage 5, sentence 3, with a name while a non-**Cb** (Betsy) is realized with a pronoun—a violation of the rule stated above.

The second discourse phenomenon addressed by centering has to do with the transitions of centers across a pair of utterances. Three kinds of transitions are defined: *continue, retain,* and *shift*. In a *continue transition,* the **Cb** of an utterance (utt_n) is the same as the **Cb** of the previous utterance (utt_{n-1}). In a *retain transition,* the **Cb** of an utterance (utt_n) is again the **Cb** of the previous utterance (utt_{n-1}), but its ranking in the **Cf** list of utt_n means that it is unlikely to be the **Cb** of the next utterance (utt_{n+1}). In a *shift transition,* the **Cb** of an utterance (utt_n) is not the same as the **Cb** of the previous utterance (utt_{n-1})[3]. The relative processing demands of these three kinds of transitions are: continue easier than retain easier than shift.

Experimental tests of centering theory (Gordon et al., 1993), using self-paced reading time methodology, have provided support for three of its principle claims, that there is a strong preference to have the **Cb** realized as a pronoun, that an utterance only contains one **Cb**, and that the **Cf** is a set whose members are ordered by prominence.

The most basic experiment manipulated pronominalization of entities in passages like Passages 4 and 5. In these passages, the first utterance introduces two individuals by name. One of these ("Susan" in the examples) appears as grammatical subject in surface-initial position throughout the passage. These factors are taken to ensure that that entity is both the **Cb** and the highest ranking member of the **Cf** throughout the pas-

---

[3] More formal definitions of the three kinds of center transitions, as well as the constraint on manner of realization that was described above, are given in Grosz et al., (1986) and are repeated in Gordon et al. (1993). The current definitions are sufficient to convey their basic content.

sage. The manner of realization (pronoun vs. name) of both named entities is manipulated after the introductory sentence. The most basic finding is that reading times are significantly elevated when the **Cb** is realized by a name rather than a pronoun—a finding dubbed the "repeated-name penalty." Differences in reading time are not observed as a function of whether the non-**Cb** is realized as a pronoun or a name. This result supports the essence of centering theory's contention that the **Cb** must be realized as a pronoun for an utterance to be coherent with a discourse segment. However, the original formulation limited this contention to cases where a non-**Cb** was realized by a pronoun. The experimental results demonstrate the importance of realizing the **Cb** as a pronoun regardless of how other entities in the utterance are realized.

Additional experiments examined linguistic factors that were responsible for an entity's being the **Cb** of an utterance, using the repeated-name penalty as a diagnostic. In particular, these experiments dissociated the factors of grammatical subject and surface-initial position by using passages such as 6 and 7 below:

Passage 6
Elizabeth read Tom's palm the other day.
According to **her/Elizabeth**, good things were in store for **him/Tom**.
Vague predictions like this usually come true.
Passage 7
Susan gave Fred a pet hamster.
In **his/Fred's** opinion, **she/Susan** shouldn't have done that.
Giving a pet as a gift is somewhat of an imposition.

The experiments manipulated the manner of realization (name vs. pronoun) of the highlighted entities in the critical second sentence of each passage. This manipulation only affected reading times for grammatical subjects (e.g., Susan in the critical sentence of Passage 7). There, realization as name led to slower reaction times than realization as a pronoun—the repeated-name penalty. No repeated-name penalties were observed for entities in any other position, including those in the fronted phrases such as "According to her" and "In his opinion." These results lead to the conclusion that the **Cb** of an utterance, if it has one, is the grammatical subject of the utterance if that is possible. This is consistent with a major contention of centering theory, that an utterance only has one **Cb**. The importance of subject status in determining the **Cb** is consistent with linguistic research (e.g., Chafe, 1976; Prince, 1981) showing that grammatical subjects play an important role in giving a discourse continuity.

The reading time procedure was also used to study the factors that determine prominence in the set of forward-looking centers (**Cf**). These studies looked at the magnitude of the repeated-name penalty for grammatical subjects (an indication of the extent to which the **Cb** provides coherence) as a function of that entity's role in the preceding utterance. Consider Passage 8 below:

Passage 8
1. George jumped out from behind a tree and frightened Debbie.
2. He was surprised at her hysterical reaction.
3. **He/George** never thinks about how others might feel.
3a. **She/Debbie** screamed loudly and ran away.
4. Practical jokes are not always fun for everyone.

The two alternative versions of the critical third sentence realize entities with different roles in Sentence 2: "George" is the subject while "Debbie" is a late-occurring part of the verb phrase. A substantial repeated-name penalty was observed for critical sentences that continued the subject of the previous sentence (e.g., Sentence 3 realizing "George"), while a small and not significant effect was observed for critical sentences that did not continue the subject (e.g., Sentence 3a realizing "Debbie"). This finding validates the construct of an ordered set of forward-looking centers (**Cf**) by showing that entities in the second sentence differ in terms of their ability to provide a strong link to the third sentence.

The factors determining the ordering of the **Cf** were further studied by dissociating status as grammatical subject from surface ordering. This was done using passages such as:

Passage 9
1. Susan gave Fred a pet hamster.
2. In his opinion, she shouldn't have done that.
3. **She/Susan** just assumed that anyone would love a hamster.
3a. **He/Fred** doesn't have anywhere to put a hamster cage.
4. Giving a pet as a gift can be somewhat of an imposition.

In the second sentence, "Susan" is the grammatical subject, but "Fred" occurs in surface-initial position. Manipulation of pronominalization in the alternative versions of the critical third sentence showed equally large repeated name penalties for the **Cb**s "Susan" (Sentence 3) and "Fred" (Sentence 3a). This indicates that status as grammatical subject and surface-initial position contribute equally to prominence in the set of forward-looking centers. The importance of surface-initial position in determining prominence is consistent with findings (Corbett & Chang, 1983; Gernsbacher & Hargeaves, 1988) which have shown that surface-initial position increases accessibility in memory. With regard to centering theory, the finding supports the dissociation between the **Cf** and the **Cb**. There is only one **Cb** while the **Cf** is a set, and the identity of the **Cb** is determined largely by status as grammatical subject while prominence in the **Cf** is determined by status as grammatical subject and by surface position in an utterance.

The discussion of centering so far has focused on the effects of names and pronouns on the coherence of discourse segments. In addition, centering also addresses the effects of discourse structure on the interpretation of syntactically ambiguous pronouns. In particular, it states that a syntactically ambiguous pronoun will be interpreted by default as realizing the highest ranked member of the set of forward-looking centers of the previous utterance until such time as that interpretation is overridden by other information. This hypothesis was tested (Gordon & Scearce, 1993) using passages such as 10 below:

Passage 10
1. Jim just appointed Don copy editor of the newspaper.
2. As a first assignment, he asked him to proofread this week's lead story.
3. **He/Jim** was nervous about * <u>delegating</u> so much responsibility so soon.
3a. **He/Don** was nervous about * <u>having</u> so much responsibility so soon.
4. It's usually best to give new editors a few weeks to practice first.

By realizing "Jim" as a surface-initial subject, the first two sentences establish that entity as the highest-ranked member of the **Cf** list. Sentence 3 continues to realize "Jim" as the subject, while the change of a single word ("having") in Sentence 3a means that its subject should be interpreted as "Don" on semantic grounds. The sentences were divided into phrases that were presented one at a time, and the critical third sentence was always divided at some point between the occurrence of its subject and the disambiguating word (as shown by the asterisk in the example). The most central finding is that reading times for the disambiguating phrase were substantially elevated for sentences that did not continue the subject (e.g., 3a) when they began with pronouns. This indicates that readers interpreted initial pronouns in the critical sentence as referring by default to the highest-ranked member of the **Cf** of Sentence 2 and then were forced to revise that interpretation when confronted with conflicting semantic information.

This result shows the importance of local discourse structure in the interpretation of pronouns, but it could be argued that structure was only important because at the time the pronoun was encountered, there was no semantic information on which to base an interpretation. Passages such as 11 below were used by Gordon and Scearce (1993) to examine pronoun interpretation when both structural and semantic information were available before the pronoun was encountered.

Passage 11
1. Kay asked Bev to sit for a portrait.
2. She warned her that such paintings take a very long time to complete.
3. After <u>painting</u> for several days, **she** was finally happy with the portrait.
3a. After <u>posing</u> for several days, **she** was finally happy with the portrait.
4. The finished product was truly beautiful.

As with the previous experiment, the first two sentences set up one individual as being particularly prominent, and the two versions of the third sentence either continued or shifted this entity as **Cb**. However, in this case, the semantically disambiguating information occurred before the critical pronoun. Sentences that continued the **Cb** (e.g., 3) with a pronoun were read more quickly than those (e.g., 3a) that shifted to a different pronominal entity. This indicates that local discourse structure influences the interpretation of a pronoun even when it conflicts with previously available semantic information. Undoubtedly, the final interpretation of the pronoun is determined by what is most sensible semantically. However, the on-line default interpretation of pronouns appears to be influenced by aspects of discourse structure that are at least partially impervious to semantic information. In addition, these aspects of discourse structure are readily retrievable from surface aspects of language, meaning that their use in pronoun interpretation is computationally advantageous.

Centering theory provides a synthesis of some previous findings about local discourse structure, as well as offering some unique predictions. It has made contributions to a number of natural language processing systems, and has also been tested as psychological theory. Its predictions about how manner of realization influences local discourse coherence and about how assumptions about discourse structure influence pronoun interpretation have proven very accurate. The experimental studies have also included some tests of centering theory's predictions about the relative ease of processing the three kinds of transitions of the backward-looking center: continue, retain and shift. These tests have provided some support for the predicted relation, but the magnitude of the effects have not been large. This points to the need for revising the original formulation of center transitions, perhaps so that it spans sequences of utterances larger than pairs. Further development of centering theory requires addressing a variety of issues such as the nature of the interaction between discourse constraints and intra-sentential constraints on pronoun use, algorithms that incorporate the findings of the psychological studies of centering, and further formalization of how discourse centers create semantic coherence in a discourse segment.

CONCLUSION

It should be clear that the characteristics of local discourse structure are much better understood than those of global discourse structure, so much so that arguments that at the global level there is no discourse structure per se do not seem viable at the local level. A principle reason for this is that the basic components of structure at the local level, referring expressions, can be easily identified and classified. The basic components of structure that are thought to be operative at the global level, be they goals or intentions, are considerably harder to recognize. Obviously, the strength of a theoretical structure depends greatly on its building blocks.

Even though the building blocks of structure at the local level are clear, it does not seem likely that traditional linguistic methods of analyzing intuitions about the structure of a discourse and about the relation between discourses will be successful in revealing the detailed characteristics of discourse structure at that level. This point is illustrated by the development of centering theory, where important information about effects of pronominalization and the identity of the backward-looking center only emerged through psychological experimentation. It remains an open question whether such objective methods can be developed for more rigorously demonstrating the characteristics of discourse structure at the global level.

ACKNOWLEDGMENT

Preparation of this chapter was supported by a grant from the National Science Foundation (IRI-90-09018) to Harvard University, Barbara J. Grosz, and Peter C. Gordon, Principal Investigators.

REFERENCES

Alba, J. W., & Hasher, L. (1983). Is memory schematic? *Psychological Bulletin, 93,* 203–231.
Anderson, A., Garrod, S., & Sanford, A. (1977). The accessibility of pronominal antecedents as a function of episode shifts in narrative text. *Quarterly Journal of Experimental Psychology, 35A,* 427–440.

Austin, J. L. (1962). *How to do things with words.* Oxford, England: Clarendon Press.
Bartlett, F. C. (1932) *Remembering: A study in experimental and social psychology.* Cambridge, England: Cambridge University Press.
Black, J. B., & Wilensky, R. (1979). An evaluation of story grammars. *Cognitive Science, 3,* 213–230.
Butterworth, B. (1975). Hesitation and semantic planning in speech. Journal of *Psycholinguistic Research, 4,* 75–7.
Caramazza, A., Grober, E., & Garvey, C. (1977). Comprehension of anaphoric pronouns. *Journal of Verbal Learning and Verbal Behavior, 16,* 601–609.
Chafe, W. L. (1976). Givenness, contrastiveness, definiteness, subjects, topics, and points of view. In C. N. Li (Ed.), *Subject and topic* (pp. 26–55). New York: Academic Press.
Corbett, A. T., & Chang, F. R. (1983). Pronoun disambiguation: Accessing potential antecedents. *Memory & Cognition, 11,* 283–294.
Fletcher, C. R. (1984). Markedness and topic continuity in discourse processing. *Journal of Verbal Learning and Verbal Behavior, 23,* 487–493.
Frederiksen, J. R. (1981). Understanding anaphora: Rules used by readers in assigning pronominal referents. *Discourse Processes, 4,* 323–347.
Frisch, A. M., & Perlis, D. (1982). A re-evaluation of story grammars. *Cognitive Science, 5,* 79–86.
Garnham, A. (1983). What's wrong with story grammars. *Cognition, 15,* 145–154.
Gernsbacher, M. A., & Hargreaves, D. (1988). Accessing sentence participants: The advantage of first mention. *Journal of Memory and Language, 27,* 699–717.
Glenberg, A. M., Meyer, M., & Lindem, K. (1987). Mental models contribute to foregrounding during text comprehension. *Journal of Memory and Language, 26,* 69–83.
Gordon, P. C., & Scearce, K. A. (1993). Pronominalization and discourse coherence, discourse coherence and pronoun interpretation. Paper submitted for publication.
Gordon, P. C., Grosz, B. J., & Gilliom, L. A. (1993). Pronouns, names, and the centering of attention in discourse. *Cognitive Science, 17.*
Grice, H. P. (1969). Utterer's meaning and intentions. *Philosophical Review, 68,* 147–177.
Grosz, B. J. (1977). *The representation and use of focus in dialogue understanding* (Technical Rep. No. 151). Menlo Park, CA: Artificial Intelligence Center, SRI International.
Grosz, B. J., Joshi, A. K., & Weinstein, S. (1983). Providing a unified account of definite noun phrases in discourse. *Proceedings of the 21st Annual Meeting of the Association for Computational Linguistics.*
Grosz, B. J., Joshi, A. K., & Weinstein, S. (1986). *Towards a computational theory of discourse interpretation.* Unpublished manuscript.
Grosz, B. J., & Sidner, C. L. (1986). Attention, intentions, and the structure of discourse. *Computational Linguistics, 12,* 175–204.
Grosz, B. J., & Sidner, C. L. (1990). Plans for discourse. In P. R. Cohen, J. Morgan, & M. E. Pollack (Eds.), *Intentions in communication* (pp. 417–444). Cambridge, MA: MIT Press.
Haberlandt, K., Berian, C., & Sandson, J. (1980). The episode schema in story processing. *Journal of Verbal Learning and Verbal Behavior, 19,* 635–650.
Halliday, M. A., & Hassan, R. (1976). *Cohesion in English.* London, England: Longman.
Haviland, S. E., & Clark, H. H. (1974). What's new? Acquiring new information as a process in comprehension. *Journal of Verbal Learning and Verbal Behavior, 13,* 512–521.

Hirschberg, J., & Litman, D. (1987). Now let's talk about 'now': Identifying cue phrases intonationally. *Proceedings of the 25th Annual Meeting of the Association for Computational Linguistics.*

Hirschberg, J., & Pierrehumbert, J. (1986). The intonational structuring of discourse. *Proceedings of the 24th Annual Meeting of the Association for Computational Linguistics.*

Hobbs, J. R. (1979). Coherence and co-reference. *Cognitive Science, 3,* 67–90.

Johnson-Laird, P. N. (1983). *Mental models: Toward a cognitive science of language, inference and consciousness.* Cambridge, MA: Harvard University Press.

Kintsch, W., Kozminsky, E., Streby, W. J., McKoon, F., & Keenan, J. M. (1975). Comprehension and recall of text as a function of content variables. *Journal of Verbal Learning and Verbal Behavior, 14,* 196–214.

Kintsch, W., & van Dijk, T. A. (1978). Toward a model of text comprehension and production. *Psychological Review, 85,* 363–394.

Lehiste, I. (1979). Perception of sentence and paragraph boundaries. In B. Lindblom & S. Ohman (Eds.), *Frontiers of Speech Research* (pp. 191–201). London, England: Academic Press.

Lesgold, A. M., Roth, S. F., & Curtis, M. E. (1979). Foregrounding effects in discourse comprehension. *Journal of Verbal Learning and Verbal Behavior, 18,* 291–308.

Levelt, W. J. M. (1989). *Speaking: From intention to articulation.* Cambridge, MA: MIT Press.

Mandler, J. M., & Goodman, M. S. (1982). On the psychological validity of story structure. *Journal of Verbal Learning and Verbal Behavior, 21,* 507–523.

Mandler, J. M., & Johnson, N. S. (1977). Remembrance of things parsed: Story structure and recall. *Cognitive Psychology, 9,* 111–151.

Mandler, J. M., & Johnson, N. S. (1980). On throwing out the baby with the bathwater: A reply to Black and Wilensky's evaluation of story grammars. *Cognitive Science, 4,* 305–312.

Manelis, L., & Yekovich, F. R. (1976). Repetition of propositional arguments in sentences. *Journal of Verbal Learning and Verbal Behavior, 15,* 301–312.

Marr, D. (1982). *Vision.* New York: W. H. Freeman.

Marslen-Wilson, W., Levy, W., & Tyler, L. K. (1982). Producing interpretable discourse: The establishment and maintenance of reference. In R. Jarvella & W. Klein (Eds.), *Speech, Place, and Action* (pp. 339–378) New York: John Wiley & Sons.

O'Brien, E. J. (1987). Antecedent search processes and the structure of text. *Journal of Experimental Psychology: Learning, Memory, and Cognition, 13,* 278–290.

Prince, E. F. (1981). Toward a taxonomy of given-new information. *Radical Pragmatics,* 223–255.

Rayner, K., & Pollatsek, A. (1989). *The psychology of reading.* Englewood Cliffs, NJ: Prentice Hall.

Rumelhart, D. E. (1975). Notes on a schema for stories. In D. G. Bobrow & A. Collins (Eds.), *Representation and understanding* (pp. 211–236). New York: Academic Press.

Rumelhart, D. E. (1977). Understanding and summarizing brief stories. In D. LaBerge & S. J. Samuels (Eds.), *Basic processes in reading: Perception and comprehension* (pp. 265–303). Hillsdale, NJ: Lawrence Erlbaum.

Rumelhart, D. E. (1980). On evaluating story grammars. *Cognitive Science, 4,* 313–316.

Schank, R. C., & Abelson, R. P. (1977). *Scripts, plans, goals, and understanding: An inquiry into human knowledge structures.* Hillsdale, NJ: Lawrence Erlbaum.

Searle, J. (1969). *Speech acts*. Cambridge, England: Cambridge University Press.

Sheldon, A. (1974). The role of parallel function in the acquisition of relative clauses in English. *Journal of Verbal Learning and Verbal Behavior, 13*, 272–281.

Sidner, C. L. (1979). *A computational model of co-reference comprehension in English*. Unpublished doctoral dissertation, Massachusetts Institute of Technology, Cambridge, MA.

Silverman, K. E. A. (1987). *The structure and processing of fundamental frequency contours*. Unpublished doctoral dissertation, University of Cambridge, Cambridge, England.

Thorndyke, P. W. (1977). Cognitive structures in comprehension and memory of narrative discourse. *Cognitive Psychology, 9*, 77–110.

Trabasso, T., & van den Broek, P. (1985). Causal thinking and the representation of narrative events. *Journal of Memory and Language, 24*, 612–630.

van Dijk, T. A., & Kintsch, W. (1983). *Strategies of discourse comprehension*. New York: Academic Press.

CHAPTER 3

A Neurosemiotic Perspective on Text Processing

PETER GRZYBEK

The notion of "text" is central to many neuropsychological studies attempting to understand discourse processing either in normal populations or in particular groups of neurologically impaired patients. In many of these studies, the term "discourse" is used as a synonym for "text," though neither term is theoretically defined. Instead, both terms have been used as vague umbrella terms, connoting any kind of verbal performance beyond the mere sentence level. Moreover, extremely different types of texts are subsumed under the general term "discourse": such divergent text types as jokes, stories, descriptions, indirect speech acts, idioms, and proverbs are often labeled either "discourse" or "text." To further complicate things, the manner of presentation of these different text types varies significantly in neuropsychological studies: Oral presentations are not distinguished from visual representations, and authentic communicative situations are not distinguished from hypothetical ones.

Consequently, insufficient attention has been paid to additional specifics related to any of these textual genres or to their manners of representation; to date, even the basic notions of "text" and "discourse" have not been clearly defined. This overall lack of theoretical specificity often makes it difficult, if not impossible, to interpret the results reported in neuropsychological studies.

Partly as an attempt to resolve this terminological fuzziness, this chapter explores the following topics:

1. relevant neuropsychological research on the role of the right hemisphere (RH) in text processing, since this hemisphere has repeatedly been observed to play an important role in discourse processing;
2. a general—theoretical discussion of the notion of "text," focusing on the semiotic status of the text, that is, on its sign character, in order to provide a framework for categorizing the many text types discussed in the neuropsychological literature;
3. results of studies that attempt to define exactly what a text is, that is, what renders the text a text. In this context, the achievements and shortcomings of studies from various disciplines—text linguistics, psycholinguistics, or psychology of text processing, and neuropsychology of text processing—are reviewed.
4. relate more recent approaches in the field of text theory to neuropsychological findings in order to integrate them into a broader "neurosemiotic" interpretation. Particular attention is paid to the mental model theory of text construction and to the semiotic modeling of world knowledge involved in this process.

TEXT PROCESSING AND THE RIGHT HEMISPHERE

Neuropsychological studies on discourse and text processing commenced in the 1980s. Before then, neuropsychology had focused almost exclusively on language processing on a word and sentence level, not sufficiently taking into account that, under normal circumstances, communication involves larger contexts. Thus, neuropsychology parallelled earlier developments in both linguistics and psycholinguistics, which also shifted their initially lexical perspectives to an emphasis on sentence-based processing and finally arrived at the study of sentence sequences and complex texts.

Not until the late 1970s did neuropsychology begin to consider studies of text processing in brain-damaged people a fruitful subject for analysis. Following pioneering studies on text processing in left hemisphere-damaged (LHD) aphasics (Engel, 1977; Stachowiak, Huber, Poeck & Kerschensteiner, 1977), it emerged, rather surprisingly, that right hemisphere-damaged (RHD) patients displayed significant impairments in the processing of more complex linguistic material, irrespective of the otherwise quite normally preserved linguistic competence in such persons. Thus, Moscovitch (1983) reported that RHD patients "seem to have no difficulty comprehending individual sentences, but they do have difficulty relating a sentence to a larger context" (p. 69), and Gardner, Brownell, Wapner, and Michelow (1983) noted that such patients "have seemingly normal syntax and phonology" (p. 172), but still are "markedly impaired in their ability to organize sentences into coherent narratives" (p. 183). By the end of the 1980s, "a growing body of research" revealed that "RHD patients, despite their largely intact linguistic skills, are compromised in their performance at the discourse level" (Weylman, Brownell, Roman, & Gardner, 1989, p. 582).

One of the first studies of discourse processing in RHD patients was conducted by Delis (1980); in this study, subjects were asked to arrange the mixed-up sentences of stories. The results revealed that the RHD patients made significantly more errors than normals in arranging the sentences. The author arrived at the conclusion that "processes attributed to the right hemisphere play an important role in the production of coherent discourse" (p. 40), though he was not able to isolate the specific processes involved. He also concluded that patients with RH insults are "unable to establish or maintain a stable mental representation of a situation—one that simultaneously keeps in perspective all of the situation's dimensions and nuances" (Delis, 1980, p. 42). This interpretation is basically in line with subsequent findings that the "ability to integrate complex units into a coherent whole appears to be a deficit of RHD patients" (Delis, Wapner, Gardner, & Moses, 1983, p. 48). Similarly, Wapner, Hamby, and Gardner (1981), arrived at the conclusion that RHD patients "had difficulty both in integrating the elements of a story and in appreciating the 'narrative form' of a story" (p. 27). Foldi, Cicone, and Gardner (1983) also found that, while able to recall important facts, RHD patients "have difficulty in apprehending the overall structure of the narrative" (p. 80), that is, that these patients may have problems appreciating the framework of a narrative text. Quite convergent results were presented by Brownell, Potter, Bihrle, and Gardner (1986) who also found that RHD patients "are able to process individual sentences, but they are unable to combine information across sentences as is required for normal comprehension" (p. 311). The authors assume that the patients' behavior results from an inability to make intersentential connections; they conclude: "Where normal listeners are concerned to weave a coherent interpretation of an entire discourse so that each component jibes with the broader reality, RHD patients are often stuck with, or are satisfied with, a limited and piecemeal understanding" (Brownell et al.,

1986, p. 319). It would be a lack of correct linguistic inferencing then, which is responsible for what Baker (1986), on the basis of her own studies, calls the "lack of coherence which typically marks the narrative discourse performance of right brain damaged individuals" (p. vii).

In light of this research, a number of important questions arise. The predominant question is: Is there some kind of "additional" competence which, in addition to "linguistic competence" as such (if we assume "linguistic competence" exists) is a prerequisite for the processing of text and discourse? It goes without saying that an answer to this question would have important implications for neuropsychology as a whole and for the theory of text processing, in particular.

Although the answer to the question of the specificity of different text types cannot be answered in one chapter, further groundwork can be laid for its eventual solution by discussing the general notion of text, keeping in mind, as a starting point, that there is some right hemisphere involvement in text processing, which seems to go beyond the level of basic linguistic competences and which is necessary for the construction of coherent texts. The following section, then, examines and clarifies the theoretical status of the term "text" from a semiotic perspective.

THE SEMIOTIC STATUS OF THE TEXT

When using the term text, we usually intend to refer to verbal texts alone. In the contemporary humanities, however, there is a tendency to understand the term text in a broader and more encompassing manner. According to this understanding, a text is no longer a verbally realized text only; rather, it is "any coherent complex of signs," as Mikhail M. Bakhtin (1959–61, p. 297) phrased it. Verbally encoded texts thus represent only part of the texts of a culture in general; rather, a movie, a cartoon, a cave painting, and many other cultural manifestations may be regarded as a text, as well. Consequently, not only linguistics, but other disciplines, too, such as archeology, ethnography, science of art, and others, may deal with texts in this broad understanding of the term.

To make these different notions of text comparable to each other, a general theory is needed which includes both the specifics of each text type and the traits common to all text types. Based on the assumption that all text types display a specific sign character, it seems quite reasonable to assume that **semiotics**, the general theory of signs, sign systems, and the conditions of their usage and development, might provide a general theoretical framework. A semiotic approach turns out to be useful with regard to verbal texts as well, as soon as one accepts text processing to be more than the mere object of text linguistics.

The semiotic approach to verbal texts adequately takes into consideration the important cultural dimensions of a text. What is meant by this distinction is that a text, as a cultural phenomenon, comes into being only by way of the particular cultural code underlying it. Consequently, two readings of the term text must be distinguished, as far as verbal texts are concerned: a linguistic and a cultural understanding. A distinction is thus made between an utterance and a text—a distinction which might at first seem counterintuitive, since we tend to regard any utterance as a text in the everyday understanding of this term.

We will not deal with the cultural dimension of texts in detail. Instead, we will focus on linguistic texts as one particular type of cultural text. At least one major problem remains unsolved, then, right from the beginning: How can the semiotic status of the text be explained if a verbal text may be either *only* an utterance, in one case, or a text, in another case? Bakhtin (1959–61) offers the following solution: According to him, two poles must be distinguished in a text; one of these two poles presupposes a commonly known system of signs, or an underlying "code," which is also called a "language." Within a text, everything that is repeated (repeatable) or reproduced (reproducible), corresponds to the "language." Bakhtin (1970–71) himself would call only that discipline which studies the codes of various sign systems, semiotics. The search for the invariant codes underlying different sign systems is the object of only one branch of semiotics, however, namely so-called "code-oriented" semiotics. There is a second tradition in semiotics which studies what Bakhtin calls the second pole of the text. It might be termed "process-oriented" because it focuses on the process of generating an utterance. A basic assumption of this direction of research is that "each text (as an utterance) is individual, unique, and unrepeatable" (Bakhtin 1959–61, p. 105). Process-oriented semiotics thus directs its main attention to the process of sign generation—it does not study the ready-made code of a text, but rather focuses on the process of its generation.

This second aspect of the term text has long been completely neglected. Since the late 1970s, however, the notion of text has been reconsidered and modified within formerly code-oriented semiotics. This reorientation can be clearly seen in the semiotic writings of Yurij M. Lotman, for example, a major theoretician of text and culture in contemporary semiotics.

According to Lotman (1983), the humanities in general, and semiotics in particular, have been characterized by two major tendencies since the 1920s: first, by the conviction that "science considers only repeating phenomena and invariant models thereof" (p. 24), and second, by the assumption that "the objective of any communication is the maximally exact transmission of a particular invariant meaning" (p. 24). Along with these methodological preconditions and based on a Saussurian, code-oriented semiotics went a notion of text, which was, in Bakhtinian terms, characterized by an orientation toward only the first pole of a text. As Lotman (1986) puts it, a text was predominantly regarded as material in which the laws of a particular "language" manifested themselves (p. 104).

A text, then, has been understood as the manifestation of *one* language: It is, in essence, homostructural and homogeneous. Later, following Lotman (1981b), this homostructural notion of text was submitted to an essential transformation: now, a text came to be regarded as a "generator of meaning" (p. 3), which, according to Lotman (1986) turns out to be "principally heterogeneous and heterostructural" and which, consequently, is "a simultaneous manifestation of several languages" (p. 106).

For Lotman (1983) natural language is characterized by the above-mentioned "principal semiotic heterogeneity" (p. 26). This definition of heterogeneity is different from what van Lancker (1975, 1987) terms the "heterogeneity of language": She refers to the distinction between automatic (reproduced) and propositional (newly generated) speech. Rather, Lotman (1983) means that "every natural language text is a text in different languages, or, more exactly, is an amalgam of languages with a complex system of relations between them" (p. 26). As soon as one agrees with this premise, one must "part from the assumption that natural language is a homogeneous semiotic system and to acknowledge its inevitable heterogeneity and heterostructurality". In this case, a "text in a modern understanding" therefore ceases to be "a passive carrier of meaning"; instead, it turns out to be "a dynamic, intrinsically contradictory phenomenon" (Lotman, 1986, p. 107).

Keeping in mind the Bakhtinian view of the two textual poles, one would have to acknowledge that not only one, but both poles are semiotic in nature. Consequently, semiotics must deal with both of them: Whereas code-oriented semiotics studies the language behind the text (i.e., its cultural code), process-oriented semiotics studies the text as an utterance (i.e., the process of semiosis).

There remains one major problem, however; if we take for granted that a text may be studied from two different perspectives, it remains nevertheless unresolved what exactly renders the text a text. In other words, the notion of text itself as a precondition and starting point for analysis remains ultimately undetermined. Taking into consideration Bakhtin's (1959–61) definition of text as "any coherent semiotic complex," a definition of "text" emerges in which the only necessary criterion for textuality is the presence of several semiotic elements which are somehow connected to each other. But what exactly constitutes the connectedness of these elements, and how is this connectedness achieved?

As far as verbal texts are concerned, this question has been discussed predominantly by text linguistics and by psycholinguistics (i.e., psychology of text processing) and neuropsychology. The following section considers the question of "textual coherence" from the points of view of all three fields.

IN SEARCH OF TEXTUAL COHERENCE

TEXT LINGUISTICS

Generally speaking, text linguistics, which emerged in the 1960s and had its heyday in the 1970s, began at an important point: It abandoned the examination of single signs and isolated sentences, and it attempted instead to define the relation(s) between signs or between sentences in a more detailed way.

Text linguistics began with a very Bakhtinian understanding of text, defining it as a "coherent sequence of verbal signs and/or sign complexes [. . .], which is not a priori embedded in another (more comprehensive) verbal entity" (Brinker, 1979, p. 7).

In fact, "coherence" became a key term in various aspects of text linguistics. Studies of *grammatical-lexical* coherence, for example, yielded important results about anaphoric and cataphoric processes, pronominalization, and tense structures; studies of *thematic-semantic* coherence worked to describe coherence in terms of propositional complexes; and from a *pragmatic* perspective, researchers made much progress in explaining coherence in terms of its embededness in a communicative situation. Still, despite the important steps taken by text linguistics, central concept of coherence has not yet been satisfactorily defined (cf. Viehweger, 1989, p. 256).

A significant step forward was the fruitful distinction between "coherence" and "cohesion", first proposed by Halliday and Hasan (1976), and which later became generally accepted (cf. van de Velde (1981), de Beaugrande and Dressler (1981)). In this distinction, all those functions of a text which denote relations between elements of the surface structure are embraced under the term cohesion; in contradistinction, the notion of coherence, takes into account that a text does not result in any meaning by and from itself, but only by way of an interaction between the TEXT KNOWLEDGE and the STORED WORLD KNOWLEDGE of language users (de Beaugrande & Dressler, 1981).

In distinguishing between cohesion and coherence, text linguists succeeded in shifting their theoretical focus away from a merely text-oriented perspective. They recognized that the coherence of a text is not a by-product of the text alone, and that "sufficient cohesion is only a small and unsatisfactory part of discourse reception as a whole" (van de Velde, 1984, p. 10). Instead, they emphasized the important role of the text recipient's activity in the processing of text. This partial change of perspective is quite adequately expressed by Charolles (1983), who writes:

No text is inherently coherent or incoherent. In the end, it all depends on the receiver, and on his ability to interpret the indications present in the discourse so that, finally, he manages to understand it in a way which seems coherent to him—in a way which corresponds with his idea of what it is that makes a series of actions into an integrated whole. (p. 91)

This kind of approach offers various possibilities to relate the notion of textual coherence to psychological concepts of information processing. Taking into account Hoermann's (1976) concept of "sense constancy," for example, de Beaugrande and Dressler (1981) postulate "sense continuity" as "the basis of coherence" (p. 88). In doing this, they stressed that understanding a text is not a simple process of receiving information; rather, it is an active process in which information is selected, eliminated, elaborated and, in part, newly generated on the basis of incoming information and in interaction with prior knowledge, so that the result is a text that is meaningful for the interpreter in question.

Thus, within text linguistics the opinion has gained ground that text construction (from the point of view of both reception and production) is not possible without inferences. Planalp (1986), for example, speaks of the "importance of world knowledge for making inferences and deriving gists" (p. 112), emphasizing that the content of inferences depends on world knowledge; in a similar way, van de Velde (1989) states: "man does not organize the world of verbal texts without inferencing" (p. 559). But still, what constitutes this world knowledge remains undetermined. Planalp (1986), for example, asserts rather fuzzily that "world knowledge ... entails everything that people know" (p. 113). Viehweger's (1989) definition seems at first glance more elaborate. According to him, the kind of world knowledge necessary for making inferences while processing texts can be understood as a "systematic knowledge of states-of-affairs of natural and social environment and of their interrelations, of contexts and their properties ... , of the action processes underlying certain events, etc., which people have acquired and instrumentalize in certain techniques and strategies of problem solving," and as "the entirety of the knowledge and experience gained by society which is more or less systematically acquired by an individual," or, finally, as "so-called common knowledge as well as the results of scientific insights much deeper in dimension" (p. 259).

Although these definitions of world knowledge are far from concrete, text linguists seem to agree the importance of inferencing in text construction, as well as on the important role world knowledge plays in the inferencing process. It remains unclear exactly how inferences interact with world knowledge, on the one hand, and, on another, exactly how world knowledge itself is organized. We can draw one uncontestable conclusion from the above-mentioned research, however: Given the important role world knowledge plays in the generation of texts, the study of textual coherence must not confine itself to the study of linguistic means of coherence, alone: it must take into account extralinguistic and extratextual factors if it is to progress. Consequently, Petöfi (1989), for example, argues in favor of a broader, semiotic approach to texts, noting that "a semiotic analysis of texts . . . requires a close cooperation between different disciplines" (p. 508). Petöfi therefore confirms van de Velde's (1981) earlier view that the study of coherence is an interdisciplinary task which considers data from neuroscience and psychology. In fact, an interdisciplinary consideration of psychological and neuropsychological insights might have led to new developments in text linguistics earlier.

PSYCHOLINGUISTICS OF TEXT PROCESSING

An essential starting point in the psychology of text processing is the assumption that textual coherence cannot be described by linguistic means alone and that any process of text construction goes beyond given textual information. Thus, unlike most approaches in text linguistics, the psycholinguistics of text processing began with an empirically oriented notion of text; this approach assumes that an understanding of text will be achieved only when our knowledge of text processing progresses (Rickheit & Strohner, 1985, p. 4).

Generally speaking, theoretical development in the psycholinguistics of text processing began in the early 1970s, when a group of American psychologists directed attention toward the constructive character of text processing. One of the group's starting points was the assumption that a sentence must be viewed as a piece of information used to construct semantic descriptions which can contain more information than the original linguistic input. The following example, which, since its original publication in 1972, has become one of the most quoted examples in studies of text processing, aptly illustrates the assumptions underlying the so-called "constructive theory of text processing":

Example 1
1a. Three turtles rested beside a floating log, and a fish swam beneath them.
1b. Three turtles rested on a floating log, and a fish swam beneath them.

Linguistically speaking, both sentences display an identical deep structure; they differ only in their usage of two different prepositions (beside vs. on); also, both sentences contain information about a fish swimming under three turtles. However, sentence 1b contains some potentially different information: In addition to the information that the turtles rested on the log, and that the fish swam beneath them, one would usually conclude that the fish did not only swim beneath the turtles, but beneath the log as well. This information, however, was not explicitly given in the input; instead, "it had to come from one's general cognitive knowledge of the world" (Bransford, Barclay, & Franks, 1972, p. 195).

In an effort to empirically support the claim that the interpretation of sentences 1a and 1b calls on a subject's world knowledge rather than on his or her ability to analyze linguistic units, Bransford et al. presented subjects an additional test sentence, after they heard either sentence 1a or 1b; in this test sentence (see 1c below), only the pronoun at the end of the sentence differed from the information in the initial sentence:

1c. Three turtles rested beside/on a floating log, and a fish swam beneath it.

Bransford et al. (1972) concluded that, if subjects had stored only linguistic information, they were likely, after having heard either 1a or 1b, to notice the difference between sentence 1c and sentences 1a and 1b. If, however, subjects constructed a semantic description oriented towards general world knowledge, they were expected to reject 1c as being not identical with 1a, since it was not equivalent with either the original input sentence or with the semantic description to be constructed. Being presented with 1b as initial sentence, however, subjects were highly unlikely to consider 1c as nonequivalent, because they would base their interpretation on the construction of a semantic description. The empirical results confirmed these assumptions; therefore, Bransford et al. (1972) arrived at the overall conclusion that

linguistic inputs merely act as cues which people can use to recreate and modify their previous knowledge of the world. What is comprehended and remembered depends on an individual's general knowledge of his environment. (p. 207)

The general insight gained, then, was that text processing cannot be adequately understood without going "beyond the information given" explicitly in the text. In a sense, the results and theoretical insights achieved by these studies, foreshadowed what would only later, from the early 1980s onward, be discussed in terms of "scenario" or "mental model" (see below). During the 1970s, however, the psychology of text processing was still following an earlier path. In this context, the notion of "inference" assumed central importance, a development much paralleled in text linguistics, as we have seen above.

One of the most general definitions of inference is put forth by Harris (1981); according to him, an inference is "any construction of meaning that a hearer or reader draws from a passage when he or she goes beyond what is explicitly given" (p. 88). As Harris sees it, inferences have two major functions: First, they establish relationships between the propositions in the input as well as between those propositions and already available knowledge; and second, they fill the gaps in the overall structure of the input.

Harris's definition acknowledged that the meaning of a text cannot be described by recourse to text structure (or linguistic input) alone; rather, the meaning results from a combination of the linguistic content of the text *plus* those inferences made by the reader, which make the text comprehensible, and guarantee text coherence.

Thus, inferences were considered to be necessary whenever coherence cannot be obtained otherwise; inferences were understood as additional propositions generated during text processing; they were thought to "bridge" the gaps between explicitly given propositions, that is, to "provide missing links" in the explicitly given text base. Inferences were "regarded as necessary when, and *only* when, they were "interpretation conditions" (Kintsch & van Dijk, 1978, p. 365), that is, when the text lacked information necessary for the recipient to construct a coherent text.

As to the source of inferences, it was referred to as, among other things, "general world knowledge" (Kintsch & van Dijk, 1978, p. 392); Thorndyke's (1976) summary of the role of inferences in text processing conveys the predominant attitude of the time:

A major function of inferences in discourse comprehension is to provide an integrating context for the interpretation of incoming information in order to establish coherence and continuity in the text. A person's ability to extract relevant information and make necessary inferences depends on a wide variety of stored information, including knowledge of the world. (p. 437)

Once again, we encounter the notion that some undefined "world knowledge" is necessary to ensure textual coherence; and as long as it remains unclear how this world knowledge is organized, and how exactly it comes into play in text processing, we cannot adequately understand the important function of inferencing. Abbott, Black, and Smith (1985) recently brought up this issue. They argue:

People use what they know about the real world to understand both actual events and events in stories. That people have such knowledge is hardly controversial. What is debatable is how this knowledge is organized in memory. (p. 179)

Abbott et al. thus confirm an earlier critique of inference research by van Dijk and Kintsch (1983), who found that "our knowledge about inferences in comprehension is as yet quite inadequate" (p. 52). To better understand the role and functioning of inferences, Rickheit, Schnotz, and Strohner (1985) recently raised a number of methodological issues, distinguishing between "on-line" and "off-line" methods in the study of inferences. On-line methods would comprise studies like time measurements, eye movements, thinking aloud during reading, psychophysiological measurements, and so forth. Off-line methods would include free or directed memory tasks, answering questions, and so on. The authors did not consider one additional method, however, namely the analysis of pathological cases, when the ability to make inferences seems to be impaired and can be neuropsychologically interpreted.

It is precisely in this area that a number of studies have been undertaken in the last few years—some of these were cited earlier in the chapter—which have not been adequately examined by text linguistics or by cognitive psychology. It is mainly those studies which attempt to understand text processing with regard to functional brain asymmetry, and which have demonstrated that the right hemisphere seems to play a significant role in this regard.

NEUROPSYCHOLOGY AND TEXT PROCESSING

As far as the problem of inferences is concerned, there are two important studies that directly attempt to relate the problem of inferences to RH capacities. In a study by Brownell et al. (1986), a group of RHD subjects and a control group were sequentially presented with 32 pairs of two sentences (see Example 2, sentences 1 and 2), which the subjects were instructed to understand as "minimal stories." After the subjects read them, these two sentences were removed from view, and two test items (see Example 2, sentences 3 and 4) were presented: One of them included a correct inference (expressing the relationship between sentences 1 and 2), the other one included an incorrect inference, referring to the contents of only sentence 1 or 2. Two additional true/false items (see Example 2, sentences 5 and 6) were constructed for each sentence pair in order to assess subjects' memory for the factual information alone. These additional items referred to only one of the initial sentences, and answering them did not require integration of information across sentences; compare:

Example 2
1. Barbara became too bored to finish the history book.
2. She had already spent five years writing it.

3. Barbara became bored writing a history book.
4. Reading the history book bored Barbara.
5. Barbara grew tired of watching movies.
6. She had been writing it for five years.

It turned out that the RHD patients, in fact, performed worse than the controls, and they had significantly more difficulties with inferencing than with comprehension and retention of factual information. This result is particularly interesting because another study from the same year by McDonald and Wales (1986), devoted to the same problem, arrived at contradictory results. In this study, too, a group of RHD subjects and a control group were presented with a set of initial sentences (see Example 3, sentences 1–3); after a brief interval, four test items were given: both a true and a false premise (i.e., a sentence heard before; see 4 and 6 below), and a true and a false inference (i.e., a sentence that was not heard before, but which had to be inferred from the information given; see 5 and 7 below); compare:

Example 3
1. The bird is in the cage.   (Premise 1)
2. The cage is under the table.   (Premise 2)
3. The bird is yellow.   (Filler item)
4. The cage is under the table.   (True premise)
5. The bird is under the table.   (True inference)
6. The cage is on the table.   (False premise)
7. The bird is on the table.   (False inference)

Subsequent to the presentation of sentences 1–3, and after a short interval, subjects were presented sentences 4–7 and asked to answer "yes" and "no" as to whether they heard it before.

As a result, McDonald and Wales (1986) arrived at the conclusion that their results "did not support the hypothesis that right hemisphere brain damage disturbs the ability to make inferences" (p. 78). One additional result was obtained in this study, however: It turned out that the RHD patients were as 'competent as normal controls at recognizing *true* statements (both premises and inferences), whereas they were significantly poorer than controls at correctly identifying a *false* statement as *not* heard before. Bearing this seemingly curious result in mind, it seems worthwhile taking a second glance at the previous study by Brownell et al. (1986). In fact, a similar tendency was observed in Brownell et al.'s study: It turned out that the RHD group's deficit in inferencing was due to "difficulties in dealing with *incorrect inferences* rather than with correct inferences.

This important issue is brought up by Joanette and Goulet (1987) in their attempt to explain the seemingly divergent results of the studies reported. They additionally direct attention to an important point with regard to the Brownell et al.'s study: In it, some of the initially presented items require an inference per se, as in the following sentences:

Example 4
1. Sally brought a pen and paper with her to meet the famous movie star.
2. The article would include comments on nuclear power by well-known people.

As Joanette and Goulet (1987) correctly point out, in Example 4, the first premise in itself induces an inference: reading only sentence 1, it would seem almost plausible to infer that Sally wanted to have an autograph. The second premise, sentence 2, however, draws the reader back from this inference; instead, she or he is re-oriented toward the fact that Sally is writing an article for which she needs to interview the star.

In other words: The overall task, in this case, not only requires inferencing between sentences 1 and 2; it additionally might require the subject to reject an initial inference, that is, to re-structure its entire content on the basis of a previously made inference.

A similar interpretation might hold true, then, for the McDonald and Wales (1986) study, which also implies that inferencing per se is not impaired. Difficulties arise only when the new information does not coincide with prior information, or when it is necessary to modify a previously constructed interpretation due to an incongruous new piece of information.

Given the overall difficulties RHD subjects experience in processing coherent texts, on the one hand, and taking into account that it might not be inferencing per se which is affected in these patients, on the other hand, one question quite naturally arises, namely: What kind of text theory might then be able to explain this group's problems in constructing coherent texts, and which kind of theory might then, consequently, explain the phenomenon of coherence in general?

MODELS OF TEXT(S) AND WORLD(S)

TEXTS AS MODELS

It seems obvious that an additive-linear model of text processing will not be able to fully solve the question of coherence. In fact, two basic approaches to text processing, which have been termed "elementaristic-additive" on the one hand, and "holistic," on the other hand, were distinguished in the 1980s (Schnotz 1985, 1987a, 1987b, 1988). Within each of these two approaches, the inferencing function works differently.

In the elementaristic-additive approach, the content of a text is described as a set of discrete semantic units or elements (as, e.g., propositions of a text, or, on a different level, epidodes of a story grammar). Comprehension is consequently perceived as an addition of these elements; inferences—which quite logically are reduced to a minimum necessary for text comprehension—are seen to have the function of bridging coherence gaps within the text, and they are seen to be strongly dependent on the coherence of the text itself: inferencing is strongly text-dependent.

In contradistinction to this view, holistic approaches to text processing assume that from the beginning, a holistic mental structure, or mental model, is constructed. This mental model is a dynamic representation, which is incrementally constructed (Oakhill, Garnham, & Vonk, 1989) and which, as information grows, is specified, evaluated, and, if necessary, revised on the basis of the text. According to this view, inferences are not considered to be entirely text-dependent; in fact, they do not predominantly serve the coherence structure of the text as such, but instead are generated to satisfy the requirements of the mental model being constructed. Inferences thus do not serve to fill coherence gaps in a text, but are used as a means of generating, enriching and elaborating a mental model.

The following example, given by Collins, Brown, and Larkin (1980) lent credence to the "holistic" line of research; it nicely demonstrates the strong argument in favor of the mental model theory.

Example 5
He plunked down $5 at the window. She tried to give him $2.50, but he refused to take it. So when they got inside, she bought him a large bag of popcorn. (p. 387)

Without any problem, this text should be analyzable into a propositional structure; according to an additive-elementaristic approach, no inference would be necessary for text understanding, since each proposition of the text can be related to at least one other proposition. Although the processing of this text should provide no problems, most readers face serious difficulties in actually understanding this text: More often than not, readers initially imagine a scene in front of a movie or a theater, and they assume that "she" is a woman in a ticket office, a betting window, or something similar; being astonished that "he" refuses to take the $2.50 (which is the supposed change), and being surprised that "they" went in ("he" and the woman behind the window?) they re-interpret the whole scene and arrive at a different situation.

As Example 5 shows, text processing indeed seems to involve the immediate construction of an initial holistic model which depends on the available information, and which is then progressively refined. It supports the claim that there is a distinction between "elementaristic-additive" and "holistic" text processing.

To a great extent, this distinction is based on Johnson-Laird's and Garnham's research on "mental models" (especially Garnham 1981, 1982, 1983, 1987; Johnson-Laird 1980, 1981, 1983). One of the basic assumptions of this line of research is, "that there are two kinds of representation for discourse, a superficial propositional format close to linguistic form, and a mental model that is close to the structure of events or states of affairs that are described in the discourse" (Johnson-Laird, 1983, p. 377). The logic of this approach is convincing: According to Johnson-Laird (1980), a propositional representation is a description which is neither true nor false without respect to the world (p. 98). Because our apprehension of the world is not direct (we possess only an internal representation of it), a propositional representation is only true or false with respect to a model of the world. And from the further assumptions that "all knowledge of the world depends upon our ability to construct models of it" (Johnson-Laird 1983, p. 402), and that the perception of the world is model-based, it follows that discourse about the world must be model-based, too (Johnson-Laird, 1983). Propositional and model-like representations, thus, are heterogeneous in nature (Johnson-Laird 1983):

Unlike a propositional representation, a mental model does not have an arbitrary chosen syntactic structure, but one that plays a direct representational role since it is analogous to the structure of the corresponding state of affairs in the world—as we perceive or conceive it.

Two points need to be emphasized here: First, the analogical character of mental models, and second, their status in relation to truth conditions. The first point refers back to the point of the heterogeneity of semiotic processes in general, and of text processing in particular. It turns out that the structure of a mental model, as opposed to a propositional description, is not arbitrary, but instead "represents information analogically" (Johnson-Laird, 1980, p. 108), that is, it is "structurally similar to parts of real or imaginary worlds that are described in the texts from which they derive" (Garnham, 1981, p. 564).

This leads to the second important point, the status of the mental model in relation to truth value. According to the proponents of the mental model concept, a mental model need not be veridical in nature—the processes by which fictitious discourse is produced or understood are not strikingly different from those by which true assertions are produced (Johnson-Laird, 1981, p. 361). A mental model thus is a representation of that part of the real or an imaginary world which is relevant to the interpretation of a text or discourse "(Garnham, 19, p. 2). What is crucial, then, is that "there should be something in a mental model to which the expression refers" (Johnson-Laird, 1981, p. 361). Thus, a necessary condition for the coherence of discourse is that its constituent sentences should have a common set of referents (Ehrlich & Johnson-Laird, 1982, p. 297).

It is important to note that the mental model approach is quite different from what logicians such as Hintikka, Kripke, and others, would do within the framework of possible world semantics, where the real world is only one member of the set of all possible worlds (cf. Johnson-Laird, 1983, p. 172). For Johnson-Laird (1983), an assertion is true if it corresponds to reality (p. 438); that is, it can be judged to be true (or false) by evaluating it in relation to a model of the world or by establishing that it follows necessarily from other assertions known to be true. Within the mental model approach, the actual world thus is not interpreted as one possible world among others, but as the mental model of the world the individual has internalized in the course of his or her life.[1] In this respect, it seems most reasonable to side with Johnson-Laird's (1981) distinction between a mental representation of discourse, i.e., a "discourse model" as some kind of "intermediary model" between propositional language, on the one hand, and a model that is a complete representation of the world (i.e., a "world model"), on the other hand. This distinction allows for a clearer definition as to the truth value of a given text (Johnson-Laird, 1981):

> A text represented in a discourse model is true provided there is a proper embedding of the discourse model in the real world model, i.e. a mapping of the individuals and events in the discourse model onto the individuals and events in the real world model in a way that preserves the same properties and relations. (p. 370)

As Johnson-Laird (1981) correctly points out, there remains one pervasive problem: the ontological status of the real world model into which discourse models are embeddable. It seems most practical, in this regard, to agree with him that our knowledge of reality is nothing more than another mental model. Ultimately, there seems to be no way to determine the truth value of a given text; a text and a corresponding discourse model constructed on its basis can only be related to what we know, or seem to know, about the real world. Johnson-Laird (1981), therefore, is quite right to maintain, that "there is much work to be done to account for the organization and mobilization of knowledge that underlies the plausibility of discourse" (p. 368).

---

[1] In this context, we will not further dwell on how this "world model" is different from what has been termed a world model in cultural semiotics (cf. Grzybek, 1993c).

At this point, we confront the extremely important notion of "plausibility" which will lead us a step further in understanding the observed impairment of RHD patients in processing coherent discourse. There are good reasons to assume that the mental model theory in general, and the related concept of plausibility, in particular, can explain these patients' difficulties in arriving at a coherent text.

The question at stake may be phrased as follows: If mental models are constructed on the basis of incoming information, on the one hand, and by reference to a general model of the world, on the other hand, how then, exactly, does this general world knowledge come into play? What causes the reader of Example 5, for example, to assume—at least initially—that the text seems to be about a man at the ticketoffice of a movie theater, for example, and to suspect that he is dealing with the cashier?

In his presentation of findings on mental model research, Schnotz (1988) brings up an important issue, assuming that it is real-world knowledge that causes the reader to construct "some kind of a *prototypical* situation which might represent something like the "best fit" guess to construct an initial model:

When mental models are constructed on the basis of cognitive schemata, and of the assumptions about the section of reality contained in them, one should expect, that these models correspond to some kind of prototype of the situation in question, or, that they represent the most probable state of affairs. However, there are neither any theoretical nor empirical analyses as to this topic thus far. (p. 326)

What comes into play, then, is an experience-driven decision about probability, an issue that has been discussed under the term of "plausibility" in mental model research. As Johnson-Laird (1981, 1983) argues in favor of a clear-cut distinction between "coherence" and "plausibility," asserting that "coherence must be distinguished from *plausibility*, since a discourse may be perfectly coherent yet recount a bizarre sequence of events" (1983, p. 370), Garnham (1983), too, in a general critique of story grammar approaches, maintains that two principal factors influence text processing: referential continuity and plausibility. In a more general discussion of this topic, Black, Freeman, and Johnson-Laird (1986) argue in favor of a mutual interdependence between referential coherence (as a property of discourse, based on "bridging" inferences) and overall plausibility (Black et al. 1986), understood as some kind of "statistical approximation" based on knowledge (p. 52f.). It seems most likely, then, that a clarification of the concept of plausibility implies a specification of what has been generally termed "world knowledge."

Interestingly enough, the notion of "plausibility" has been explored in neuropsychology as well—quite independently from mental model theory—in in effort to explain RHD patients' difficulties in text processing. Wapner et al. (1981) invoke the notion of a "plausibility metric" (p. 30), for example, as one way of conceptualizing these patients' difficulties in processing coherent discourse. According to these authors, normal individuals can assess, with reference to a given element, whether that element is appropriate to a given context. It is the ability to assess plausibility which seems to be vitiated in many right-hemisphere damaged patients (cf. Gardner et al., 1983, p. 186); similarly, Foldi et al. (1983) found that "these patients experienced difficulty in judging the plausibility of individual events within the context of the narrative" (p. 80). More recently, Joanette, Goulet, and Hannequin (1990) confirmed this interpretation; in their opinion, RHD subjects "seem to have problems with evaluating the plausibility of an event within a given context ('plausibility metrics')" (p. 166).

At first glance there seems to be a parallel between developments in mental model theory and neuropsychology, as to the function of plausibility in text processing. One major problem arises with this reading of the notion of "plausibility," however: If plausibility is defined as a factor which is relevant only "within a given context," then it must 'be understood as a kind of **intrinsic plausibility**, valid only within the limits of a particular text. Yet, this definition does not explain, for example, why a reader typically assumes that "she" in Example 5 is the cashier; both variants—that "she" is the cashier or an accompanying friend—are equally "plausible", though not with regard to the initial model, but "in retrospect. Both interpretations are not equally **probable**, however; that is, they do not display the same degree of **extrinsic plausibility**, or probability, based on general world knowledge.[2] Therefore, Joanette et al.'s (1990) definition of "plausibility" seems to be far more exact, referring to "the pragmatic probability of occurrence of an event given the general knowledge of the world as the specific knowledge shared by two or more individuals" (p. 176). As the authors correctly point out with regard to Example 4, it is important to determine whether incorrect inferences were accepted by the RHD subjects in Brownell et al.'s (1986) study in accordance with their degree of plausibility.

[2] This juxtaposition of "context-oriented" (intrinsic) and "world-knowledge-oriented" (extrinsic) plausibility, or probability, depends somewhat on the reading of the term context, as it is used in psychology and neuropsychology. More often than not, this term—like the term pragmatics, too—is not sharply defined, and because it is used differently from its stricter semiotic readings paves the way for misunderstandings (cf., e.g., Joanette et al., 1990, p. 160ff.). In a semiotic view, "context" may either refer to the linguistic context of a given text, or to the situational circumstances in which the text is uttered—but "context" would not be used to denominate internalized knowledge. The same holds true for the notion of pragmatics, which, in semiotics, is used to refer to external conditions of sign usage only (the relation between sign and sign user, in Morris' 1938 concept). To prevent misunderstandings, it would be reasonable to use these terms in a more sharply defined manner in psychology and neuropsychology as well.

RH information processing might, then, be strongly based in general world knowledge and be characterized by a probability-orientation with respect to it. Evidence supporting this view has emerged from studies on the processing of syllogisms after unilateral electroconvulsive shock therapy (Černigovskaja & Deglin 1986; Černigovskaja, in press; Deglin, in press). One experiment attempted to study subjects' reasoning under the conditions of a relatively autonomously working single hemisphere; to this end, subjects were presented a set of syllogisms. Usually, the task of solving a syllogism presupposes that "one remains within the framework of the given task, and relates particular elements of the task to other elements of it, instead of turning to the reality the task is about" (Tulviste, 1988, p. 247). This "theoretical" strategy allows a subject to solve the task "independent of his/her knowledge about reality, and independent of the fact if s/he believes in the premises and conclusions" (p. 244).

To test if the two cerebral hemispheres differed in strategy, some of the syllogisms employed by Černigovskaja and Deglin (1986) were related to the subjects' personal experience (therefore they were expected to known the answers a priori; compare Example 6 below), and some of them were solvable only by way of logical conclusions based on the given premises (compare Example 7):

Example 6
1. Fish can be found in all rivers where fishermen throw out nets.
2. Nets are thrown out into the river Neva.
3. Are there fish in the river Neva or not?

Example 7
1. All states have flags.
2. Zambia is a state.
3. Does Zambia have a flag or doesn't it?

In their analyses of the results, the authors did not direct as much attention toward the correctness of the answers given as to the type of reasoning the patients used to justify their answers. Still, under the control conditions, subjects gave mainly correct answers; these were predominantly of a formal-theoretical motivation. After RH treatment, this tendency to give rather "theoretical" reasons even increased. As opposed to this, after LH treatment (i.e., with predominant RH functioning), the number of "empirical" answers increased significantly (e.g., "Formerly, there were many fish in the river Neva, but now that they have poisoned the river, the fish have disappeared"); when patients did not know the answer, they no longer tried to arrive at the solution by relating the premises to each other, but instead tried to explain or define as much as they could about the realia of the syllogism in question (e.g., "Does a state such as Zambia exist, after all? Where is it? Who lives there?"; or "What Nonsense! Such a state does not exist!").

Evidently two different strategies are employed by the two hemispheres in solving the syllogisms: a theoretical-formal strategy, characteristic of the LH, which relies on logical reasoning, and an empirical strategy, which is based on the individual's personal experience and his or her world knowledge, characteristic of the RH. This finding seems to be in line with the RH's assumed involvement in general world knowledge, as discussed above. But wasn't it the (LH) theoretical-formal approach which seemed to be dominant in these tasks? To demonstrate that this is not actually the case, Černigovskaja and Deglin (1986) constructed a second series of syllogisms involving false premises, such as the following:

Example 8
1. Apes can jump through trees.
2. Porcupines are apes.
3. Can porcupines jump through trees or not?

In this case, after LH treatment, patients emphatically refused to be told lies, identifying the false premise by pointing out that porcupines are not apes (e.g., "A porcupine? It can jump through trees? It's not an ape. It has spines, like a hedgehog. No, this is not true."). On the other hand, after RH treatment, patients did not arrive at correct solutions, not relating the contents of the syllogism to their general world knowledge, but remaining within the syllogism's framework (e.g., " A porcupine jumps through the trees, if it is an ape . . . . If the porcupine is an ape, then it jumps through trees. This is what is written here.").

Irrespective of the conclusion's obvious absurdity, the LH seems to be inclined to intrinsic, intensional logic and semantics, whereas the RH processes information with reference to a previously internalized model of the world. In contradistinction to the LH, for which there seem to exist only "possible worlds" which represent intrinsically plausible models, the RH is oriented toward experience: It generates extrinsically plausible models, which are, in this sense "probable worlds."[3]

This conclusion converges with observations about RHD patients' inability to discern the world of fiction from real world events; Wapner et al. (1981), for example, found that their patients constantly violated the boundary of the stories and "seemed uncertain about the difference

---

[3] The neuropsychological results obtained in this study might explain what has been termed "belief bias effects" in syllogistic reasoning (cf. Oakhill, Garnham, & Johnson-Laird, 1990).

between what could happen and what actually did happen" (p. 24); moreover, these patients seemed "unable to honor the world of the fictive, the imaginary . . ." (p. 30).

To summarize, these insights about the reported RH functions relate not only to what generally has been termed "world knowledge." They also provide a concrete definition of Hoermann's concept of "sense constancy," and thus a theoretical and empirical framework for the phenomenon of text coherence. Now, is there a way to further specify the character of this undefined "world knowledge"?

MODELING WORLD KNOWLEDGE

Attempts to model human world knowledge emerged in the domain of artificial intelligence in the mid-1970s and, subsequently, in the realm of psychology. Such attempts have spawned terms like frame, schema, or script. Schank and Abelson (1977), for example, speak of a "world knowledge store" (p. 9), and of "implicit real-world knowledge" (p. 24). Based on these concepts, Roman, Brownell, Potter, Seibold, and Gardner (1987) attempted to test the hypothesis that the observed RH deficit in processing coherent texts is related to or dependent on a reduced access to scripts; this hypothesis seemed reasonable, since other studies with LHD (aphasic) patients showed that this group's otherwise well-structured speech production may be guided by the activation of such scripts (Ulatowska, Freedman-Stern, Weiss Doyel, & Macaluso-Haynes, 1983). However, the study by Roman et al. (1987) demonstrated a "general preservation in script knowledge in RHD patients" (p. 167); their results, then, argued against a loss of script knowledge as such in RHD patients (cf. Joanette & Goulet, 1990).

A logical conclusion resolving these seemingly contradictory results would be that scripts are not the only possible way of organizing or representing world knowledge. In other words: If access to world knowledge is impaired in RHD patients, but script knowledge is not affected, then there must exist a different way of mentally organizing world knowledge—one which does not involve scripts! When we compare the script- or frame-oriented organizational approach to the mental model approach delineated above, it becomes clear that attempts to define world knowledge in terms of scripts or frames do not take into account the important analogical components of world knowledge. A mental model, on the other hand, is used to construct a world model, which in turn plays a crucial role in the construction of a so-called discourse model. Studies measuring only subjects' script constructing abilities concequently ignore the important role of analogical components in both world and discourse models.

From a semiotic point of view, it seems reasonable to understand scripts either as the formalization of a symbolically coded world model, or as the symbolic translation (or transcoding) of otherwise analogically or iconically coded world knowledge (cf. Grzybek, 1991b). A comparable interpretation has been achieved by Schnotz (1985, 1988) with respect to mental models. As he correctly emphasizes, a mental model, as opposed to a propositional representation of discourse, does not consist of digital units, but represents discourse in an analogical form. A mental model is thus characterized by a different quality than a propositional description, although a mental model may be, at least in part, *described* in terms of digital units or symbols (such as the phrases of a text or the corresponding propositions)—but a description of a mental model is not, of course, the mental model itself.

Attempts to model world knowledge in terms of scripts or frames, and the empirical studies based on those attempts, have thus relied exclusively on an arbitrary (symbolic) code, dismissing the important function of iconic elements in all semiotic processes. Here, the relevance of a comprehensive semiotic theory which might improve neuropsychological interpretations of text processing becomes obvious. This approach quite logically results in a need for relevant *neurosemiotic* concepts.

CONCLUSION

A comprehensive neurosemiotic theory requires, first, specific hypotheses concerning the processing of both symbolic and iconic components by the two cerebral hemispheres. A good starting point might be the hypothesis put forth by Deglin, Balonov, and Dolinina (1983), who speak of the "iconic world model" (p. 41) the RH contributes to communicative processes. It would be incorrect, of course, to interpret neurosemiotic interpretations as a simple-minded projection of the problem of coherence or "textuality" from the semiotic level onto the neurological level. In further elaborating specific neurosemiotic hypotheses, it is important that the relationship between symbolic and iconic processes is not oversimplified.

Also, it would be banal to say that signs are generated in the brain; and it would be oversimplistic to unproblematically equate symbolic processes with the LH, and iconic processes with the RH. Clearly, however, a more exact neurosemiotic interpretation of what Lotman terms the "heterogeneity" of semiosis is needed.

It goes without saying that the quality of any attempt to relate semiotic concepts to neuropsychological findings depends on the semiotic categories employed. To this purpose, it would be useful to employ not only the commonly known categories of signs, that is, symbols, icons, and indexes, but to reconsider the original definition of each of these terms, disregarding later modifications which reinterpret them on the basis of specific theoretical assumptions.[4] One might consider, for example, that Charles S. Peirce's original semiotic theory stresses the fact that the processing of any symbol necessarily involves iconic components; in contradistinction to many more recent "re-interpretations" of his sign typology, which ignore this iconic element, his concept describes a constant overlapping of symbolic and iconic components (cf. Grzybek 1989, 1991a, 1991b, 1993a).

Given Peirce's more comprehensive semiotic theory, which forsees Lotman's concept of heterogeneity from a slightly different perspective, we can anticipate pioneering studies in text processing, which try to establish the actual role of the RH in these processes. The most recent developments in the neuropsychology of text processing already offer closer parallels to the text-theoretical studies of Bakhtin and Lotman. Parallels to Bakhtin (mainly to his references to the "second pole" of a text) are unmistakable: Neuropsychologists such as Deglin et al. (1983) write that the RH "determines the orientation of speech toward extralinguistic reality and to individual, irreproducible personal experience" (p. 38). Further convergencies with Lotman's views on the principal heterogeneity of semiotic processes also emerge—the more so because Lotman himself, in his ruminations on text theory, mentions the concept of functional brain asymmetry (1977, 1981a, 1983).

A consideration of the asymmetrical functions of the left and right hemispheres is clearly germaine to developments in both (textual) semiotics and in the cognitive sciences in general. We have yet to find out precisely how the heterogeneity of semiosis is engendered by the two hemispheres, and how heterogeneous semiotic processes are then integrated by the human brain. A thorough semiotic theory can contribute to a more adequate investigation of these and other neuropsychological questions, whereas neuropsychological findings can assist semioticians in evaluating their own theoretical categories.

ACKNOWLEDGMENT

I am sincerely grateful for Hiram H. Brownell's, Yves Joanette's, and Brigitte Stemmer's valuable comments on an earlier version of this text. As usual, P. Rachael Wilson has done an admirable job in editing the text.

---

[4] The few neuropsychological studies which employ this basic sign typology to semiotically interpret their findings, are mainly based on Roman Jakobson's modifications of it, rather than on Peirce's original definitions.

REFERENCES

Abbott, V., Black, J. B., & Smith, E. E. (1985). The representation of scripts in memory. *Journal of Memory and Language, 24,* 179–199.

Bakhtin, M. M. (1959–61). The problem of text in linguistics, philology, and the human sciences. In M. M. Bakhtin, *Speech genres and other late essays* (pp. 103–131). Edited by C. Emerson & M. Holquist, 1986. Austin, TX: University of Texas Press.

Bakhtin, M. M. (1970–71). From notes made in 1970–71. In M. M. Bakhtin, *Speech genres and other late essay* (pp. 103–131). Edited by C. Emerson and M. Holquist, 1986. Austin, TX: University of Texas Press.

Baker, R. A. (1986). *Narrative discourse performance in right hemisphere lesioned stroke patients.* Unpublished doctoral dissertation, The University of Texas at Dallas.

Black, A., Freeman, P., & Johnson-Laird, P. N. (1986). Plausibility and the comprehension of text. *British Journal of Psychology, 77,* 51–72.

Bransford, J. D., Barclay, J. R., & Franks, J. J. (1972). Sentence memory: A constructive versus interpretive approach. *Cognitive Psychology, 3,* 193–209.

Brinker, K. (1979). Zur Gegenstandsbestimmung und Aufgabenstellung der Textlinguistik. In J. S. Peöfi (Ed.), *Text vs sentence. Basic questions of text linguistics* (pp. 3–12). Hamburg, FRG: Buske.

Brownell, H. H., Potter, H. H., & Bihrle, A. M. (1986). Inference deficits in right brain-damaged patients. *Brain and Language, 27,* 310–321.

Černigovskaja, T. V. (in press). Die Heterogenität des verbalen Denkens als cerebrale Asymmetrie. In P. Grzybek (Ed.), *Semiotics—Psychosemiotics—Neurosemiotics.* Bochum, FRG: Brockmeyer.

Černigovskaja, T. V., & Deglin, L. Ja. (1986). Metaforičeskoe sillogističeskoe myšlenie kak projavlenie funkcional'noj a simmetrii mozga. *Trudy po znakovym sistemam, 19,* 68–84.

Charolles, M. (1983). Coherence as a principle in the interpretation of discourse. *Text, 3,* 71–97.

Collins, A., Brown, J. S., & Larkin, K. M. (1980). Inference in Text Understanding. In R. J. Spiro, B. C. Bruce, & W. F. Brewer (Eds.), *Theoretical issues in reading comprehension* (pp. 385–407). Hillsdale, NJ: Lawrence Erlbaum.

de Beaugrande, R., & Dressler, W.U. (1981). *Einführung in die Textlinguistik.* Tübingen, FRG: Niemeyer.

Deglin, V. L. (in press). "Die paradoxe Mentalität oder Warum Fiktionen die Realität ersetzen." In Grzybek, P. (Ed.), *Semiotics—Psychosemiotics—Neurosemiotics.* Bochum, FRG: Brockmeyer.

Deglin, V. L., Balonov, L. Ja., & Dolinina, L. B. (1983). Jazyk i funkcional'naja asimmetrija mozga. *Trudy po znakovym sistemam, 16,* 31–42.

Delis, D. C. (1980). *Hemispheric processing of discourse.* Unpublished doctoral dissertation, University of Wyoming, Laramie.

Delis, D. C., Wapner, W., Gardner, H., & Moses, J. A. (1983). The contribution of the right hemisphere to the organization of paragraphs. *Cortex, 19,* 43–50.

Ehrlich, K., & Johnson-Laird, P. N. (1982). Spatial descriptions and referential continuity. *Journal of Verbal Learning and Verbal Behavior, 21,* 296

Engel, D. (1977). *Textexperimente mit Aphatikern.* Tübingen, FRG: Narr.

Foldi, N. S., Cicone, M., & Gardner, H. (1983). Pragmatic aspects of communication in brain-damaged patients. In S. J. Segalowitz (Ed.), *Language functions and brain organization* (pp. 51–86). New York: Academic Press.

Gardner, H., Brownell, H. H., Wapner, W., & Michelow, D. (1983). Missing the point: The role of the right hemisphere in the processing of linguistic materials. In E. Perecman (Ed.), *Cognitive processing in the right hemisphere* (pp. 169–191). New York: Academic Press.

Garnham, A. (1981). Mental models as representations of text. *Memory and Cognition, 9*, 560–565.

Garnham, A. (1982). *On-line construction of representations of the content of texts.* Bloomington: Indiana University Linguistics Club.

Garnham, A. (1983). What's wrong with story grammars. *Cognition, 15*, 145–154.

Garnham, A. (1987). *Mental models as representations of discourse and text.* Chichester: Ellis Horwood.

Grzybek, P. (1989). *Studien zum Zeichenbegriff der sowjetischen Semiotik (Moskauer und Tartuer Schule).* Bochum, FRG: Brockmeyer.

Grzybek, P. (1991a). Neurosemiotik—Kultursemiotik. Ein integratives Konzept. In K. Eimermacher, & P. Grzybek (Eds.), *Zeichen—Text—Kultur* (pp. 97–186). Bochum, FRG: Brockmeyer.

Grzybek, P. (1991b). Textsemiotik: Semiotik des Textes? In *Problemy lingvistiki teksta* (pp. 4–34). Minsk.

Grzybek, P. (1993a). A semiotic re-interpretation of the 19th century concept of 'asymbolia.' In P. Grzybek (Ed.), *Semiotics—Psychosemiotics—Neurosemiotics.* Bochum, FRG: Brockmeyer. [In press]

Grzybek, P. (1993b). Bakhtinian semiotics and the semiotics of the Moscow-Tartu school. In B. Kosanovic & M. Radovic (Eds.), *Studies on M. M. Bakhtin.* Novi Sad. [In press]

Grzybek, P. (1993c). The notion of 'model' in Soviet semiotics. In J. Andrew, Ch. Pike, & R. Reid (Eds.), *Russian culture: Structure and tradition.* Keele, GB. [In press]

Halliday, M. A. K., & Hasan, R. (1976). *Cohesion in English.* London: Longman.

Harris, R. J. (1981). Inferences in information processing. In G. H. Bower (Ed.), *The psychology of learning and motivation* (vol. 15, pp. 81–128). New York: Academic Press.

Hoermann, H. (1976). *To mean—To understand.* Problems of psychological semantics. Heidelberg: Springer [1981].

Joanette, Y., & Goulet, P. (1987). *Inference deficits in right brain-damaged right-handers: Absence of evidence.* Paper presented at the Tenth European Conference of the International Neuropsychological Society. Barcelona, Spain.

Joanette, Y., & Goulet, P. (1990). Narrative discourse in right-brain-damaged right-handers. In Y. Joanette & H. H. Brownell (Eds.), *Discourse ability and brain damage: Theoretical and empirical perspectives* (pp. 131–153). New York: Springer.

Joanette, Y., Goulet, P., & Hannequin, D. (1990). *Right hemisphere and verbal communication.* New York: Springer.

Johnson-Laird, P. N. (1980). Mental models in cognitive science. *Cognitive Science, 4*, 71–115.

Johnson-Laird, P. N. (1981). Comprehension as the construction of mental models. *Philosophical Transactions of the Royal Society of London, B–295*, 353–374.

Johnson-Laird, P. N. (1983). Mental models. *Towards a cognitive science of language, inference, and consciousness*. Cambridge, MA: Cambridge University Press.
Kintsch, W., & van Dijk, T. A. (1978). Toward a model of text comprehension and production. *Psychological Review, 85*, 363–394.
Lotman, Ju. M. (1977). Kul'tura kak kollektivnyj intellekt i problemy iskusstvennogo razuma. Moskva: Akademija nauk.
Lotman, Ju. M. (1981a). Mozg—tekst—kul'tura—iskusstvennyj intellekt. In *Semiotika i informatika, 17*, 3–1
Lotman, Ju. M. (1981b). Semiotika kul'tury i ponjatie teksta. In Trudy po znakovym sistemam, 12, 3–7.
Lotman, Ju. M. (1983). Kul'tura i tekst kak generatory smysla. In *Kibernetičeskaja lingvistika* (pp. 23–30). Moskva: Nauka.
Lotman, Ju. M. (1986). K sovremennomu ponjatiju teksta. In *Učenye zapiski Tartuskogo gosudarstvennogo universiteta, vyp. 736*, 104–108.
McDonald, S., & Wales, R. (1986). An investigation of the ability to process inferences in language following right hemisphere brain damage. *Brain and Language, 29*, 68–80.
Morris, Ch. W. (1938). *Foundations of a theory of signs*. Chicago, IL: The University of Chicago Press.
Moscovitch, M. (1983). The linguistic and emotional functions of the normal right hemisphere. In E. Perecman (Ed.), *Cognitive processing in the right hemisphere* (pp. 57–82). New York: Academic Press.
Oakhill, J., Garnham, A., & Johnson–Laird, P. N. (1990). Belief bias effects in syllogistic reasoning. In K. J. Gilhooly, M T. G. Keane, R. H. Logie, & G. Erdos (Eds.), *Lines of thinking: Reflections on the psychology of thought. Vol. 1: Representation, reasoning, analogy and decision making* (pp. 125–138). Chichester: John Wiley & Sons.
Oakhill, J., Garnham, A., & Vonk, W. (1989). The on-line construction of discourse models. *Language and Cognitive Processes, 4*, 263–286.
Petöfi, J. S. (1989). Constitution and meaning: A semiotic text-theoretical approach. In M.-A. Conte, J. S. Petöfi & E. Sözer (Eds.), *Text and discourse connectedness* (pp. 507–542). Amsterdam/Philadelphia: John Benjamins.
Planalp, S. (1986). Scripts, story grammars, and causal schemas. In D. G. Ellis (Ed.), *Contemporary issues in language and discourse processes* (pp. 111–125). Hillsdale, NJ: Lawrence Erlbaum.
Rickheit, G., Schnotz, W., & Strohner, H. (1985). The concept of inferences in discourse comprehension. In G. Rickheit, & H. Strohner (Eds.), *Inferences in text processing* (pp. 3–49). Amsterdam: North-Holland.
Rickheit, G., & Strohner, H. (1985). Psycholinguistik der Textverarbeitung. *Studium Linguistik, 17/18*, 1–78.
Roman, M., Brownell, H. H., Potter, H. H., Seibold, M. S., & Gardner, H. (1987). Script knowledge in right hemisphere-damaged and in normal elderly adults. *Brain and Language, 31*, 151–170.
Schank, R. C., & Abelson, R. P. (1977). *Scripts, plans, goals and understanding. An inquiry into human knowledge structures*. Hillsdale, NJ: Lawrence Erlbaum.
Schnotz, W. (1985). *Elementaristische und holistische Theorieansätze zum Textverstehen*. Deutsches Institut für Fernstudien an der Universität Tübingen, Forschungsberichte 35.

Schnotz, W. (1987a). *Mentale Kohärenzbildung beim Textverstehen*. Deutsches Institut für Fernstudien an der Universität Tübingen, Forschungsberichte 42.
Schnotz, W. (1987b). New directions in text comprehension. In E. de Corte, H. Lodewijks, R. Parmentier, & P. Span (Eds.), *Studia paedagogica: Learning and instruction* (pp. 321–338). Oxford: Pergamon Press.
Schnotz, W. (1988). Textverstehen als Aufbau mentaler Modelle. In H. Mandl & H. Spada (Eds.), *Wissenspsychologie* (pp. 299–330). München/Weinheim: Psychologie Verlags Union.
Stachowiak, F. J., Huber, W., Poeck, W., & Kerschensteiner, M. (1977). Text comprehension in aphasia. *Brain and Language, 4,* 177–195.
Thorndyke, P. W. (1976). The role of inferences in discourse comprehension. *Journal of Verbal Learning and Verbal Behavior, 15,* 437–446.
Tul'viste, P. (1988). *Kul'turno-istoričeskoe razvitie verbal'nogo myšlenija*. Tallin: Valgus.
Ulatowska, H. K., Freedman-Stern, R., Weiss Doyel, A., & Macaluso-Haynes, S. (1983). Production of narrative discourse in aphasia. *Brain and Language, 19,* 317-334.
van de Velde, R. G. (1981). *Interpretation, Kohärenz und Inferenz*. Hamburg: Buske.
van de Velde, R. G. (1984). *Prolegomena to inferential discourse processing*. Amsterdam/Philadelphia: John Benjamins.
van de Velde, R. G. (1989). The role of inferences in text organization. In M.-A. Conte, J. S. Petöfi, & E. Sözer (Eds.), *Text and discourse connectedness* (pp. 543–562). Amsterdam/Philadelphia: John Benjamins.
van Dijk, T. A., & Kintsch, W. (1983). *Strategies of discourse comprehension*. London: Academic Press.
Van Lancker, D. (1975). *Heterogeneity in language and speech: Neurolinguistic studies*. Los Angeles. [UCLA Working Papers in Phonetics, #29].
Van Lancker, D. (1987). Nonpropositional speech: Neurolinguistic studies. In A. W. Ellis (Ed.), *Progress in the psychology of language*, (vol. 3, pp. 49–118). London/Hillsdale, NJ: Lawrence Erlbaum.
Viehweger, D. (1989). Coherence—Interaction of modules. In W. Heydrich, F. Neubauer, J. S. Petöfi, & E. Sözer, (Eds.), *Connexity and coherence. Analysis of text and discourse* (pp. 256–274). Berlin/New York: de Gruyter.
Wapner, W., Hamby, S., & Gardner, H. (1981). The role of the right hemisphere in the apprehension of complex linguistic materials. *Brain and Language, 14,* 15–33.
Weylman, S. T., Brownell, H. H., Roman, M., & Gardner, H. (1989). Appreciation of indirect requests by left- and right-brain-damaged patients: The effects of verbal context and conventionality of wording. *Brain and Language, 36,* 580–591.

PART II

*Narrative Capacities
of Healthy Elderly Subjects*

CHAPTER 4

Assessment of Intraindividual Change in Text Recall of Elderly Adults

ROGER A. DIXON, CHRISTOPHER HERTZOG,
INGRID C. FRIESEN, AND DAVID F. HULTSCH

During the last several decades, research examining memory performance in normal adults has shown substantial age-related differences on a variety of memory tasks (Craik, 1977; Hultsch & Dixon, 1984). With few exceptions, normal young adults perform better than normal older adults on tasks requiring verbal recall of supraspan lists of digits, symbols, and other stimuli, both in terms of number of items recalled and the speed of retrieval of such information from memory. Generally, this pattern is found in studies of discourse processing and comprehension, although the extent and degree of age differences depends on a number of factors. The investigation of memory (as a specific category of information processing and comprehension) for text materials (as a subset of discourse) has both benefitted from and influenced research in the area of discourse processing (e.g., Kintsch, 1974; van Dijk & Kintsch, 1983; Meyer, 1975). In general, the text is viewed as being composed of smaller units (e.g., words, sentences, or semantic propositions) which are coded by the reader and evaluated semantically on the basis of a larger context of discourse, knowledge, schemata, or situation models (van Dijk & Kintsch, 1983). Some interindividual or group-related differences in text recall performance may be affected by the familiarity or ecological relevance of the testing conditions or text materials, for example, by the ease with which an appropriate schema or situation model can be invoked (Dixon & Hertzog, 1988; van Dijk & Kintsch, 1983).

Research on normal aging and memory for text materials has addressed a host of potential influences on individual differences in performance. For example, recent studies have investigated such influences on adult age-related differences in text recall performance as verbal and other cognitive abilities (e.g., Dixon, Hultsch, Simon, & von Eye, 1984; Hartley, 1986; Hultsch, Hertzog, & Dixon, 1990), familiarity (e.g., Byrd, 1986-87), text structure (e.g., Stine & Wingfield, 1987; Zelinski, Light, & Gilewski, 1984), and metamemory (e.g., Dixon & Hultsch, 1983). In general, the results support the contention that differential predictive patterns are observed for young and old adults (for reviews see Hultsch & Dixon, 1984; Zelinski & Gilewski, 1988). Although most recent studies have reported age-related deficits in text memory which conform to the general pattern observed in verbatim recall of word lists, some have found that, under certain conditions, selected older adults may be adept at remembering information contained in text. Consistent with recent trends in cognitive psychology, the ecological relevance of the tasks (texts) and the criterial measures (e.g., gist recall) is an issue for further consideration.

There are numerous complications in reaching conclusions about patterns of—much less explanations for—age differences in text processing. In addition to the common difficulties of comparing samples on any of a variety of subject characteristics, three methodological complications may be highlighted. First, although text recall and aging research has been conducted in a growing number of laboratories, there are few common instructions, materials, or operational definitions of subject variables. Second, the absence of rules for comparing results obtained with different theoretical frameworks for representing the meaning of text renders some important comparisons problematic. A third complication is related to the design of most studies in cognitive aging and neuropsychology. Specifically, because most studies of text processing and aging are cross-sectional in nature, it is not possible to evaluate change in performance across time.

This chapter has three major goals. First, we discuss the general value of studying within-person change in discourse processing in addition to between-person differences. Because we are interested in both theoretical and applied issues, we explore the potential advantages of intraindividual assessment in both cognitive aging and neuropsychology. Second, we describe some of the special methodological requirements of longitudinal or intraindividual research designs. As noted earlier, these include issues of materials, frameworks for representing text, and replicability. To this end, we focus on a set of 25 equivalent texts we have produced explicitly for use in multiple-occasion designs (Dixon, Hultsch, & Hertzog, 1989). Third, we offer two examples of research on intraindividual changes in text recall performance. In two studies, we have followed: (a) a set of seven older women across as many as 90 weekly occasions and (b) a set of 10 older women and one Alzheimer's patient across 10 weekly occasions.

GENERAL VALUE OF INTRAINDIVIDUAL ASSESSMENT

Memory for prose has played an increasingly important role in research on normative and pathological changes in verbal memory in adults. In neuropsychological assessment, memory for paragraphs has been successfully used to discriminate normal adults from populations with clinical syndromes, such as amnesiacs (Kopelman, Wilson, & Baddeley, 1989), Alzheimer's disease (Flicker, Ferris, Crook, Bartus, & Reisberg, 1986), multiple sclerosis (Grant, McDonald, Trimble, Smith, & Reed, 1984; Rao, Leo, & St. Aubin-Faubert, 1989), Huntington's disease (Caine, Banford, Schiffer, Shoulson, & Levy, 1987), and brain-damaged patients (Rehak et al., 1992). Several researchers have recommended inclusion of text memory measures in general neuropsychological assessment batteries (e.g., Egelko et al., 1988; Kopelman, 1986; Wilson, 1987).

The Wechsler Memory Scale-Revised Logical Memory (LM) scale is a frequently used measure of story recall (Erickson & Scott, 1977). It contains two simple paragraphs, each with 25 segments. Performance on this task is measured in terms of the total number of segments recalled verbatim, although some investigators give partial credit for gist recall. The LM scale has several advantages in clinical applications. It is easy to administer and score, and its widespread use has generated considerable normative data on performance levels in different populations. (Normative information is not so well established for very old adults.) Nevertheless, the scale also has important limitations. The idea units of LM scale stories are not grounded in any formal theory of text representation in memory (such as those articulated by such cognitive psychologists as Kintsch, 1974). Consequently, rules governing the segmentation of the text are not explicitly stated, the differences across segments in terms of importance for the story's theme are unknown, and the scoring criteria regarding verbatim and gist recall do not necessarily reflect the nature of propositional units stored in memory. Moreover, the brief length and structural simplicity of the stories may not afford optimal differentiation of subtle distinctions in memory dysfunction in clinical populations.

Several authors have commented on the value of integrating recent trends in cognitive psychology—and, in particular, cognitive discourse analysis—with neuropsychology and cognitive aging (e.g., Kahn, Joanette, Ska, & Goulet, 1990). We are aware, however, of relatively few efforts to compare performance on the LM test with performance on texts for which scoring systems are based on theories of text representation. It would be valuable to explore these comparisons for several reasons. First, although the LM test has proven quite useful, it is possible that more subtle differentiations of discourse memory skill may be made on the basis of longer texts with finer distinctions in level of recall. Second, because of their brevity and simplicity, the LM stories may have somewhat limited value for more than one occasion of testing. Participants may remember crucial portions of the stories from a previous testing, especially if the test sessions are relatively close in time. Third, texts that are somewhat longer and which have theoretically derived representation schemes typically allow for scoring recall of the various levels of information contained in any story. These levels range hierarchically from the main ideas of the story to the smallest details. Therefore, not only is it possible to score overall gist or verbatim recall, but it is also possible to score the profile of recall across the hierarchy of information contained in the text (Dall'Ora, Della Sala, & Spinnler, 1989; Dixon et al., 1984; Rehak et al., 1992; Schultz, Schmitt, Logue, & Rubin, 1986). Differential recall of central ideas versus details may contribute to classification of persons into different clinical populations.

Although individual differences in cognitive performance have received a significant amount of study, the issue of intraindividual (within-person) variability over time is rarely addressed. Intraindividual assessment has several potential advantages, especially in older populations, given informal observations of clinicians that there are fluctuations in the functional competence of elderly individuals. As Kaszniak (1990) has noted, lack of consistency over time in certain behaviors and constructs can be expected for elderly persons. How much intraindividual consistency or inconsistency can be expected of normal or special population elderly persons is both an open and important question. It is an open question, in part, simply because relatively little pertinent data (i.e., more than two occasions of measurement) have been typically collected. It is an important question because if the range of intraindividual variability is substantial, then single occasion assessments may not provide accurate or valid estimates of "true" competence. The greater the inconsistency in memory performance across time, the more one must qualify the interpretations of a single-occasion assessment.

Consider the following illustration. A normal elderly adult performs significantly below the norm for his or her age group on a set of assessment tests administered on one occasion. This low level of performance, however, may be within the normal range of his or her own across-time variability of performance. That is, if this hypothetical individual were to be tested on equivalent forms of the same tests over multiple occasions, his or her performances might range from more than one standard deviation above to more than one standard deviation below the age group norm. The issue for assessment becomes one of evaluating how much of the potential (if unmeasured) or actual (if measured) intraindividual variability to consider in qualifying the inferences drawn from a single norm-referenced assessment. In other words, the issue is how extensively to use group norms instead of estimating directly the individual's own baseline of performance. If intraindividual variability for given tasks is appreciable, then one must be aware of the potentially thorny problems inherent in balancing the use of age group norms against intraindividual baselines.

Unfortunately, it is not possible to evaluate the extent of fluctuation for a given individual with a single occasion of testing. Furthermore, the extent to which the population distribution used to generate norms represents combined interindividual differences in intraindividual performance averages and variability is unknown. Therefore, norm-based inferences about where the observed performance of the individual may be located in his or her own (hypothetical) distribution of performances (across time and conditions) simply are not possible. Instead, one must assume that intraindividual variability is sufficiently small that it can be ignored. It should also be noted that the extent of fluctuation in performance for individuals belonging to a variety of clinical populations is not known, although the expected degree of fluctuation may vary by severity of the condition. This latter point is illustrated in Figure 4–1. For a given condition, the range of performance on a given set of indicators may be greater for a "true" normal (Person A) than for a "true" case with a mild degree of impairment (Person B). Both may be greater than for a person actually at a severe level of impairment (Person C). Norm-based assessment will, therefore, generally be accurate. Sometimes, however, Person A would be judged as probably impaired and Person B would be judged as probably normal. Of course, the degree of overlap may be even more substantial than illustrated in Figure 4–1, and the number of occasions in which Person A is below, and Person B is above, the normative cut-off may be greater than indicated in the schematiza-

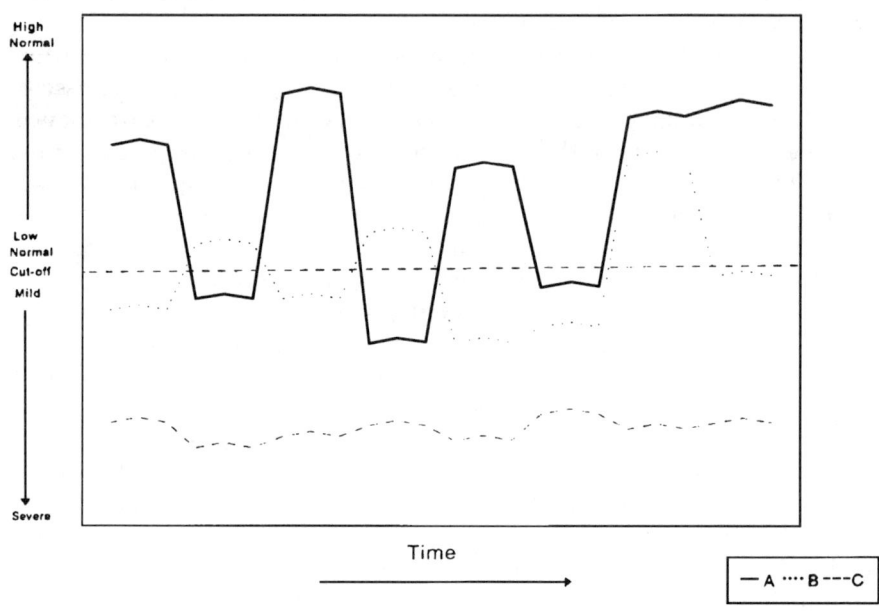

Figure 4–1. Range of intraindividual variability may vary by severity of clinical condition.

tion. Interestingly, it is possible (although not illustrated) that extremely proficient performers may also show somewhat reduced intraindividual variability, although at the opposite (upper) end of the performance scale.

SELECTED METHODOLOGICAL ISSUES

Such intraindividual variability could be due to a variety of factors, some of which are methodological in nature, some of which may themselves be clinically relevant, and some of which are related to other normally fluctuating processes. According to Nesselroade (1991), such intraindividual variation in performance may not be merely a reflection of unreliability in the task. Rather, it is determined both by imprecision of measurement and lawful but unstable influences on performance. Nesselroade's (e.g., 1988, 1991; Nesselroade & Ford, 1985) work on intraindividual designs has done much to clarify key conceptual and empirical issues. He has emphasized, for example, the advantages of distinguishing between states and traits (Nesselroade, 1988). States are endogenously (e.g., hormonal) or exogenously (e.g., social) produced and may vary across situations and occasions. Traits, on the other hand, connote temporal and cross-situational stability. Often psychologists intend to measure the latter with a given instrument or battery, but tap into some aspects of the former. As Nesselroade (1988) notes, state variation can even influence interindividual performance differences of presumably stable personality traits such as locus of control (Roberts & Nesselroade, 1986) and temperament (Hooker, Nesselroade, Nesselroade, & Lerner, 1987). Both traits have been found to exhibit both relatively stable interindividual (trait-like) variability and fluctuant (state-like) intraindividual variability.

The implications for research are numerous, but include the following (Nesselroade, 1988). First, the power of putative trait measures to predict other behaviors or to reflect underlying clinical conditions may be reduced by confounding to an unknown extent with conceptually similar state variation (e.g., trait anxiety confounded with state anxiety). Second, observations on putative trait measures may also be influenced (contaminated) to an unknown extent by conceptually distinct state variation (e.g., trait depression influenced by state illness or anxiety). Third, it is critical to develop measures that are sensitive to variability and change, and that can be used on multiple occasions, for it is only through such designs that the trait-state distinction for a given process can be clarified.

Perhaps the most frequently used research design in normal cognitive aging research is the cross-sectional design, in which two or more age groups are compared on one occasion. A variant of this design, in which clinical groups and populations are compared, often with young and old adult normal controls, is perhaps the most frequently used design in neuropsychological aging research. There are several assumptions attendant to these designs regarding the level (low) and potential impact (small) of intraindividual change. However, fluctuations in intraindividual performance levels will influence individual differences as measured in such cross-sectional designs. In the case of memory performance, systematic intraindividual variability may occur as a function of intraindividual state changes and shifting environmental influences (Dixon & Hertzog, 1988). Individual differences in memory performance within a population will reflect (a) stable individual differences in memory ability, (b) current status of the individual (e.g., health, mood), and (c) random measurement error. Studies of cognition and aging typically assume that the magnitude of within-group error in older samples reflects sources (a) and (c), but not (b).

As we have posed the question elsewhere (Hertzog, Dixon, & Hultsch, 1992), what if it were the case, however, that a meaningful proportion of between-persons variance in memory was due to intraindividual influences that were unstable over time? Researchers examining mood states have shown that substantial proportions of variance in state measures are in fact unstable, such that test-retest correlations are low even though the reliability of the measures is relatively high (e.g., Nesselroade, Pruchno, & Jacobs, 1986; Spielberger, 1977). Indeed, several studies of intraindividual variation in affect suggest coherent patterns of flux in mood that relate to variables such as perceived stress and social behavior (Watson, 1988; Zevon & Tellegen, 1982). There is evidence for effects of physiological and psychological states on cognition, including mood (e.g., Broadbent, Broadbent, & Jones, 1989; Clark & Teasdale, 1982; Eich & Metcalfe, 1989). Intraindividual variation in mood and other variables may, therefore, produce intraindividual variation in memory performance.

Substantial intraindividual variability in discourse memory performance could have implications for clinical memory assessment. It could increase the variance within normal control groups, reducing statistical power and requiring larger sample sizes to obtain sensitive tests of patient group differences. More important, intraindividual variability could harm the validity of cross-sectional, age-stratified norms on tests like the LM scale for assessment of memory impairment in the elderly. Benign senescent forgetting, or the more recently proposed syndrome of age-associated memory impairment (AAMI) (Crook et al., 1986), is characterized by poor memory performance that is not secondary to a pathological physical process (e.g., Alzheimer's disease or cerebral infarct). One proposed criterion for AAMI is memory task performance that is one standard deviation below norms for young adults (Crook et al., 1986). As illustrated in Figure 4-1, intraindividual variation in performance might cause an elderly individual to be classified as having AAMI one day, but to be judged to have normal memory functioning another day (Hertzog et al., 1992).

Use of between-persons group norms for standardized memory tests to aid in the diagnosis of AAMI or other age-related, progressive pathologies of memory requires the assumption that low norm-referenced performance indicates within-person decline (Hertzog et al., 1992). It is true that the expected value of an individual's performance is the age-group mean, and that performance below the cutoff has a higher probability of being influenced by age-related decline, but there are other influences on performance. Reports from the Baltimore Longitudinal Study of Aging show significant age changes in mean levels of visual and verbal memory performance, but individual differences in the amount of longitudinal change are not highly correlated with initial status (Alder, Adam, & Arenberg, 1990). Moreover, the estimated magnitude of mean intraindividual changes with increasing age in those studies is relatively small when scaled against the distribution of individual differences. One cannot be certain that an individual exhibiting low performance has actually declined over time if one has not directly or indirectly estimated change from pre-morbid status. Alternatively, age-related decline in an individual with high pre-morbid memory ability might go undetected if assessment were based only on between-subjects norms.

Given these concerns, short- and long-term longitudinal case studies may be a valuable method for assessing both normative and pathological decline in older persons' memory function. In such designs each individual serves as his or her own control, and change over time can be evaluated against a standard error of measurement based on observed intraindividual variability in performance (Hertzog & Schear, 1989). There are, however, two major potential obstacles to implementation of such designs in assessment contexts. The first problem involves the magnitude of intraindividual variability relative to true, long-term intraindividual change (Nesselroade, 1991). To the extent that variability in performance is large, long periods of observation may be required to detect statistically reliable decrement (Salthouse, Kausler, & Saults, 1986). The second obstacle is the high likelihood of practice effects on memory task performance, even in the elderly. This problem would be especially acute if the same instrument were repeatedly administered over short time periods. In the extreme, practice effects could lead to ceiling effects in performance, especially on measures of memory for simple materials, such as short paragraphs. One could, therefore, wonder whether longitudinal case-study designs are feasible for evaluating change in cognitive performance in the elderly and whether the pattern of decline across multiple cognitive attributes has diagnostic value (with respect to either etiology or long-term prognosis).

MULTIPLE EQUIVALENT TEXTS FOR INTRAINDIVIDUAL DESIGNS

As described above, among the prominent methodological issues in intraindividual designs is the potential for re-test or practice effects. Some evidence for possible practice effects has been reported in analyses of reliability of the Wechsler Memory Scale, typically over a 4- to 7-week interval. Is it useful or advisable to use the Logical Memory scale with both shorter test intervals and more frequent testing? Although more extensive data are needed on this issue, we have been developing the position that multiple occasions of assessment may be advisable for selected theoretical and clinical purposes. Moreover, by "multiple" we mean both more than two and at more frequent intervals than 6 months. Frequent testing intervals probably require multiple equivalent stimuli, the characteristics of which are well-known and documented. Whereas this is relatively simple to accomplish for word lists, it is for more complicated for discourse. To this end, we have developed a set of 25 narrative texts designed to be equivalent in a variety of important characteristics. In this section we describe these narrative texts and their characteristics. These texts have been made available through a technical report (Dixon et al., 1989) to a number of researchers. We summarize some other features in subsequent sections.

STRUCTURAL FEATURES OF THE 25 STORIES

The 25 narrative texts described in this chapter were designed to be structurally and semantically equivalent. With respect to structural features they are all approximately 300 words (in exactly 24 sentences) long. An overview of the structural features of the texts is presented in Table 4–1. The propositional system of Kintsch (1974) was used to represent the meaning of the texts.

One unique feature is that each text is three-tiered. That is, each one contains not only a 300-word version (all 24 sentences), but a 165-word version (first 13 sentences) and a 100-word version (first 8 sentences). The target values for each tier were closely approximated: The average number of words for Tier 1 is 103.6 (range: 97–110), the average for Tier 2 is 164.7 (range: 159–170), and the average for Tier 3 (total story) is 303.1 (range: 298–308). Furthermore, the mean number of words per sentence across the 25 stories is similar (range: 9.8–15.2). Thus, the texts may be used as either 25 short (100-word) texts, 25 somewhat longer (165-word) texts, or 25 relatively long (300-word) texts, depending on the research questions of the investigator. Approximately 160 propositions are contained in each narrative. The average number of propositions for Tier 1 is 53.8 (range = 47–63), the average for Tier 2 is 86.6 (range = 78–100), and the average for the total story is 159.5 (range = 146–178). Across the 24 sentences of each story the number of propositions per sentence is similar (range = 5.32–7.92).

The stories are designed to be well-organized; that is, they possess high structural clarity. Each text presents the main idea (the major event and the main character(s)) in the first sentence. Each text also contains propositions ranging from main ideas (level 1) to intermediate ideas (levels 2 and 3) to details (levels 4–7). The proportion of propositions in each level of information to total number of propositions contained in a passage is another indicator of text structure. Overall, the stories are quite similar in their distributions of propositions across levels of information. For example, as would be expected in well-structured texts, a small proportion of the propositions are main ideas (1%), with larger

Table 4–1. Selected structural and readability characteristics of the 25 stories

Story No./Title	Number of Words			Number of Propositions			Flesch-Kincaid (grade)
	First Tier	Second Tier	Third Tier	First Tier	Second Tier	Third Tier	
1. A Visit to the Doctor	101	163	298	50	83	147	6.91
2. Running	110	168	305	51	81	146	7.08
3. A Concerned Husband	104	164	308	46	90	165	6.96
4. A Change in Life	102	166	304	52	88	159	6.35
5. Retiring from the Bank	106	166	303	47	81	153	7.21
6. A Vacation	105	168	302	51	83	148	6.70
7. Another Grandchild	102	166	302	63	100	162	6.51
8. A Trip Abroad	105	165	299	59	92	166	7.03
9. A Move	102	163	307	55	92	173	5.66
10. A Purchase	105	166	308	54	85	158	6.23
11. A Graduation	105	168	300	59	95	160	6.87
12. An Important Event	106	166	302	55	87	158	6.90
13. A Celebration	97	159	299	51	84	165	6.98
14. Hunting	105	160	302	59	86	164	5.38
15. Camping	99	159	304	54	78	162	6.70
16. First Flight	102	163	302	49	81	147	6.35
17. Playing Cards	101	162	302	55	90	178	6.67
18. Fishing	106	162	305	54	82	163	4.96
19. A Pilot	104	170	305	54	89	163	6.81
20. Working in the Yard	105	167	304	48	80	153	5.19
21. A Picnic	106	164	301	53	83	154	6.82
22. An Annual Celebration	100	167	303	48	84	155	7.60
23. A Rodeo	105	165	300	60	90	164	7.14
24. A Holiday	103	166	307	51	94	161	6.77
25. A Visitor from France	103	164	302	56	88	163	7.33
M	103.6	164.7	303.0	53.8	86.6	159.5	6.6
SD	2.74	2.84	2.76	4.11	5.38	7.87	.66

proportions being somewhat subordinate ideas (about 14% level 2s and 42% level 3s), and with the remainder of the propositions categorized as details (levels 4–7). In sum, relatively high equivalence on a number of structural indicators has been achieved.

READABILITY OF THE STORIES

Each of the 25 stories was evaluated in terms of readability according to three prominent scales. The scales were: (a) the Fry readability graph, (b) the Flesch readability score, and (c) the Flesch-Kincaid readability score

(Schuyler, 1980). These scales use indicators of readability such as sentence length and word length and then weight them in a given formula to arrive at an estimate of ease of readability. All stories are rated, according to the Fry graph, as being at the sixth to eighth grade level (M = grade 7.04). The Flesch scores for these stories range from 62.9 to 82.1 (M = 70.0). Seventeen of the stories were rated between 60 and 70; such ratings are characterized as a standard style (between fairly difficult and fairly easy), typical of digests (which are easier to read than "quality" magazines but more difficult than "slick fiction"). Six of the stories were rated between 70 and 80; such ratings are characterized as fairly easy to read, typical of slick fiction. Two of the stories were rated in the 80 to 90 range (80.4 and 82.1); such ratings are characterized as easy to read, typical of pulp fiction. According to the Flesch-Kincaid scale, the average grade level of the 25 stories was 6.6 (see Table 4–1). In sum, these data indicate that the 25 stories are consistently "standard" to "fairly easy" in style, with reading demands at about the Grade 7 level. All of these stories should be accessible to most normal young, middle-aged, and older adults, and nearly all to adults with mild to moderate cognitive impairments.

FEATURES OF THE CONTENTS OF THE STORIES

We present selected characteristics of the content of the stories in Table 4–2. As can be seen in Table 4–2, the 25 stories feature protagonists that are evenly divided by gender (nine female, nine male, and seven female-male couples). In addition, although it is always evident that the protagonists are older adults, this evidence is often subtle. That is, the age of the protagonist is usually indicated through their roles and activities rather than simply reporting their age. The stories are set in various locations across North America. The following areas of North America are represented: (a) two in eastern United States; (b) four in midwestern United States; (c) two in southern United States; (d) four in western United States; (e) two in Canada; (f) four involve trips (eastern United States to Europe, eastern United States to the midwest, eastern United States to the west, midwestern United States to the west); (g) two are located in small towns; and (h) five occur in unspecified locations. Other features are as follows.

1. They are all narrative stories describing a single event, or series of closely related events, in the life of (an) older protagonist(s).
2. The description includes the intentions, plans, evaluations, outcomes, behavior, complications, and ruminations of the protagonists, as well as the context of the event.

Table 4–2. Some characteristics of the content of the 25 stories

Story No./Title	Gender of Protagonist	Indication of Age	Location of Story
1. A Visit to the Doctor	F	widow	small town
2. Running	M	61	small town
3. A Concerned Husband	M	grandparent	Louisville, KY
4. A Change in Life	F	retired	Wisconsin
5. Retiring from the Bank	M	retired	Idaho
6. A Vacation	M	retired	Grand Canyon
7. Another Grandchild	C	grandparents	unspecified
8. A Trip Abroad	C	unspecified	Boston-Ireland
9. A Move	F	older widow	unspecified
10. A Purchase	C	parents of adults	Calgary, Canada
11. A Graduation	F	62	Iowa-Midwest
12. An Important Event	F	grandmother	Tennessee
13. A Celebration	F	90	Kansas
14. Hunting	M	father of adult	Colorado
15. Camping	C	older couple	Pittsburgh-Michigan
16. First Flight	F	mother of adult	Connecticut-Seattle
17. Playing Cards	C	married 45 years	unspecified
18. Fishing	M	retired	Western New York
19. A Pilot	M	widower	Western Texas
20. Working in the Yard	F	widow	unspecified
21. A Picnic	C	senior citizens	unspecified
22. An Annual Celebration	C	parents of adults	Washington, DC
23. A Rodeo	F	older widow	Wyoming
24. A Holiday	M	grandparent	Minneapolis, MN
25. A Visitor From France	M	64	Montreal, Canada

F = Female, M = Male, C = Couple

3. In each case, the event is normative (typical) for a given life course and it is relatively concrete.
4. In the interest of ecological validity, an effort was made to set the emotional content of the stories so as to range from moderate disappointment or apprehension, through optimistic ambivalence, to contentment and happiness, with most stories situated at the positive end of the continuum.

In sum, they were designed to present generally familiar themes to North American adults, without including declarative information that could influence the performance of particular segments of the population. The texts were generally rated as interesting to listen to or read.

USING THE TEXTS

Researchers may employ either a reading or listening paradigm to investigate free recall, recognition, or comprehension.

Free Recall

As described earlier, the number of words and propositions per tier (across the 25 stories) is similar. We adopted the propositional analysis system of Kintsch (1974) to represent the meaning of the texts. The text bases for scoring propositional recall are available in Dixon et al. (1989). Included in these text bases are levels of analysis (of the hierarchical organization of the texts). Also included in the report are recommendations for scoring free recall.

Recognition

Recognition items pertaining to the full-length version of each story are available. Eight items in each of three categories were developed ($n = 24$). The three categories are: (a) *True Gist Paraphrases*, which are statements contained in and consistent with the story; (b) *False Gist Paraphrases*, which are statements containing at least one component that is incorrect and inconsistent with the story; and (c) *Elaborations*, which are statements or inferences consistent with the story (or world knowledge) but not contained in the story (and thus scored false).

Comprehension Questions

For some research purposes, testing comprehension may be preferable to either free recall or recognition. Calogero, Hunt, and Kerr (1987) produced five short-answer comprehension questions for each of these 25 stories. Each of the questions addresses a specific but different aspect of the content of the stories, such as particular predicates, references, causal statements, and temporal information. The information queried in these questions is located in various parts of each text. Therefore, using these comprehension questions requires that the full-length version of the text(s) be administered.

RESEARCH EXAMPLES

In this section we briefly describe two examples of research on intraindividual variability in text recall performance by older adults. First, we summarize the main purpose and findings of a study conducted by Hertzog et al. (1992), which investigated the recall performance of seven older adults for as many as 90 weekly occasions. Second, we summarize selected initial observations from a recent study in which five young-old adults, five old-old adults, and one Alzheimer's disease patient were tested for text recall on 10 weekly occasions. In both studies our initial goals were: (a) to assess whether such multiple occasion testing could be conducted on very old adults, (b) to examine the extent of intraindividual variability in performance, and (c) to evaluate whether weekly testing results in uniformly improved performance, and perhaps reduced variability, for the individuals.

RESEARCH EXAMPLE 1

We began this study (see Hertzog et al., 1992, for more information) with seven women who were over age 65 at the time of initial assessment ($M = 75.4$ years). Each of the women had an extensive health examination prior to testing, and they reported themselves to be relatively healthy and suffering no major effects from any health conditions or medications. The goal was to test them weekly for as long as possible and up to 90 weeks. The minimum number of sessions completed was one subject who finished 25 occasions, which is about 6 months of testing. This subject withdrew for reasons pertaining to her spouse's condition (he had Alzheimer's disease). The remaining six subjects lasted past occasion 60, with four of them reaching about 90 weeks of participation. There may well have been some skepticism about whether adults of this age could participate for over a year of rigorous psychological testing or, put differently, up to 90 successive occasions. Our observation is that, despite a number of changes in their lives during the period of testing, long-term intraindividual panel designs can be successfully implemented with older persons. Were these participants unusual for the age group? Our evidence suggested that they were normal in a variety of ways, including health, vocabulary, and performance on other standardized cognitive tasks (see Hertzog et al., 1992).

Before examining intraindividual variability, it is useful to characterize the extent of interindividual variability in performance. We measured text recall in this study by using the full versions of the 25 equivalent texts (Dixon et al., 1989). We administered the 25 stories in blocks, such that the order of the 25 stories within each block was random, with the constraint that the same story could not be at the beginning of one block and the end of the previous block. One story was administered in each session. Subjects were asked to read the story and write their free recall on lined paper we provided. We scored the free recall according to the criteria described earlier, that is, whether a gist representation of each proposition was present or not. We examined both overall free recall (collapsing across stories and occasions) and recall of the hierarchical organization of the text. Regarding the former, the individual differences were substantial; for example, one participant recalled about 56% of the information in the stories, whereas another recalled only about 21%. Regarding the latter, the participants generally were able to identify and remember the main ideas of the stories. They reproduced the typical effect of a greater proportion of higher- than lower-level propositions.

How extensive was intraindividual variability in performance? Examining the plots of text recall performance across occasions it was clear that there was substantial intraindividual variability in performance for all subjects. One subject's performance, for example, ranged from 14% on one occasion to 64% on another. Identifying substantial intraindividual variability is notable, but it might be possible that all subjects varied in much the same way. Quite the opposite was true. The trends of performance across time varied significantly between subjects. Correlating performance with occasion of measurement resulted in significant positive correlations for two of the subjects and significant negative correlations for two other subjects. Whereas the former suggest a general increase in performance across time, the latter suggest a general decline in performance. Figures 4–2 and 4–3 illustrate these trends for two of the panel members. Note the general upward trend to P01 and the general downward trend to P03. Note also, however, that there is a great deal of variability for both subjects, both of whom recorded repeated peaks and valleys in their intraindividual trajectories.

Finally, there was little evidence for strong practice effects. No subjects improved to or near ceiling, and there was no suggestion of reduced variability late in the series of sessions. We, of course, cannot argue that the same pattern would occur for different materials, much less materials that are repeated frequently. It appears that several factors may have reduced the likelihood of practice effects. First, the availability of a large set of texts which were both equivalent and complex, as well as a design that minimized (or randomized) the possibility that a given passage would be read and recalled during neighboring sessions, may have worked to lessen potential practice effects. Second, the texts themselves were long (300 words) and complex, making it unlikely that individuals could remember substantial portions of a given story from one exposure to the next. In contrast to the possible ceiling effects of such a study, we observed a mixture of positive gains and negative losses that may have been due to a host of factors, including mood swings, changes in the family, temporary illnesses, active phases of chronic diseases,

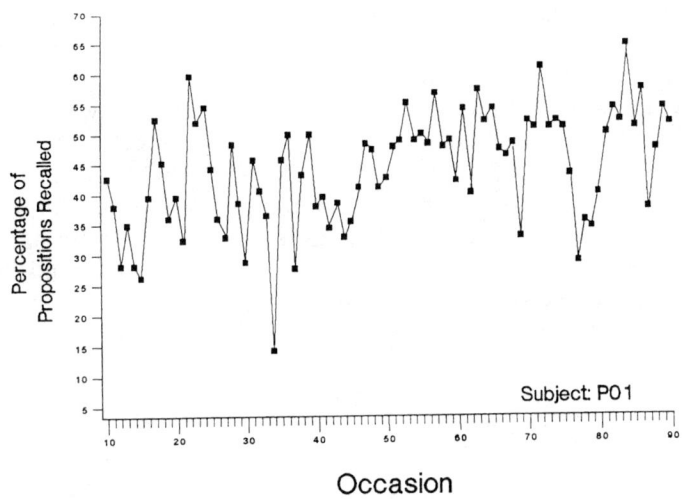

Figure 4–2. Selected subject (P01) who demonstrated substantial intraindividual variability and a general upward trend in performance (From Hertzog, C., Dixon, R. A., & Hultsch, D. F. [1992]. Intraindividual change in text recall of the elderly. *Brain and Language, 42,* 248–269, used by permission.).

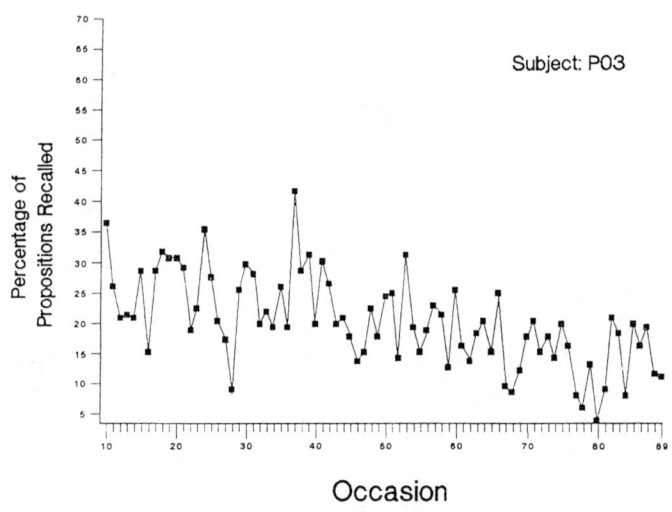

Figure 4–3. Selected subject (P03) who demonstrated substantial intraindividual variability and a general downward trend in performance (From Hertzog, C., Dixon, R. A., & Hultsch, D. F. [1992]. Intraindividual change in text recall of the elderly. *Brain and Language, 42,* 248–269, used by permission.).

medication changes, enthusiasm, familiarity or interest in some of the stories, shifting senses of self-efficacy or control, and even variability in memory ability. The improvements for two of the subjects may indeed have been subtle reflections of practice or at least learning-to-learn, but these effects do not overwhelm the general picture of intraindividual variability. The declines for two of the subjects may have been indicative of the effects of a disease process or terminal drop. Indeed, it is possible that, without some learning to learn effects, the declines may have been even more substantial. For this reason, the declines observed in such panel studies may have substantial clinical significance.

RESEARCH EXAMPLE 2

A second study, which is still in progress, was designed to examine several issues, including (a) the extent of intraindividual variability on shorter texts, (b) the potential for practice on shorter texts, (c) comparisons with standardized neuropsychological tasks, and (d) selected factors that may be related to intraindividual variability in performance on a given task. In this ongoing study, authors Friesen and Dixon collected data on 10 weekly occasions. Participants were five normal young-old adult women (M age = 68.2 years), five normal old-old adult women (M age = 82 years), and one woman diagnosed with probable Alzheimer's disease (age = 75 years). Although several tests of mood, depression, and standard neuropsychological functioning were included in the design, we focus here on the story recall tasks. We included two relevant tasks: the LM subtest of the Wechsler Memory Scale-Revised and 10 short versions of the stories from the Dixon et al. (1989) collection (DHH). To minimize potential practice effects, the two stories from the LM subtest (Anna Thompson and Robert Miller) were alternated (i.e., presented every second occasion, or once every 2 weeks). The short version (about 100 words) of the DHH texts were presented to be more comparable to the LM stories. Because there are 25 stories in this collection we were able to select 10 different passages for use in this study. Therefore, no DHH story was repeated.

As in the earlier study, the range of performance across subjects and occasions was considerable. To illustrate our initial observations we focus here on the immediate recall condition, starting with the DHH texts. Again, as was the case in the previous research example, there were substantial interindividual differences. Recall for the young-old participants ranged from an average of 42.5% of the information overall to only 26.2%, Recall for the old-old participants ranged from an average of 44.3% of the information overall to only 11.5%. The AD subject recalled 7.8% overall (range across occasions: 0–15%). Again, the intraindividual variability was substantial, with the difference between extreme performances for some older adults being over 30% of the information in the DHH texts. Overall, the range for the young-old participants was 14–59%, and the range for old-old participants was 0–59%.

Shifting to the LM stories, we observed a similar degree of interindividual differences and substantial intraindividual variability for recall of these texts. The difference between extreme scores for some older individuals was approximately 40% of the information contained in the texts. The overall range of performance for young-old participants was 24–84%, and the range for old-old participants was even larger, 8–88%. The trends of performance vary substantially across individuals. The AD participant performed generally lower (overall $M = 14.8$; range: 4–24%) than adults from other groups, but was occasionally within one standard deviation of the mean for the old-old group. In addition, the AD subject occasionally performed as well or better than selected old-old subjects on immediate recall for both the DHH and the LM stories.

Figure 4–4 presents the profiles of performance on the DHH texts for the AD subject, as well as three selected young-old and old-old individuals. Figure 4–5 presents the profiles for performance on the LM stories for the same seven individuals. It is notable that the highest scores for the two sets of stories are considerably different. Whereas the top score for the DHH texts is slightly less than 60%, there are about 30 scores for the Logical Memory stories that are over 60%, and a few of these exceed 80%. Nevertheless, for the LM stories, subjects do not hit 80% consistently until after the seventh occasion, and then only three do so. It is notable that one young-old subject (211) hits 80% by the seventh occasion then shows step-like decline over the next three occasions. One might assume that this indicates some change in functional capacity were it not for the fact that her performance on the more complex DHH texts continues to fluctuate during this period. The AD subject seems to have more difficulty with the DHH texts, although her highest performance is only slightly above 20%, which is less than the 20th percentile. Her profile is separated from that of the normals. For these texts, there are fewer instances of overlap with normals, and the performance is generally lower. The performance of two of the normals, however, is just as low on some occasions. Case 309 remembers as much as 40% of the information in the second LM story, which for an old-old individual is about the 50–60th percentile, and as little as 10% for the same story (less than the 5th percentile). Although these data do not appear in the figures, there was also considerable fluctuation for the delay conditions for both sets of stories.

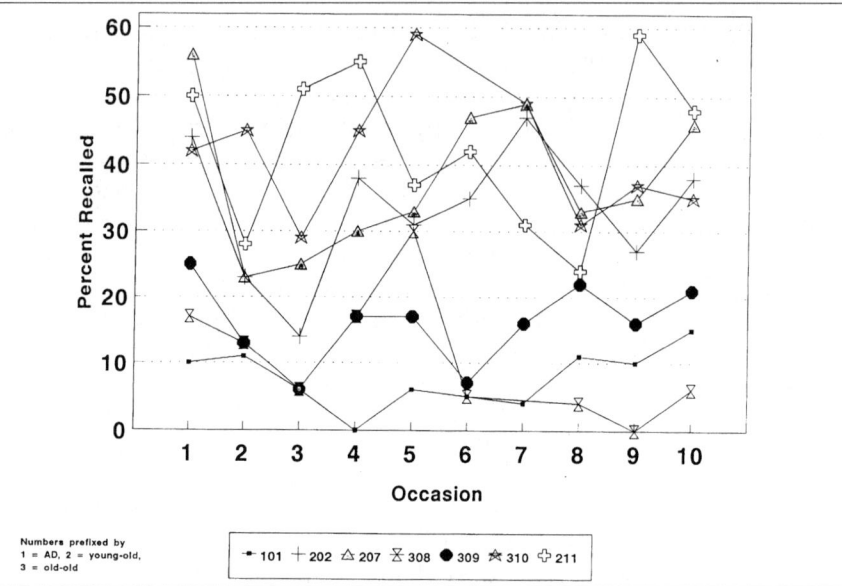

Figure 4–4. Selected intraindividual performance profiles for the short version of the Dixon et al. (1989) stories. Case numbers prefixed by 1 = AD, 2 = young-old, and 3 = old-old.

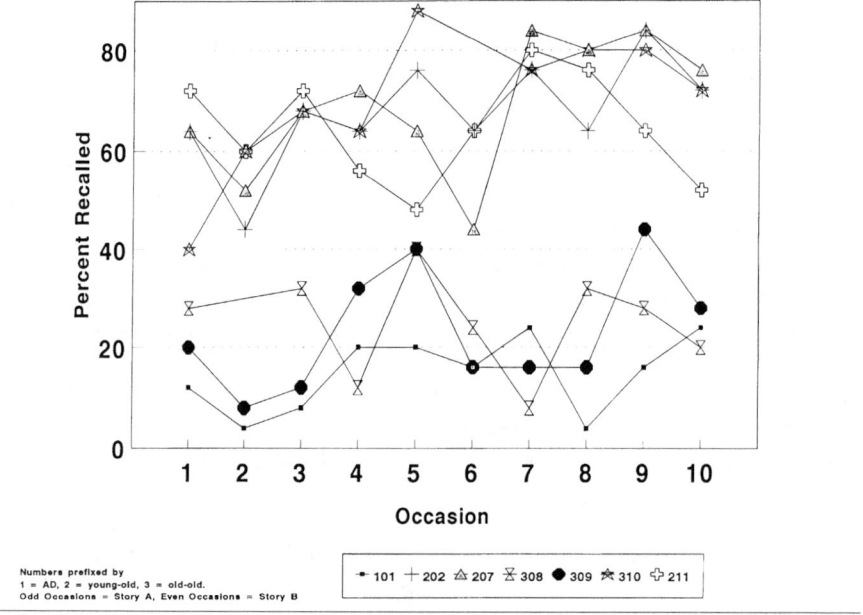

Figure 4–5. Selected intraindividual performance profiles for the Logical Memory stories. Case numbers prefixed by 1 = AD, 2 = young-old, and 3 = old-old.

Practice effects could be indicated by strong positive correlations between performance and occasion. Although neither set of stories provided robust evidence for practice effects, there was a slight difference between the two. Overall, for the DHH texts the correlation between occasion and performance was zero for both young-old and old-old adults. For the LM stories, the correlation for both the young-old and the old-old participants was low and positive ($r = .23$ and $.15$, respectively). Practice effects are small, but more noticeable for the LM texts. Two possible reasons for this are that (a) the LM stories were of necessity repeated (although on alternate weeks), and (b) they were shorter and less complex. Again, the substantial intraindividual variability may have been due to a variety of factors, and further research on the mechanism(s) through which these influences operate would be useful.

Although the results of this study are preliminary, they tend to support and extend those of Hertzog et al. (1992). In both studies—with both long and short versions of DHH stories—substantial intraindividual variability in recall on multiple weekly occasions was observed. Such intraindividual variability was also observed in this study for recall performance on the LM stories. Interestingly, despite the weekly testing sessions, recall performance on the LM stories did not hit ceiling. Individual performance continued to fluctuate throughout the 10 occasions. Both studies illustrate the potential hazards of using normed assessment of recall performance for normal older adults. For the AD patient in the second study, however, this would not have presented a problem, for she did not perform at a level that would have mistakenly indicated the absence of cognitive impairment. Further research may clarify the level of cognitive impairment at which relatively little fluctuation in performance may be expected.

CONCLUSION

In this chapter we have attempted (a) to discuss the general value of investigating intraindividual change in text memory skills in older adults, (b) to describe some of the special methodological issues and requirements of intraindividual designs, (c) to propose some solutions and tools for carrying out such research, and (d) to illustrate the technique and results of intraindividual panel designs. Clinicians have noted anecdotally that there are fluctuations in the functional competence of elderly individuals. Similarly, researchers have demonstrated with growing frequency that there is great within-person variability in mood, personality, and cognitive performance. We explored the extent to which such intraindividual inconsistency (a) is real and not solely a product of measurement error, (b) is a characteristic of a wide variety of processes and constructs, and (c) extensive (not minuscule) and long-lasting. To the extent that intraindividual variability for a given process has the above three characteristics, single session assessments supplemented with comparisons to normative averages are at risk for over- or underestimating the "true" competence of a given individual.

We suggest two possibilities. First, in many cases it may be useful for an individual's performance to be compared to his or her own baseline of performance, in addition to the interindividual averaged norms. Assessment is viewed, therefore, as a long-term prospective enterprise. In this context, designs such as those we have described in this chapter cost more in terms of time and effort, but they provide a benefit that may be substantial in some cases. Second, it may also be useful to supplement published norms with cautions concerning—if not observed estimates of—intraindividual variability. Our conclusions regarding these issues are consistent with a growing body of literature regarding older adults. There is a considerable degree of intraindividual fluctuation in cognitive performance that is due to a host of factors, few of which are observable in single-occasion assessments. Certainly more research is required on (a) the extent of measures that demonstrate intraindividual fluctuation, (b) the degree of intraindividual variability for each of these measures, (c) the populations displaying such variability in given tasks, and (d) the mechanisms responsible for short-term within-person change. With extensive intraindividual variability as an emerging backdrop to assessment of normal older adults and some as-yet-unknown portion of clinical populations, the accuracy of evaluations depends on the extent to which future research sheds light on these issues.

ACKNOWLEDGMENTS

The first author acknowledges grant support from the Natural Sciences and Engineering Research Council of Canada and from the Canadian Aging Research Network (CARNET).

REFERENCES

Alder, A. G., Adam, J., & Arenberg, D. (1990). An individual differences assessment of the relationship between change in and initial level of adult cognitive functioning. *Psychology and Aging, 5,* 560–568.

Broadbent, D. E., Broadbent, M. H. P., & Jones, J. L. (1989). Time of day as an instrument for the analysis of attention. *European Journal of Cognitive Psychology, 1*, 69–94.

Byrd, M. (1986-87). The effects of previously acquired knowledge on memory for textual information. *International Journal of Aging and Human Development, 24*, 231–240.

Calogero, M., Hunt, E., & Kerr, B. (1987). Unpublished data on text comprehension. Department of Psychology, University of Washington, Seattle.

Caine, E. D., Banford, K. A., Schiffer, R. B., Shoulson, I., & Levy, S. (1987). A controlled neuropsychological comparison of Huntington's disease and multiple sclerosis. *Archives of Neurology, 43*, 249–254.

Clark, D. M., & Teasdale, J. D. (1982). Diurnal variations in clinical depression and accessibility of memories of positive and negative experiences. *Journal of Abnormal Psychology, 91*, 87–95.

Craik, F. I. M. (1977). Age differences in human memory. In J. E. Birren & K. W. Schaie (Eds.), *Handbook of the psychology of aging* (pp. 384–420). Princeton, NJ: Van Nostrand Reinhold.

Crook, T., Bartus, R. T., Ferris, S. H., Whitehouse, P., Cohen, G. D., & Gershon, S. (1986). Age-associated memory impairment: Proposed diagnostic criteria and measures of clinical change-report of a National Institute of Mental Health work group. *Developmental Neuropsychology, 2*, 261–276.

Dall'Ora, P., Della Sala, S., & Spinnler, H. (1989). Autobiographical memory: Its impairment in amnesic syndromes. *Cortex, 25*, 197–217.

Dixon, R. A., & Hertzog, C. (1988). A functional approach to memory and metamemory development in adulthood. In F. E. Weinert & M. Perlmutter (Eds.), *Memory development: Universal changes and individual differences* (pp. 293–330). Hillsdale, NJ: Lawrence Erlbaum.

Dixon, R. A., & Hultsch, D. F. (1983). Metamemory and memory for text relationships in adulthood: A cross-validation study. *Journal of Gerontology, 38*, 689–694.

Dixon, R. A., Hultsch, D. F., & Hertzog, C. (1989). *A manual of twenty-five three-tiered structurally equivalent texts for use in aging research* (2nd ed.; Technical Report No. 2). Victoria, B.C., Canada/Atlanta, GA: Collaborative Research Group on Cognitive Aging.

Dixon, R. A., Hultsch, D. F., Simon, E. W., & von Eye, A. (1984). Verbal ability and text structure effects on adult age differences in text recall. *Journal of Verbal Learning and Verbal Behavior, 23*, 569–578.

Egelko, S., Gordon, W. A., Hibbard, M. R., Diller, L., Lieberman, A., Holliday, R., Ragnarsson, K., Shaver, M. S., & Orazem. J. (1988). Relationship among CT scans, neurological exam, and neuropsychological test performance in right-brain-damaged stroke patients. *Journal of Clinical and Experimental Neuropsychology, 10*, 539–564.

Eich, E., & Metcalfe, J. (1989). Mood dependent memory for internal versus external events. Journal of Experimental Psychology: *Learning, Memory and Cognition, 15*, 443–455.

Erickson, R. C., & Scott, M. L. (1977). Clinical memory testing: A review. *Psychological Bulletin, 84*, 1130–1149.

Flicker, C., Ferris, S. H., Crook, T., Bartus, R. T., & Reisberg, B. (1986). Cognitive decline in advanced age: Future directions for psychometric differentiation of normal and pathological age changes in cognitive function. *Developmental Neuropsychology, 2,* 309–322.

Grant, I., McDonald, W. I., Trimble, M. R., Smith, E., & Reed, R. (1984). Deficient learning and memory in early and middle phases of multiple sclerosis. *Journal of Neurology, Neurosurgery, and Psychiatry, 47,* 250–255.

Hartley, J. T. (1986). Reader and text variables as determinants of discourse memory in adulthood. *Psychology and Aging, 1,* 150–158.

Hertzog, C., & Schear, J. M. (1989). Psychometric considerations in testing the older person. In T. Hunt & C. J. Lindley (Eds.), *Testing the older person: A reference guide for geropsychological assessments* (pp. 24–50). Austin, TX: Pro-Ed.

Hertzog, C., Dixon, R. A., & Hultsch, D. F. (1992). Intraindividual change in text recall of the elderly. *Brain and Language, 42,* 248–269.

Hooker, K., Nesselroade, D. W., Nesselroade, J. R., & Lerner, R. M. (1987). The structure of intraindividual temperament in the context of mother-child dyads: P-technique factor analyses of short-term change. *Developmental Psychology, 23,* 332–346.

Hultsch, D. F., & Dixon, R. A. (1984). Memory for text materials in adulthood. In P.B. Baltes & O. G. Brim, Jr. (Eds.), *Lifespan development and behavior* (Vol. 6, pp. 77–108). New York: Academic Press.

Hultsch, D. F., Hertzog, C., & Dixon, R. A. (1990). Ability correlates of memory performance in adulthood and aging. *Psychology and Aging, 5,* 356–368.

Kahn, H. J., Joanette, Y., Ska, B., & Goulet, P. (1990). Discourse analysis in neuropsychology: Comment on Chapman and Ulatowski. *Brain and Language, 38,* 454–461.

Kaszniak, A. W., (1990). Psychological assessment of the aging individual. In J.E. Birren & K. W. Schaie (Eds.), *Handbook of the psychology of aging* (3rd ed., pp. 427–445). San Diego, CA: Academic Press.

Kintsch, W. (1974). *The representation of meaning in memory.* Hillsdale, NJ: Lawrence Erlbaum.

Kopelman, M. D., (1986). Clinical tests of memory. *British Journal of Psychiatry, 148,* 517–525.

Kopelman, M. D., Wilson, B. A., & Baddeley, A. D. (1989). The autobiographical memory interview: A new assessment of autobiographical and personal semantic memory in amnesic patients. *Journal of Clinical and Experimental Neuropsychology, 11,* 724–744.

Meyer, B. J. F. (1975). *The organization of prose and its effects on memory.* Amsterdam: North-Holland.

Nesselroade, J. R. (1988). Some implications of the trait-state distinction for the study of development over the life span: The case of personality. In P. B. Baltes, D. L. Featherman, & R. M. Lerner (Eds.), *Life-span development and behaviour* (Vol. 8, pp. 163–189). Hillsdale, NJ: Erlbaum.

Nesselroade, J. R. (1991). The warp and the woof of the developmental fabric. In R. Downs, L. Liben, & R. M. Lerner (Eds.), *Visions of aesthetics, the environment, and development: The legacy of Joachim F. Wohlwill* (pp. 213–240). Hillsdale, NJ: Lawrence Erlbaum.

Nesselroade, J. R., & Ford, D. H. (1985). P-technique comes of age: Multivariate, replicated, single-subject designs for research on older adults. *Research on Aging, 7,* 46–80.

Nesselroade, J. R., Pruchno, R., & Jacobs, A. (1986). Reliability vs. stability in the measurement of psychological states: An illustration with anxiety measures. *Psychologische Beitrage, 28*, 255–264.

Rao, S. M., Leo, G. J., & St. Aubin-Faubert, P. (1989). On the nature of memory disturbance in multiple sclerosis. *Journal of Clinical and Experimental Neuropsychology, 11*, 699–712.

Rehak, A., Kaplan, J. A., Weylman, S. T., Kelly, B., Brownell, H. H., & Gardner, H. (1992). Story processing in right-hemisphere brain-damaged patients. *Brain and Language, 42*, 320–336.

Roberts, M. L., & Nesselroade, J. R. (1986). Intraindividual variability in perceived locus of control in adults: P-technique factor analyses of short-term change. *Journal of Research in Personality, 20*, 529–545.

Salthouse, T. A., Kausler, D. H., & Saults, J. S. (1986). Groups versus individuals as the comparison unit in cognitive aging research. *Developmental Neuropsychology, 2*, 363–372.

Schultz, K. A., Schmitt, F. A., Logue, P. E., & Rubin, D. C. (1986). Unit analysis of prose memory in clinical and elderly populations. *Developmental Neuropsychology, 2*, 77–87.

Schuyler, M. R. (1980). A readability formula program for use on microcomputers. *Journal of Reading, 25*, 260–291.

Spielberger, C. D. (1977). State-trait anxiety and interactional psychology. In D. Magnusson & N. S. Endler (Eds.), *Personality at the crossroads: Current issues in interactional psychology* (pp. 173–183). Hillsdale, NJ: Lawrence Erlbaum.

Stine, E. A. L., & Wingfield, A. (1987). Levels upon levels: Predicting age differences in text recall. *Experimental Aging Research, 13*, 179–183.

Watson, D. (1988). Intraindividual and interindividual analyses of positive and negative affect: Their relation to health complaints, perceived stress, and daily activities. *Journal of Personality and Social Psychology, 54*, 1020–1030.

Wilson, B. A. (1987). *Rehabilitation of memory*. New York: Guilford.

van Dijk, T. A., & Kintsch, W. (1983). *Strategies of discourse comprehension*. New York: Academic Press.

Zelinski, E. M., & Gilewski, M. J. (1988). Memory for prose and aging: A meta-analysis. In M. L. Howe & C. J. Brainerd (Eds.), *Cognitive development in adulthood: Progress in cognitive development research* (pp. 133–158). New York: Springer-Verlag.

Zelinski, E. M., Light, L. L., & Gilewski, M. J. (1984). Adult age differences in memory for prose: The question of sensitivity to passage structure. *Developmental Psychology, 20*, 1181–1192.

Zevon, M. A., & Tellegen, A. (1982). The structure of mood change: An idiographic/nomothetic analysis. *Journal of Personality and Social Psychology, 43*, 111–122.

CHAPTER 5

Qualitative Differences in Working Memory and Discourse Comprehension in Normal Aging

HELEN J. KAHN AND DANIELLE CORDON

This chapter examines why older adults are able to remember some types of information better than others and how these characteristics of memory relate to the comprehension of narrative discourse. To that end, we are particularly interested in the role that working memory plays in an individual's interpretation of information during comprehension. Earlier research (Davis & Ball, 1989; Light & Anderson, 1985; Norman, Kemper, Kynette, & Cheung, 1991; Stine & Wingfield,1990; Tun, Stine, & Wingfield, 1991; Ulatowska, Cannito, Hayashi, & Fleming, 1986) has shown age-related effects of working memory on comprehension. One current explanation for such effects entails a model that incorporates the principle of allocation of mental resources—specifically, comprehension may be easier for some types of information than for others because of differences in the availability of working memory resources (Just & Carpenter, 1992).

MODELS OF WORKING MEMORY

Contemporary models of memory (Baddeley, 1986; Just & Carpenter, 1992; Salthouse, 1990) challenge the traditional structural models which emphasized only storage. In 1974, Baddeley and Hitch proposed a model that highlighted certain computational aspects of working memory. The functions of these computations in comprehension were to perform an integration of information, resolve ambiguity, and provide pronoun reference resolution among others. To more naturally capture the nature of discourse comprehension, current models hold that both storage and computation are necessary components (Just & Carpenter, 1992; Whitney, Ritchie, & Clark, 1991).

Baddeley and Hitch's original (1974) model considered working memory as a system of limited capacity which was divided between storage and processing components. Using a dual-task paradigm, their hypothesis was that an individual's performance would deteriorate if more space and processing capabilities were required than what the individual had available (Baddeley & Hitch, 1974). Baddeley's (1986) later theory describes a central executive, that is, a supervisory system, which directs attentional resources, as well as selects and operates control processes. The control processes (in Baddeley's [1992] current terminology these are identified as "slave systems") include a temporal-durational component called the "articulatory loop" and a spatial-capacity component, called the "visuospatial scratchpad."

The central executive component continues to be the subject of debate, in part because the original description by Baddeley (1986) was somewhat vague. Recently, Baddeley (1992) proposed that the role of the central executive is to coordinate the information from the two control mechanisms. Other researchers (Just & Carpenter, 1992; van Dijk & Kintsch, 1983) have proposed analogous central executive systems. For instance, van Dijk and Kintsch (1983) proposed a supervisory system whose function is to activate and update a representation in storage and then consider that representation in light of the events, actions, and persons described in the text. The representation may also incorporate prior knowledge or experiences and, simultaneously with the text interpretation, the supervisory system must also direct the integration of information from long-term memory. In short, the supervisory system oversees all information that is needed for processing. Just and Carpenter's (1992) theory of working memory and comprehension also implicates a supervisory system but unlike Baddeley (1986) they do not consider modality specific buffers (e.g., the articulatory loop and the visuospatial scratchpad). In their theory, capacity refers to the maximum amount of activation available in working memory to perform the dual functions of storage and/or computations. As long as the activation level is above some minimum threshold value, information can be processed by the computational aspects of working memory. But if the total amount of activation is less than the amount required to perform a particular task, information will decay, be deleted, or otherwise forgotten. At the heart of their theory is the trade-off between storage and computations and how such trade-offs reflect working memory capacity. Whenever task demands are high, for example, during ambiguity resolution or syntactic parsing of complex sentences, there are consequences for comprehension. If an individual slows processing time, expending more effort in the consideration of a difficult text, storage will suffer, and, therefore, information can be "held over" for later processing. If the individual continues reading the text, less prior information is available for the interpretation of subsequent text. However, if considerable effort is placed on maintaining the contents of working memory through some elaborative rehearsal strategy, new information that is difficult cannot be efficiently processed. Anytime there are trade-offs between storage and computations, because the allocation of resources are directed to tasks with high demands, comprehension will suffer.

THE ROLE OF WORKING MEMORY IN DISCOURSE COMPREHENSION

When working memory is considered in terms of discourse comprehension, it is usually within the framework of processing constraints. The view that van Dijk and Kintsch (1983) hold is that memory is a natural by-product of discourse processing and that capacity has inherent limitations, in both the allocation of resources and the amount of information to-be-processed. The amount of information that can be processed is constrained whenever an individual simply does not have the capacity to efficiently process that information. Resource limitations, however, occur because demands on the individual are high enough that processing capabilities become overloaded.

In 1983, van Dijk and Kintsch suggested that research on constraints in discourse processing would become a major focus in the coming years. It appears that their prediction has been realized since, in recent years, there has been a great deal of interest in processing constraints, particularly as the concept applies to working memory (Erlich & Delafoy, 1990; King & Just, 1991; Lee, William, & Whitney, 1991; MacDonald, Just, & Carpenter,1992). Marcel Just, Patricia Carpenter, and their colleagues have published a series of articles over the past few years that discuss a capacity theory of language comprehension (Carpenter & Just, 1983; Carpenter & Just, 1989; Just & Carpenter, 1980; Just & Carpenter, 1987) with particular emphasis on how some people demonstrate more capacity constraints than others. The focus of their research has been on manipulating the context of a text so that an individual must adjust his or her allocation of resources to adapt to the difficulty of the task. Their subject pool has been primarily college-age students who, according to the Reading Span Test (Daneman & Carpenter, 1980) (see below) differ in the amount of available working memory resources. MacDonald et al. (1992) have shown that when an individual must retain more than one possible interpretation of a text, that is, multiple meanings, working memory resources are taxed. Their hypothesis is that readers with high memory spans are better able to handle difficult tasks, or maintain multiple interpretations of text, than low memory span readers.

To investigate individual difference in working memory capacity, Just and Carpenter have used the Reading Span Test (Daneman & Carpenter, 1980). The test requires that a subject read a series of sentences while trying to remember the final word of each sentence until asked to recall them. The final score reflects the maximum number of sentences in a set that a subject can reliably recall and is referred to as reading span. According to Daneman and Carpenter's (1980) study, subjects with high reading span scores recall text more accurately than subjects with low reading span scores. Reading span measures correlate highly with other measures of reading comprehension (Daneman & Carpenter, 1980; Just & Carpenter, 1992; Masson & Miller, 1983). Further, the Reading Span Test is more sensitive to the computational and storage requirements of comprehension than traditional short-term memory tasks that emphasize storage only.

In our research, we are interested in how constraints on working memory change with age and, in particular, the amount of available mental resources and how individuals allocate those resources to adjust for difficult types of texts. In the following section, we will show evidence for patterns of individual differences in working memory capacity in later adulthood.

DISCOURSE COMPREHENSION, WORKING MEMORY, AND AGING

In the last decade, various hypotheses have been advanced to account for the decline in discourse comprehension associated with normal aging. One line of work suggests that discourse comprehension is affected by not only **how much** older adults are asked to remember but also what **type** of information they are asked to remember. In this connection, we conducted a series of studies in which we considered the role played by prior knowledge in memory for text. (Kahn, 1990; Kahn, 1991; Kahn & Till, 1991). The pronoun is a convenient tool for this type of research because it invokes two types of memory: memory for preceding discourse and memory for prior knowledge. Prior knowledge, sometimes referred to as world knowledge, semantic, or long-term memory, is described as the internal representation of how people typically act, what they do, and how events occur in the world (Just & Carpenter,1987).

Consider the following sentences:

1a. The accountant added the figures while the client signed the tax forms.
1b. He used a calculator.

Note that there there are pragmatic constraints within the noun reference phrases of Sentence 1a such that accountants ordinarily do the figuring and clients ordinarily sign forms during the tax season. Further, there is a contextual relationship between the noun referent phrase "added the figures" in Sentence 1a and "He used the calculator" in Sentence 1b. It is apparent that whoever does the adding needs a calculator. These contextual constraints are based on the expectations associated with prior knowledge concerning accountants and clients and who would ordinarily use a calculator during tax computation.

We hypothesized that the degree of "expectedness," that is, the degree to which prior knowledge is invoked, would influence the accuracy of pronoun reference. When the degree of expectedness is **strong** within the noun referent phrase, such as in Sentence 1a, pronoun reference resolution would be facilitated, and the amount of working memory resources required would be reduced. However, when the degree of expectedness is **weakened**, pronoun resolution would be more difficult and more working memory resources would be required. We also speculated that the size of the memory load, that is, the textual distance between the noun phrase and the pronoun phrase would influence the efficiency of pronoun resolution.

Table 5–1 illustrates the stimuli that were constructed to vary according to the degree of expectedness that was manipulated in the text. For instance, in the first example in the table, the sentence "The groom took the wedding ring out of a pocket while the pastor read the wedding vows from the Bible" was considered an **expected context** because preliminary studies showed that subjects were in agreement that a groom gets ready to put the ring on the finger of his bride while a pastor performs the wedding ceremony (confirmed by our pilot data in Kahn & Till, 1991). However, a sentence such as "The model thoughtfully contemplated the canvas while the artist stood very still" was considered an **unexpected context** because most individuals we tested in our preliminary studies agreed that a model does the posing, and an artist gazes at

Table 5–1. Sample stories and questions

Expected Context (Intervening Sentences = 1)

The groom took the wedding ring out of a pocket while the pastor read the wedding vows from the Bible. The organist played the traditional wedding march when the bride entered.

Target Sentence	He looked for the bride's hand.
Comprehension Question	Was there music at the wedding?

Unexpected Context (Intervening Sentences = 2)

The model thoughtfully contemplated the canvas while the artist stood very still. An instructor walked around the class and inspected each student's work. Gaining the proper perspective takes a lot of time and patience.

Target Sentence	He considered the next stroke.
Comprehension Question	Was the artist alone in the studio?

Neutral Context (Intervening Sentences = 3)

The tourist spotted the dangerous shark while the swimmer ran from the water. The sight of people running created panic on the beach. It was announced over a bullhorn that everyone should remain calm. The advice was to move slowly and make little movement in the water.

Target sentence	He looked through the binoculars.
Comprehension Question	Was the crowd on the shoreline tranquil?

Source: From Kahn, H., & Till, R. A. (1991). Pronoun reference and aging. *Developmental Neuropsychology, 7*, 459–475, reprinted by permission.

---

the canvas. The context, while not entirely contradictory, does not fit prior knowledge. "The tourist spotted the dangerous shark while the swimmer ran from the water," was considered a **neutral context** because either individual could have spotted the shark or ran from the water—both are neutral with respect to prior knowledge.

We tested 36 younger (mean age 21.3) and 36 older (mean age 67.19) adults. Subjects were matched for years of education and vocabulary and were in good general health. A computer presented passages one sentence at a time with the subjects self-controlling the rate of presentation. The computer recorded the accuracy of response and reading times for each sentence. To achieve counterbalancing, a given passage appeared equally often in the three conditions of expectedness (Expected, Unexpected, or Neutral) and memory load (Intervening Sentences, 1, 2, or 3).

After a training session on sample passages, subjects were instructed that they would be asked to read passages varying in length and that the final sentence would begin with a pronoun. Their task was to decide the referent for that pronoun from the first sentence that they had read. To ensure that the subjects read the entire paragraph, a comprehension question concerning the main idea of the paragraph appeared an average of every third trial.

The results indicated that young subjects showed little effect of expectedness for their responses to the pronoun reference statements (mean rates of accuracy were 91% for expected context, 87% for unexpected, and 84% for neutral context). In contrast, the older subjects showed a highly significant effect of expectedness (mean rates of accuracy were 84% for expected context, 68% for unexpected context, and 74% for neutral context). Memory load, that is, the number of sentences intervening between the noun reference sentence and the target sentence, produced an effect according to expectedness, but not according to age. For all subjects, memory load influenced the accuracy of noun choice for the unexpected and neutral contexts, but was absent in the expected context. Thus, our findings are at variance with prior empirical studies (Light & Capps, 1986) that the length of text is responsible, most notably the number of sentences intervening between a pronoun and its referent noun, for less efficient recall in normal older adults.

When we analyzed reading times, we found that older adults took longer to read the passages than the younger adults, but that the degree of expectedness did not interact with age. All subjects read the expected sentences faster than the neutral sentences, which in turn were read faster than the unexpected sentences. Furthermore, target sentences that referred to expected sentences were read faster than the target sentences referring to unexpected or neutral sentences. Stine (1990) also found that younger and older adults were similar in reading times on a sentence task and that reading times for all subjects were influenced by textual factors such as word frequency and sentence boundaries.

When we analyzed the reading times for the intervening sentences, we found a significant interaction of Age by Expectedness for the first intervening sentence. Young adults read the first intervening sentences at a similar rate for all three levels of expectedness. However, the reading times for older adults were faster in the expected condition, but there was no difference in reading times for intervening sentences in the the neutral and unexpected conditions. We speculated that these differences in reading time reflect differences in the allocation of resources for working memory. When the initial sentences in a passage were in an expected context, fewer working memory resources were needed than when the sentences were in an unexpected or neutral context. When the initial sentences were unexpected or neutral with respect to prior knowledge, more resources were needed, requiring more processing time. It is possible that when older adults read initial sentences that were unexpected or neutral, they proceeded to the intervening sentences with the intention of rehearsing the information or performing some other equally time-consuming strategy. The younger adults may also have engaged in some rehearsal strategies, but they were not sufficiently time consuming to have increased reading time. The accuracy results further support such differential strategies by age. When faced with a forced noun choice in the unexpected condition, older adults may have responded on the basis of what they already knew, that is, their prior knowledge that was already held in long term-memory rather than the context of the text. They then selected the expected context alternative. Regardless of the rehearsal strategy invoked, it is apparent that all subjects knew they would need to spend more time processing the textual information for unexpected and neutral contexts than for expected contexts.

One explanation for our findings (Kahn & Till, 1991) may be that when the information to recall is well-known (the expected context), remembering and manipulating the information places minimal demands on working memory. Either there is little new information to store or less integration is needed because the new information corresponds to already well-ingrained prior knowledge. But when information is contradictory or bears little relationship to prior knowledge, as in the unexpected or neutral context, more demands are placed on working memory. This interpretation is supported by the Just and Carpenter (1992) model and by their earlier work in which individuals with low reading span scores are less accurate on difficult comprehension tasks than individuals with high reading span scores. Working memory capacity and available resources influence not only the amount of text that can be processed, but also the type of text that can be maintained over time, particularly when there is more than one interpretation possible. Thus, in the case where text has a strong contextual relationship to prior knowledge (the expected context), the resource demands would be minimal because only one interpretation need be maintained in working memory. However, when text has a weak contextual relationship (unexpected or neutral context) to prior knowledge, then the current text must not only be maintained, but also interpreted in light of what the individual already "knows" about the topic. For a period of time, one or more interpretations are considered, and with fewer resources available, compared to the younger group, the older group may have more difficulty maintaining these interpretations, recalling the correct interpretation when the time came or even inhibiting one interpretation over another.

There is, in fact, empirical evidence that older adults are less adept at inhibiting responses than younger adults. Hasher, Stolzfus, Zacks, and

Rympa (1991) recently proposed that although older adults are adept at searching out ideas and knowledge that pertain to a particular goal or task, they do have more difficulty inhibiting or suppressing irrelevant information. Earlier, Hasher and Zacks (1988) demonstrated that older adults are more likely than younger adults to maintain interpretations of text that have been contradicted or superseded by new, conflicting information. This finding is confirmed by neuropsychological evidence in which behavioral tests, such as the Wisconsin Card Sorting Test (a test of shifting from one strategy to another by inhibiting the former response) showed that older adults are less efficient in shifting context (Daigneault, Braun, & Whitaker, 1992).

Several studies have shown that working memory scores, according to specific measures on reading or listening span tests, are consistently lower for older adults than for younger adults, (Babcock & Salthouse, 1990; Kahn & Cordon, 1993; Stine & Wingfield, 1987). We wanted to test that notion and extend our work by adding an independent measure of working memory to our testing protocol to investigate whether constraints in working memory might account for age-related differences in accuracy of noun reference.

Twenty-two subjects (12 older adults, mean age 70.78, and 10 younger adults, mean age 22.46) read the stories from Kahn and Till (1991) in storybook form. Subjects read the passages one sentence at a time as in our former study, with each sentence appearing on one page. Subjects were told they would not be allowed to look back to previous sentences. The Reading Span Test (Daneman & Carpenter, 1980), an experimental measure of working memory capacity, was also given to each subject.

Our results showed that age interacted with degree of expectedness, thus replicating our earlier findings (Kahn & Till, 1991). In this study we again found no difference between age groups for the expected condition, but significant differences in accuracy of noun choice for the unexpected and neutral conditions. There was no effect of age on memory load, also replicating our earlier findings. For the Reading Span Test, we found that older adults scored significantly lower than the young adults (mean scores: Young 4.14, Old 3.08) (Kahn, 1991).

These results suggest that reduced resources in working memory limit the ability of older adults to retain and monitor text under some comprehension conditions more than others. A study by Tun, Wingfield, and Stine (1991) supports our findings. They found that when young and old adults were asked to listen to a spoken passage for subsequent recall, while simultaneously performing a reaction time task, there was an age-related decrease in latencies on the secondary task. This would suggest that older adults had less storage or were less able to allocate resources to the secondary task, because the primary task, listening to spoken passages, was too taxing on their mental reserves. When a subset of data was analyzed by matching younger and older subjects on memory span scores, the age-related differences in reaction time diminished. Thus, measures of working memory span can serve as good predictors of performance on tasks of varying levels of difficulty.

SUMMARY AND DIRECTIONS FOR FUTURE RESEARCH

To better understand the qualitative differences that exist between age groups, not only the capacity but also the contents of working memory should be evaluated. One promising methodology used by Olson, Duffy, and Mack (1984) and by Whitney et al. (1991) is the **think-aloud procedure**. In these studies, low-span and high-span readers were asked to produce direct verbalizations of their thoughts as they read passages. Olson et al. (1984) and Whitney et al. (1991) found qualitative differences in the think-aloud protocols between their two respective groups. Low-span readers had a tendency to determine an interpretation early in their reading and remained committed to that interpretation. High-span readers elaborated less at the beginning of a passage, and instead "reserved" judgment until they had read through the majority of a passage. It would appear that this method would be equally promising for examining the strategies and sources of knowledge involved in investigating age-related differences in discourse comprehension. The advantage of the think-aloud method in research on memory and aging is that it provides a means of studying the qualitative differences that may exist between the age groups in contrast to studying just the storage capacity of working memory alone.

CONCLUSIONS

Research on how working memory resources change throughout the lifespan, particularly with respect to discourse comprehension, will be useful in developing further research on the qualitative and quantitative changes in memory capabilities with advancing age. This type of data will be useful to clinicians (physicians, neuropsychologists, speech-language pathologists) who evaluate and treat memory complaints of older adults (typically over the age of 65). The fields of neuropsychology and speech-language pathology, for instance, have responded to the need for assessment tools and empirical information on memory in pathological populations (Alzheimer's disease and other types of dementias), but unfortunately, there is little information concerning the control population, the normal older adult. Cross-sectional experimental designs, where two age groups are compared on a task hypothesized to vary with age, are especially useful for providing such basic research. Experimental work, such as the studies discussed in this chapter, may demonstrate that older adults do have age-related changes in working memory resources, but only under some conditions, for example, when the information to be processed is not familiar to them or does not relate well to their prior knowledge or is otherwise difficult. In general, it is no longer enough to ask **if** memory changes with age, but rather **how** memory changes with age.

REFERENCES

Babcock, R. L., & Salthouse, T. A. (1990). Effects of increased processing demands on age differences in working memory. *Psychology and Aging, 5,* 421–428.

Baddeley, A. (1986). *Working memory.* London, England: Oxford University Press.

Baddeley, A. (1992). Working memory. *Science, 255,* 556–559.

Baddeley, A., & Hitch. G. J. (1974). *Working memory.* In G. H. Bower (Ed.), *The psychology of learning and motivation,* (vol. 8, pp. 47–90). New York: Academic Press.

Carpenter, P. A., & Just, M .A. (1983). What your eyes do while your mind is reading. In K. Rayner (Ed.), *Eye movements in reading: Perceptual and language processes.* (pp. 275–307). New York: Academic Press.

Carpenter, P. A., & Just, M .A. (1989). The role of working memory in language comprehension. In D. Klahr & K. Kotovsky (Eds.), *Complex information processing: The impact of Herbert A. Simon* (pp. 31–68). Hillsdale, NJ: Lawrence Erlbaum.

Daigneault, S., Braun, C .M. J., & Whitaker, H. A. (1992). Early effects of normal aging on perseverative and non-perseverative prefrontal measures. *Developmental Neuropsychology, 8,* 99–114.

Daneman, M., & Carpenter, P .A. (1980). Individual differences in working memory and reading. *Journal of Verbal Learning and Verbal Behavior, 19,* 450–466.

Davis, G. A., & Ball, H. E. (1989). Effects of age on comprehension of complex sentences in adulthood. *Journal of Speech and Hearing Research, 32,* 143–150.

Erlich, M., & Delafoy, M. (1990). La mémoire de travail: Structure, functionnement, capacité (Working memory: Structure, function and capacity). *Année Psychologique, 90,* 403–427.

Hasher, L., & Zacks, R. T. (1988). Working memory, comprehension and aging: A review and a new view. In G. H. Bower (Ed.), *The psychology of learning and motivation,* (Volume 22, pp. 193–225). San Diego, CA: Academic Press.

Hasher, L., Stolzfus, E. R., Zacks, R. T., & Rympa, B. (1991). Age and inhibition. *Journal of Experimental Psychology: Learning, Memory and Cognition, 17,* 163–169.

Just, M. A., & Carpenter, P. A. (1980). A theory of reading: From eye fixations to comprehension. *Psychological Review, 87,* 329–354.

Just, M. A., & Carpenter, P. A. (1987). *The psychology of reading and language comprehension.* Newton, MA: Allyn and Bacon.

Just, M. A., & Carpenter, P. A. (1992). A capacity theory of comprehension: Individual differences in working memory. *Journal of Experimental Psychology: General, 111,* 228–238.

Kahn, H. (1990). *The effect of prior knowledge on discourse comprehension and aging.* Paper presented at Theoretical and Experimental Neuropsychology: Neuropsychologie Expérimentale et Théorique (TENNET), Montréal, Québec, Canada.

Kahn, H. (1991). *The role of working memory in discourse comprehension and aging.* Paper presented at Theoretical and Experimental Neuropsychology: Neuropsychologie Expérimentale et Théorique (TENNET), Montréal, Québec, Canada.

Kahn, H. J., & Cordon, D. (1993). *Relationship of working memory and long-term memory in aging.* Paper presented at Conference on Memory in Normal Aging and Dementia, Third Annual Rotman Research Institute Conference, Toronto, Ontario, Canada.

Kahn, H., & Till, R. A. (1991). Pronoun reference and aging. *Developmental Neuropsychology, 7*, 459–475.

King, J., & Just, M. A. (1991). Individual differences in syntactic processing: The role of working memory. *Journal of Memory and Language, 30*, 580–602.

Lee, S., William, H., & Whitney, P. (1991). Reading perspectives and memory for text: An individual differences analysis. *Journal of Experimental Psychology: Learning, Memory and Cognition, 17*, 1074–1081.

Light, L. L., & Anderson, P. A. (1985). Working-memory capacity, age and memory for discourse. *Journal of Gerontology, 40*, 737–747.

Light, L. L., & Capps, J. L. (1986). Comprehension of pronouns in young and older adults. *Developmental Psychology, 22*, 580–585.

MacDonald, M. C., Just, M. A., & Carpenter, P. A. (1992). Working memory constraints on the processing of syntactic ambiguity. *Cognitive Psychology, 24*, 56–98.

Masson, M. E. J., & Miller, J. A. (1983). Working memory and individual differences in comprehension and memory of text. *Journal of Educational Psychology, 75*, 314–318.

Norman, S., Kemper, S., Kynette, D., & Cheung, H. (1991). Syntactic complexity and adults' running memory span. *Journals of Gerontology, 46*, 346–351.

Olson, G., Duffy, S. A., & Mack, R. L. (1984). Thinking-out-loud as a method for studying real-time comprehension processes. In D. E. Kieras & M. A. Just (Eds.), *New methods in reading comprehension research* (pp. 253–286). Hillsdale, NJ: Lawrence Erlbaum.

Salthouse, T. A. (1990). Working memory as a processing resource in cognitive aging. *Developmental Review, 10*, 101–124.

Stine, E. A. L. (1990). On-line processing of written text by younger and older adults. *Psychology and Aging, 5*, 68–78.

Stine, E. A. L., & Wingfield, A. (1987). Process and strategy in memory for speech among younger and older adults. *Psychology and Aging, 2*, 272–279.

Stine, E. A. L., & Wingfield, A. (1990). How much do working memory deficits contribute to age differences in discourse memory? *European Journal of Cognitive Psychology, 2*, 289–304.

Tun, P. A., Wingfield, A., & Stine, E. A. L. (1991). Speech-processing capacity in young and older adults: A dual-task study. *Psychology and Aging, 6*, 3–9.

Ulatowska, H., Cannito, M., Hayashi, M., & Fleming, S. (1986). Disruption of reference in aging. *Brain and Language, 28*, 24–42.

van Dijk, T. A., & Kintsch, W. (1983). *Strategies of discourse comprehension.* New York: Academic Press.

Whitney, P., Ritchie, B. G., & Clark, M. B. (1991). Working-memory capacity and the use of elaborative inferences in text comprehension. *Discourse Processes, 14*, 133–145.

CHAPTER 6

The Effect of Normal Aging on Discourse: A Sociolinguistic Approach

WILLIAM LABOV AND JULIE AUGER

This chapter is concerned with efforts to determine the effect of normal aging on the development of the language faculty, to serve as a baseline in the examination of pathological conditions, and as a way of better understanding the language faculty itself. Initial assumption about the language faculty was that it underwent rapid development in the early years of life but remained virtually unchanged throughout later life. Two lines of research have altered this view in several respects. Sociolinguistic research in speech communities has produced two general regression equations that indicate a steady continuation of language learning with advancing age. In Montreal, Sankoff and Lessard (1975) showed that vocabulary size increases steadily with age. In Philadelphia, Guy and Boyd (1990) found that speakers of a language continue to analyze morphological forms more deeply with advancing age. Cross-sectional studies of language and aging have also indicated some general developmental trends. Obler (1985) found increase in vocabulary as well as increase of pragmatic skills. However, a number of reports indicate a deterioration of language faculties with normal aging, particularly in regard to syntactic processing and production (Walker, Hardiman, Hedrick, & Holbrook, 1981). In a variety of cross-sectional studies, Kemper and her associates found a progressive decrease in syntactic complexity, particularly in the production of left-branching structures, and also a significant correlation with a decrease in short-term memory (Kemper, 1988; Kemper, Kynette, Rash, O'Brien, & Sprott, 1989; Kynette & Kemper, 1986).

LONGITUDINAL STUDIES

The present contribution is a first report on longitudinal studies of the effect of normal aging on language. These studies are based on re-interviews of subjects in the two sociolinguistic studies cited earlier. In 1971, the Montreal corpus of Quebec French was created as a stratified random sample of 120 speakers, and has since been the subject of many quantitative analyses of variation in phonology, morphology, syntax, and pragmatics (Sankoff & Sankoff, 1973). In 1984, the Montreal research group headed by Thibault restudied the community, endeavoring to locate the same subjects who were interviewed in 1971: They succeeded in obtaining re-interviews with 60 of the 120 subjects. The study of the Philadelphia community of several hundred speakers was carried out from 1973 to 1976. Individual interviews with members of social networks in 10 neighborhoods produced a base sample of 116 speakers. Re-interviewing of these speakers was begun in 1989, in research funded by the National Institute of Aging, to determine the effects of normal aging on language, focusing on the phonetic and phonological system and the structure of narrative discourse.

Sociolinguistic interviews simulate the conversational style of spontaneous speech, developing interest and emotional involvement as one way of reducing the effect of observation and recording speech that approximates the vernacular style used in everyday life (Labov, 1984). Interventions of the interviewer are designed to maximize the flow of speech as well as minimize the formality of the interview situation. Although there is no fixed set of questions, as in a sociological survey, there is a schedule of topics, often triggered by questions from the interviewer, which can be quite comparable from one interview to another. The Montreal re-interviews used such comparable topics, but with a different series of interviewers.

The Philadelphia re-interviews were designed at the outset to record speech from the same subject under conditions as close as possible to the original recording. The same interviewers were recruited for this purpose, and the original interviews were studied carefully to cover the same subjects. The methodology of the original Philadelphia neighborhood studies placed considerable emphasis on techniques for obtaining dramatized narratives of personal experience (Labov, 1984; Labov & Waletzky, 1967), and the re-interviews were designed to obtain retellings of the same events. Although the subjects were fully aware of the original interviews, they did not know which narratives had been told at that time, so the second narrative was in fact a fresh re-telling.

THE MONTREAL STUDY OF SYNTACTIC COMPLEXITY

The oldest speakers re-interviewed in Montreal were examined for evidence of changes of syntactic complexity in the production of spontaneous speech. A variety of measures of syntactic complexity have been developed over the years, and most of them prove to be highly correlated (van den Broek, 1977). To provide comparability with the Kynette and Kemper (1986) study, the same measures of syntactic complexity were used in so far as possible. Two such measures will be reported here, both based on the proportion of complex sentences per T-Unit, where a T-unit is defined as an independent clause along with all subordinate clauses that are dependent on it. These two measures are:

Subordination: the proportion of T-Units that contain at least one finite dependent clause, either left-branching or right-branching.
Left Branching: the proportion of T-Units that contain at least one instance of a left-branching dependent clause.

The direction of branching is defined relative to the main predication. A right-branching clause is one that is placed after the finite tense marker of the main predication. In sentence 1, the sentence complement *if somebody was here* is a right-branching clause that follows the main predication *like to know*.

1. I would like to know if somebody was here that cashed a check by the name of so-and-so.

In English and French, finite relative clauses always follow the noun they are dependent on; whether they are left or right branching depends on whether they follow the main predication or not. In sentence 1 *that cashed a check* is right branching in that it also follows *like to know*.

Left-branching clauses are those that are placed before the finite tensed element of the independent clause, as in sentence 2

2. In the meantime, while my brother was in the casket, they stole my-my sister-in-law's welfare check.

Here the subordinate clause *while my brother was in the casket* is left branching, because it precedes *stole*, the main finite verb of the independent clause. *In the meantime* is also left branching, but because it is not a finite clause, it is not considered in the subordination or left-branching indices. In sentence 3, the relative clause *that brought the check* is left branching because it precedes the main predication *bought*.

   3. and the one that brought the check, she bought a gallon o' oil, she bought sugar, an' she bought other little things

Relative clauses that modify the subject of a sentence are, therefore, normally left branching.

It should also be noted that direct quotations were not rated as clauses subordinated to their verbs of quotation, but were rated only as complex sentences if there was a subordinate clause within the quotation.

It can be noted that the left-branching measure is a proper subset of subordination, and indicates a subset of sentences with a higher degree of complexity in regard to sentence processing. It is generally agreed that left-branching clauses are more difficult to produce and understand than right-branching sentences (Levin & Garrett, 1990). A number of theories connect this difficulty with memory limitations (Bever & Townsend, 1979; Frazier & Fodor, 1978; Kimball, 1973). There is, therefore, considerable support for Kemper's association of decreases in sentence complexity with age and decreases in memory span (Kemper, 1988; Kynette & Kemper, 1986).

RESULTS OF THE LONGITUDINAL MONTREAL STUDY

The Montreal interviews are extended discussions ranging from 1 to 2 hours. Rather than present single indices of complexity for the entire corpus, we examined the progressive development of complexity by means of a runs analysis of the subordination index. A T-unit containing a subordinate clause run was defined as complex; one not containing such a clause was defined as simple. A run is then defined as a sequence of clauses that are all simple or all complex. Figure 6–1 shows the cumulative subordination measure for Montreal subject number 73, Roger. He is a specialized physician who was 51 years old at the time of the 1971 survey and 64 years old at the time of the 1984 study.

It can be observed that the indices for 1971 and 1984 begin with radically different values, with 1971 much lower than 1984. However, after the first 10 runs, the cumulative indices coincide for some time. They then separate sharply at run 30, with a long run of complex sentences at

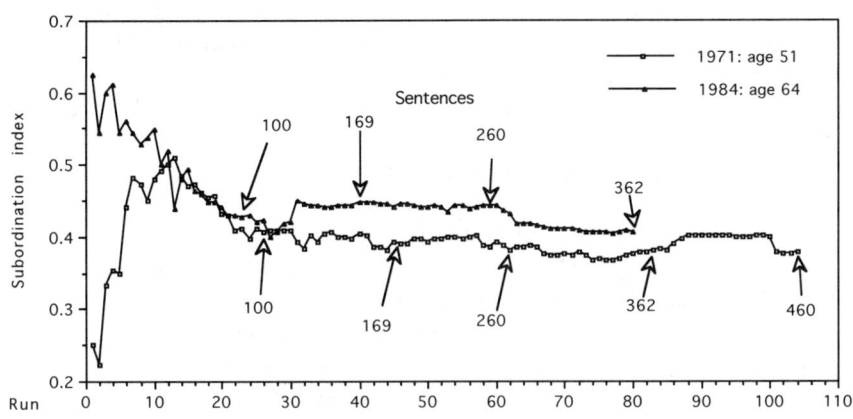

Figure 6–1. Cumulative proportion of sentences with subordinate clauses by runs analysis for Montreal subject number 73, Roger: 1971 versus 1984.

run 30 in 1984 and a long run of simple sentences at run 31 in 1971. The relative distances of the two indices are then maintained until run 60, when a series of simple sentences reduce the advantage of the 1984 interview. The difference is still maintained as the 1984 interview terminates; the 1971 interview is considerably longer. As it proceeds, the subordination index rises, until it reaches the same level as the later interview, and finally falls a few points at the end.

To give some idea of the relative length of these sequences, the cumulative number of sentences (defined as T-units) is indicated for both interviews. The total number of T-Units does not diverge for any point, since the mean length of runs is comparable.

Figure 6–2 shows a comparable runs analysis for a working-class speaker, Montreal subject number 30, Gérard. He is a retired print shop foreman, 70 years old at the time of the 1984 re-interview. The overall pattern of the two indices is similar, in that the differences between them are maintained for considerable periods of time, but ultimately converge. But in this case, it is the earlier interview which shows greater complexity. Note that the overall level of the subordination index is much lower for Gérard than Roger: This is a difference between middle-class and working-class speakers that is consistent across our data set.

This preliminary analysis indicates that one might obtain an inaccurate measure of the speaker's overall subordination index by taking less than an hour or two of speech. Two interrelated factors appear to be responsible for the fluctuations in the subordination index: the topic and narrative versus non-narrative discourse structures. *Narratives* are here defined as a mode of reporting specific past events by means of a sequence of independent clauses that follow the same order as the temporal sequence of the original events (Labov & Waletzky, 1967). Though some complex sentences occur in narrative, the main sequence of actions is represented as a series of simple independent clauses. The runs that shift the overall subordination index downward usually represent the insertion of a narrative into the conversation. On the other hand, some topics lead to a higher subordination index as, for example, the discussion of the French language. The link between the two factors is that some topics lead to a greater use of narrative, whereas others lead to a lesser use. Table 6–1 shows the subordination and left-branching indices of data from 10 Montreal subjects pooled for three topics that are represented in all 10 interviews. It is evident that the French language topic leads to higher

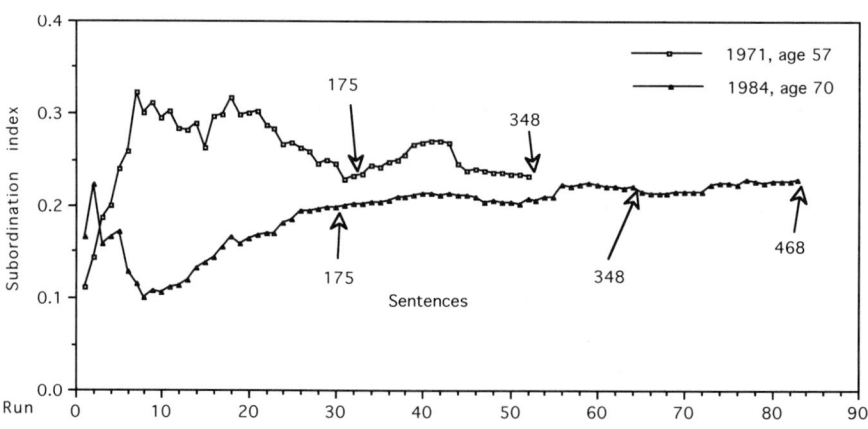

Figure 6–2. Cumulative proportion of sentences with subordinate clauses by runs analysis for Montreal subject number 30, Gérard: 1971 versus 1984.

Table 6–1. Indices of syntactic complexity by topic for 10 Montreal subjects

Topic	Subordination		Left Branching		
	Index	N	Index	N	Total N
Neighborhood	.204	249	.098	99	1007
French language	.309	692	.112	201	1789
Television	.205	158	.058	36	626

indices of syntactic complexity in both cases. For the subordination index, discussions of the neighborhood and television are at the same level. The left-branching index is considerable higher for the neighborhood topic, but none of the left-branching differences are significant. In fact, the only significant difference in this global treatment of topic is the effect of French language for the subordination index ($\chi^2 = 6.7, p = .001$).

An examination of the differentiation of topic by individual speakers shows there is a strong tendency for the left-branching index to vary with topic. Figure 6–3 shows the results for topic by age for three such subjects. The effect of topic is a strong one, as shown by the high values for French language and low values for games and children. The effect is quite consistent across time: Correlations for the three subjects are $r = +.998$ (Germaine), $+.764$ (Laurette), and $+.938$ (Eugenie). For all three subjects combined, r is $+.854$. Although topics have a strong effect on speaking style, and speakers preserve these patterns over time, individual speakers are free to choose a variety of different approaches to it. A speaker may indeed treat an abstract topic by a narrative or a concrete one by a series of hypothetical propositions. Thus, Germaine and Laurette used little left branching in discussing their neighborhoods, but Eugenie showed the reverse pattern, with the highest levels of this index for the neighborhood topic.

This individual variation is greater for left branching than for subordination, where the main effect of French language is preserved across all speakers and both times. Table 6–2 shows the significant results of a multiple regression analysis of 10 Montreal interviews, combining 1971 and 1984 data. The two dependent variables are the subordination index and the left-branching index. The independent variables included all topics represented in three or more interviews, the age and social class of the speakers, and the year interviewed. No significant effect of the year of interview appeared for either variable, nor any effect of age. The French language produced a significant effect for the subordination index, and no topic produced a reliable effect for the left-branching index.

The social class of the speaker proved to be a consistent and major determinant of complexity. Figure 6–4 shows the distribution of the two indices by the occupational status of the speaker's family. The four highest status members of the sample (a physician, an architect's wife, a retired dean, and the owner of a wholesale company) show a nonoverlapping distribution with the two lower middle-class speakers (meat inspector, receptionist). Table 6–2 mirrors this distribution, with a significant and sizable effect for the professional class for both the subordination and the left-branching index. A weaker and less significant effect differentiates the lower middle-class speakers from the working class for the subordination index.

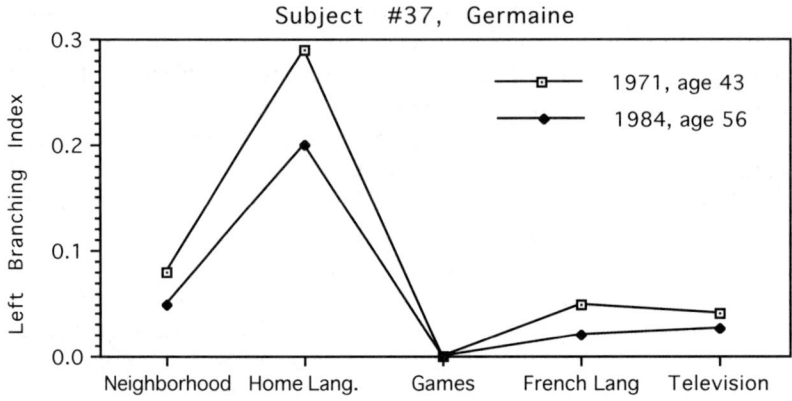
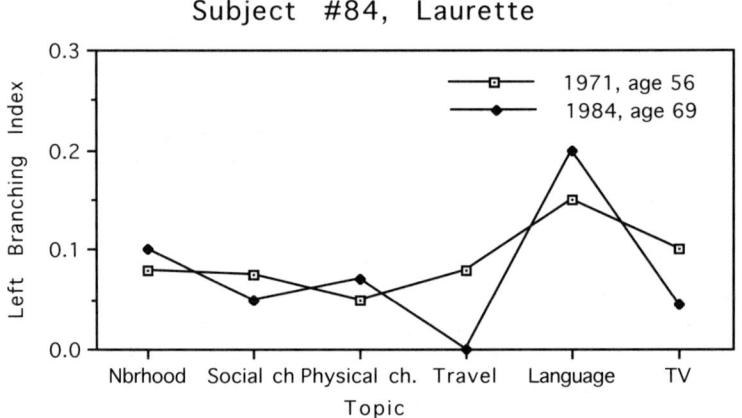
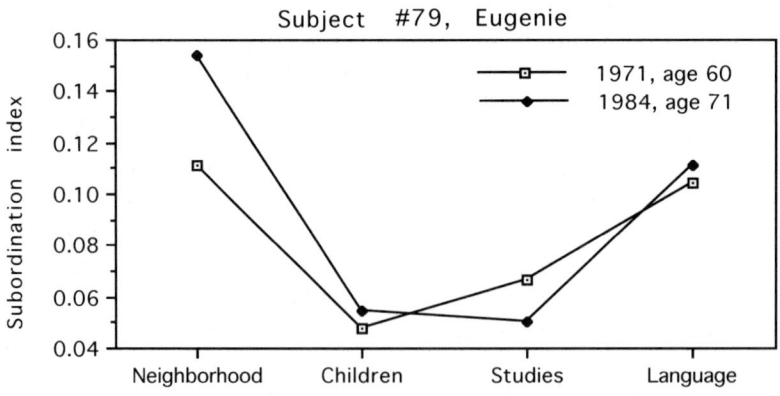

Figure 6–3. Indices of syntactic complexity by topic for three Montreal subjects.

Table 6–2. Multiple regression analysis of 10 Montreal interviews

	p (two-tailed)
Dependent variable: Subordination	
Topic: French Language	0.00
Social class: Professional	0.00
Social class: lower middle	0.04
Dependent variable: Left Branching	
Social class: Professional	0.05

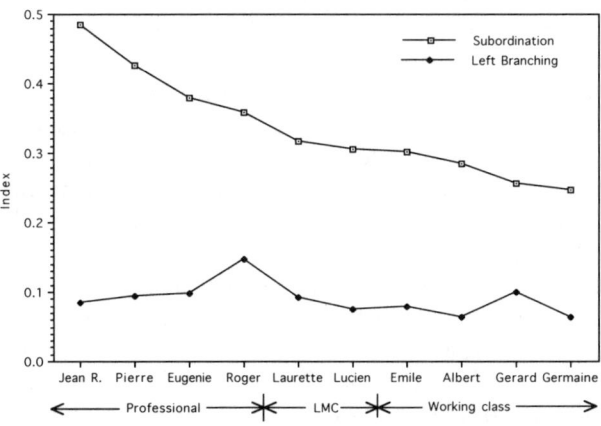

Figure 6–4. Distribution of subordination and left-branching indices by social class for 10 Montreal subjects.

RESULTS OF THE LONGITUDINAL PHILADELPHIA STUDY

The Montreal study showed no relationship between age and syntactic complexity, but a wide variation from topic to topic in the amount of complexity. The Philadelphia study permitted us to control topic as well as audience and social context since the same interviewer was recording the same person in the same context. We focused first on narratives, because these are the discourse structures that are the best understood and the most well-formed. Narratives offered us the most promise for a close comparison of the use of syntactic structures over time.

One of the first subjects re-interviewed was Jenny R., a South Philadelphian Italian-American woman who was 70 years old when she was first interviewed by Anne Bower in 1973. Jenny was one of the central figures of a social network in a stable South Philadelphia upper working-class neighborhood that was studied intensively by Bower. Jenny was well-known in the group for her sensitivity to psychic phenomena (she was born with a caul on her head). Her first interview, almost 3 hours long, includes many narratives of her personal experience of premonitions, visions of dead relatives, and religious experiences, as well as re-tellings of similar stories that her mother and grandmother had told her. In 1990, after studying all of the topics and narratives of the original interview, Bower re-interviewed Jenny who was 87.

Jenny was in excellent health, with an unremarkable medical record and no detectable changes in her articulation, fluency, or memory. An acoustic examination of the spectral features of her voice showed no overall differences in breathiness, hoarseness, or steadiness of pitch. Whether or not the term "normal aging" describes her pattern, "healthy aging" does appear to be appropriate.

Bower succeeded in obtaining a large number of narratives from Jenny, in an interview of approximately the same length as the original. Many of the original stories were re-told. Table 6–3 displays the two indices of syntactic complexity—subordination and left branching— for five of the narratives that were the most comparable for the original interview in 1973 and the re-interview in 1990.

We observe that for subordination, there are three cases where the index is higher in 1990, one where it is the same, and one where it is lower. The 1990 mean is slightly higher, but the difference is not at all significant. The situation with left branching is about the same: In four of the five cases, the 1990 value is higher, and, in one case, the 1973 value is higher. Again, there is a small but nonsignificant difference in the means favoring 1990.

Table 6–3 echoes the Montreal data in showing no evidence for a decline in syntactic complexity. If there is a trend, it is toward increasing complexity. It is also striking to note that the narratives are specific in the degree of complexity that they generate. There is a significant correlation between the indices for the two dates: .60 for subordination and .88 for left branching. This underlines the difficulty in defining consistent measures of complexity from such global stylistic categories as *narrative* or *language*. Different narratives will call for different kinds of linguistic treatment.

Table 6–4 shows a comparable table for a second South Philadelphia subject, Matt M., from the same social network. He was 66 years old at the time of the first interview and 83 when the re-interview took place. Both interviews included narratives of violent events in South Philadelphia. There were several shootings, one in which he himself was wounded. Table 6–4 again shows a small but nonsignificant increase in the subordination index, and about the same level for the left-branching index. It is apparent that Matt M.'s narratives are not as closely matched as Jenny R.'s

Table 6–3. Syntactic complexity of Jenny R. narratives retold

	Subordination		Left Branching	
	1973	1990	1973	1990
The welfare check	.133	.134	.025	.049
Her father's death	.153	.230	.057	.044
Her brother's death	.238	.250	.095	.125
Bishop Newman appears	.357	.278	.071	.111
The treasure	.187	.292	.027	.042
Mean	.214	.237	.055	.074
	$r = +.60$		$r = +.88$	

Table 6–4. Syntactic complexity of Matt M's. narratives retold

	Subordination		Left Branching	
	1973	1990	1973	1990
Primo Carnera	.107	.118	.036	.058
Five shootings on a Sunday	.173	.148	.019	.074
Getting shot	.089	.145	.060	.022
Diving off the bridge	.111	.278	.056	.000
Mean	.120	.172	.042	.039
	$r = -.08$		$r = -.92$	

since there is no correlation for the subordination index and an inverse correlation for left branching. The overall view is the same as that for Jenny R.: There is no evidence for a decline in syntactic complexity.

The figures given so far take only partial advantage of the controlled character of the data in showing mean values for entire narratives. Since the same events are being re-told, it should be possible to look more closely at syntactic structure formation at the moment where the speaker is formulating propositions into sentences. Four narratives re-told by Jenny R. were examined clause by clause, and all of the events that were represented in both versions were isolated. Each of these representations were then compared in the two versions. Figure 6–5 shows the most complex of these. It is an account of how shortly after her brother Eddie's death, his welfare check was stolen, and cashed by the thief. The family did not know where the check had been cashed, but Eddie appeared to Jenny in a dream, and told her the name and address of the

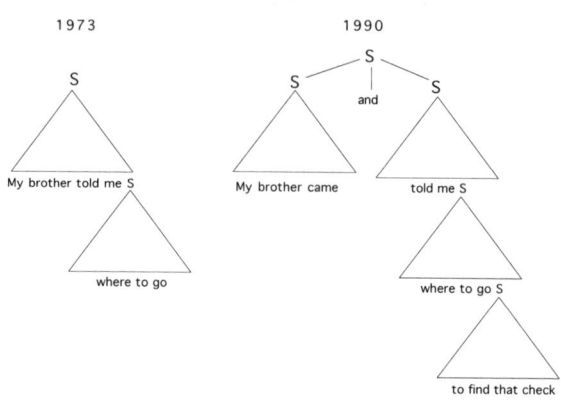

Figure 6–5. Comparative syntactic structures of sentence 29 of "The Welfare Check."

store. Jenny and her mother found the store, and the owner told them the name of the woman who had signed the check. Jenny does not name the woman (since she is now dead), but reports that she did admit that she stole the check and was sorry she had done it.

Some parts of the story are elaborated in the original version, and not represented in 1990, and other parts are more fully developed in 1990. The essential elements of the narrative can be followed through the comparable clauses in the Appendix. The two center columns represent a classification of each sentence with relative degrees of complexity ordered as follows:

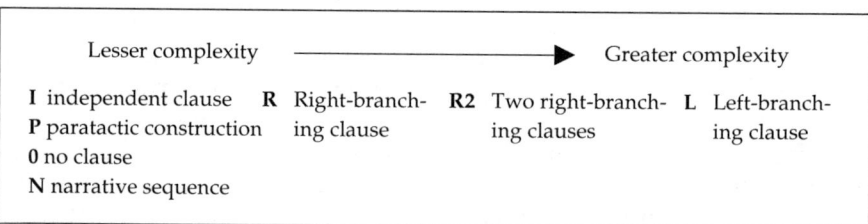

The narrative classification is used when an event is represented in one version with a sequence of narrative clauses and by a more complex syntactic construction in the other, as in the third clause of the Appendix:

1973			1990
Well, me and my—my sister-in-law we went all—we came all the way down this way here lookin', asking all the grocers, whoever had ah . . . cashed a check by a certain name.	R	N	Well, the poor girl, you know, tha . . . she . . . she was livin' with my aunt. So, after a week, she came down here. She said, "Jenny, do me a favor. Come with me to the stores. So, we came to Mister Caruso. No check. (Mmm) No-nobody by that name. We went–there was another grocery store down here at the corner.

In the 1973 version, the search for the store was narrated in a single sentence, with several right-branching structures. Since two of them (*lookin'*, *asking*) are nonfinite, they are not counted in this index. The right-branching clause, *whoever had cashed a check* is a finite complement of *asking*, and so yields the rating R. The same events are narrated in a series of eight independent clauses in 1990, a simpler construction from the syntactic point of view.

Under this classification, any row with comparable clauses may be rated as equal in complexity for the two versions, of greater complexity in the 1973 version, or of greater complexity in the 1990 version. An inspection of the columns shows that most rows show the same structure, a few have greater complexity in 1973, and a sizable number show greater complexity in 1990. Typical of these is row 22, where the syntactic contrast is immediate.

22. She says, "I wanna ask you something." She says, "You know, did a woman come here and cash a check?"	P	R2	She said, uh, to the man, she says, uh, "I would like to know if somebody was here that cashed a check by the name of so-and-so,"

Table 6–5 summarizes the results of this procedure for four of the most comparable narratives told by Jenny R. The total number of comparable

TABLE 6–5. Comparative complexity of narratives retold by Jenny R., Philadelphia

	1973 = 1990	1973 ≥ 1990	1973 ≤ 1990
The welfare check	14	2	8
Frying sausage at midnight	6	1	1
Eddie's dog bites Tony	13	2	2
The sea captain	20	2	4
Total	53	7	15

clauses is 75. Of these, 53 are the same, 7 show greater complexity in the earlier version, and 15 show greater complexity in the later version. The narrative of the Appendix, "The Welfare Check," shows the most striking difference. One other narrative shows a slight increase in complexity for the later version, and two of the shorter narratives show no difference at all.

CONCLUSION

These preliminary results of the longitudinal studies are consistent in showing no decline in syntactic complexity over the 13- to 17-year intervals of the comparison. This holds for the 10 Montreal speakers, and the 2 South Philadelphia speakers examined here. Any changes that have been observed are in the opposite direction—toward the development of greater syntactic complexity, more consistent with the increased depth of morphological analysis noted in Guy and Boyd (1990) than with the findings reported by Kemper and her associates (Kemper, 1988; Kemper et al., 1989; Kynette & Kemper, 1988).

What factors might account for the difference between these results and the findings of Kemper and associates (Kemper, 1988; Kemper et al., 1989; Kynette & Kemper, 1986)? Some of the details of the syntactic analysis are different; the Kemper and colleagues analysis was done by a computational algorithm (the LINGQUEST analysis program, Mordecai, Palin, & Palmer, 1982), with decision procedures that are not readily available. But we do not believe that it is likely that differences in analysis would produce such a difference in the result. As shown by van den Broek (1977), most such measures of complexity are highly correlated. Although it is true that our subordination index and left-branching index are not always correlated (see Figure 6–4), most of the choices made within each index do not radically affect the result. For example, a hypothetical clause without an *if* complementizer as in *You do it, you'll be sorry* was counted as a subordinate construction in English, but a paratactic, nonsubordinated construction in French, without affecting the overall results. However, if one were to count verbs of quotation (*He said*, ". . .) as main clauses with the quotation subordinated to them, there would be a radical increase in the number of complex clauses in dramatized narratives, but none in indirect narratives and general discussions. However, none of these possible differences points to an explanation for the differences in the main results of these two types of studies.

Another possibility is that the subjects we have studied are healthier than the ones selected by the cross-sectional procedure. There might indeed be a bias of selection in any longitudinal study, in that subjects who do not feel as well, or as competent, may resist the request for a reinterview. This does not seem altogether likely given the low percentage of refusals in our current work in Philadelphia and the remarkable success of the Montreal group in locating 50% of the same subjects.

A third possibility is suggested by the observations of Kemper et al. (1989) that "the elderly adults' expository statements were judged to be more interesting and clearer than the young adults' statements" (p. 64). They suggest that older adults may have learned that simpler syntax is more useful in conveying ideas: "The elderly adults may have avoided using complex syntactic constructions because they had learned that such constructions are difficult for others to understand" (p. 64). The materials we have examined are less formal than the expository statements considered here; in the course of narrative, complex syntax is used not so much for clarification as for the evaluation of the social and emotional issues involved (Labov 1972; Labov & Waletzky 1967). As remarked above, narrative syntax is simpler on the whole, although with maturation, speakers acquire the skill to use complex structures at critical points within the narrative. If the older speakers in the cross-sectional studies used more narrative, this would contribute to a lowering of their overall measures of syntactic complexity, an effect that would not appear in an analysis that compares one narrative performance with another. This possibility is consistent with the results of Kemper (1990). The diaries kept by adults over a 70-year time span showed an increase rather than a decrease in the complexity of the narratives over this period.

ACKNOWLEDGMENT

The work reported here was supported by a grant from NIH, awarded by the National Institute on Aging for "A longitudinal study of language in normal aging," Contract AG07806-02.

REFERENCES

Bever, T. G., & Townsend, D. J. (1979). Perceptual mechanisms and formal properties of main and subordinate clauses. In W. E. Cooper & E. C. T. Walker (Eds.), *Sentence processing* (pp. 159–226). Hillsdale, NJ: Lawrence Erlbaum.

Frazier, L., & Fodor, J. D. (1978). The sausage machine: A new two-stage parsing model. *Cognition, 6*, 291–325.

Guy, G., & Boyd, S. (1990). The development of a morphological class. *Language Variation and Change, 2*, 1–18.

Kemper, S. (1988). Geriatric psycholinguistics: Syntactic limitations of oral and written language. In L. Light & D. Burke (Eds.), *Language, memory and aging* (pp. 58–76). Cambridge: Cambridge University Press.

Kemper, S. (1990). Adults' diaries: Changes made to written narratives across the life span. *Discourse Processes, 13*, 207–223.

Kemper, S., Kynette, D., Rash, S., O'Brien, K., & Sprott, R. (1989). Life-span changes to adults' language: Effects of memory and genre. *Applied Psycholinguistics, 10*, 49–66.

Kimball, J. (1973). Seven principles of surface structure parsing in natural language. *Cognition, 2*, 15–47.

Kynette, D., & Kemper, S. (1986). Aging and the loss of grammatical forms: A cross-sectional study of language performance. *Language & Communication, 6*, 65–72.

Labov, W. (1972). *Language in the inner city*. Philadelphia: University of Pennsylvania Press.

Labov, W. (1984). Field methods of the Project on Linguistic Change and Variation. In J. Baugh & J. Sherzer (Eds.), *Language in use* (pp. 28–53). Englewood Cliffs, NJ: Prentice Hall.

Labov, W., & Waletzky, J. (1967). Narrative analysis. In J. Helm (Ed.), *Essays on the verbal and visual arts* (pp. 12–44). Seattle: University of Washington Press.

Levin, H., & Garrett, P. (1990). Sentence structure and formality. *Language in Society, 19*, 511–520.

Mordecai, D. R., Palin, M., & Palmer, C. (1982). LINGQUEST 1: *Language sample analysis*. Columbus, OH: Charles E. Merrill.

Obler, L. K. (1985). Language through the life-span. In J. Berko Gleason (Ed.), *The development of language* (pp. 277–306). New York: Academic Press.

Sankoff, D., & Sankoff, G. (1973). Sample survey methods and computer-assisted analysis in the study of grammatical variation. In R. Darnell (Ed.), *Canadian languages in their social context* (pp. 7–64). Edmonton, Alberta: Linguistic Research.

Sankoff, D., & Lessard, R. (1975.) Vocabulary richness: A sociolinguistic analysis. *Science, 190*, 689–690.

van den Broek, J. (1977). Class differences in syntactic complexity in the Flemish town of Maaseik. *Language in Society, 6*, 149–182.

Walker, V. G., Hardiman, C. J., Hedrick, D. L., & Holbrook, A. (1981). Speech and language characteristics of an aging population. In J. J. Lass (Ed.), *Advances in basic research and practice*, (Vol. 6, pp. 143–202). New York: Academic Press.

APPENDIX

Comparable Clauses in the Narration of "The Welfare Check"

TOLD BY JENNY R. IN 1973 AND 1990.

I = independent clause
P = paratactic construction
N = narrative construction

R = right branching
L = left branching
0 = no clause present

	Jenny R., A1209, age 70			Jenny R., B002, age 87
	Jenny R., A1209, age 70			Jenny R., B002, age 87
1	I ah, my brother had died,	I	I	And my brother passed away.
2	and somebody took his welfare. [Check] Check.	I	I	In the meantime, while my brother was in the casket, they stole my-my sister-in-law's . . . uh . . . uh . . . not he census . . . the . . . (Social Security check? er . . .) No, the other one. Welfare. The welfare. They were gettin' welfare.
3	Well, me and my—my sister-in-law we went all— we came all the way down this way here lookin", asking all the grocers, whoever had ah, [cashed their check] cashed a	R	N	Well, the poor girl, you know, tha . . . she was livin' wit' my aunt. So, after a week, she came down here. She said, "Jenny, do me a favor. Come woth me to the stores.

3	(continued). check by a certain name.			(continued). So, we came to Mister Caruso. No check. (Mmm) No-nobody by that name. We went, there was another grocery store down here at the corner.
4	Nobody knew.	I	I	Nobody ha—the check.
5	Aah-(hh) It-she s's—we—abou—It was five o'clock. I ah was wide awake. I seen my brother in the room.	N	LR	"Well, it wasn't in the morning, early in the morning, I saw my— my brother came in my door. My brother, Eddie.
6	He says, "Jenny, if you want to find, where the welfare—where the check was check—was uh— [cashed] cashed, go to 935 N-Ninth St.	L	LR	He said,"Jenny, if you want to find, where they cashed the check, go to 935 South Ninth Street, and the name of the grocery store is Lichambelli.
7	I eh came downstairs.	I	I	So, I came downstairs.
8	I says, "Mom, you know, I was in between my sleep but I seen Eddie,	P	R	I said "Ma, you know I drea— Eddie came in my dream,
9	and he tol' me to go to 935	R	R	and he told me to go 935 Ninth Street
10	and there was the—the check was cashed	R	L	He says, that's where you'll find my check.
11		0	I	and the name is Richambelli.
12	So my brother Stanley, and everybody: "Oh, you're the one that sees everything.	R	I	So, Stanley says, "Eh . . ., you and your dreams."
13	You're the, you're the main one. You listen to her, you gonna go crazy," they tell my mother.	L	I	He says, "You're always havin' dreams."
14	So my mother, when they went out, th-they went to work. She says: "Come on." It was about—then, then that night after supper she says, "Come on, get dressed	I	I	So, my mother says, "Hey, look. After supper, get—put—get dressed.
15	and we'll go to Ninth Street."	I	I	An' we go,
16	So we gotta to see if there was that 935."	L	L	and see wha—if we could find this here address."
17	So we went to Ninth Street—935.	I	I	Well, we went.

The Effect of Normal Aging on Discourse

18	We find the place.	I	P	We—walked awhile, an' there was on Ninth Street. 935."
19	And it was, the store was Richeldelli.	I	I	And the name, Richambelli.
20	We went in,	I	I	She went in,
21	and my mother, she made us, she bought sugar and coffee.	I	P	and she bought sugar, and she bought coffee.
22	She says, "I wanna ask you something." She says, "You know, did a woman come here and cash a check?"	P	R2	She said, uh, to the man, she says, uh, "I would like to know if somebody was here that cashed a check by the name of so-and-so,"
23	He says: What kind, well what's her name? Could you give me her name? Maybe, I have it here." She says certain her name, you know, she gave her name. I don't wanna mention it because she's dead. she says: well . . .	NR	LR	who it was, you know, that my sister-in-law knew who it was.
24	He says, "Let me look . . . in there."	I	I	He says, "Now wait a minute. I'll go check."
25	So he looked.	I	I	He went and checked.
26	He says: "Yes, she was here yesterday,	I	I	He says, "Yep. The check was . . . changed over here. (Son of a gun)."
27	and she bought . . . sugar, she bought coffee and she bought other things here. He says, "and I cashed a check."	P	L	He says "and the one that brought the check, she bought a gallon o'oil, she bought sugar, an' she bought other little things," you know.
28	Well, now you coulda lit candles in front of my mother. You know?	I	I	"Oh my God!" my mother said, "it's her. She's the one."
29	But there, *my brother told me where to go.*	R	R	My brother came an' told me where to go to find that check.
30	No people, if you tell this to people—people don't believe it. But eh, there's a lot of things—that I have seen. You know. But eh, people won't believe it!	L	L	That's, you know, there are things that they—now when I tell these things to the people, they don't believe it.

CHAPTER 7

Narrative Discourse Processing in Normal Aging: A Neuropsychological and Comparative Study

CLAUDIO L. N. GUIMARAES DOS SANTOS
AND JEAN-LUC NESPOULOUS

In this chapter we report some results from a long-range study of the neuropsychological basis of discourse processing in general and that of narrative discourse in particular. One focus is the use of SPECT (Single Photon Emission Tomography) to assess cerebral activity as normal subjects perform an auditory comprehension and memorization task involving three types of discourse: *descriptive without a thematic unit* (DD), *narrative* (ND), and *argumentative* (AD). Another focus is the propositional analysis of recall protocols to assess the quality of performances in normal subjects of varying ages.

INTRODUCTION

Discourse processing constitutes a branch of neuropsychology that is just emerging. Yet, a number of important works produced in the last 15 years already testify to both the incredible vitality and the amazing complexity of this expanding field. Such complexity clearly imposes on anyone who intends to undertake a study in this domain a crucial condition: to define the theoretical framework within which one plans to examine a particular topic. The necessity of such a condition is especially clear when the object of investigation happens to be not only discourse in general, but also a very particular kind of discourse, that is, narrative discourse. The reason for this is easily understood: No other type of discourse has been more extensively studied. For reviews on this subject, see Fayol (1985), Rondal and Thibaut (1987), Deschênes (1988), and Courtés (1991). Indeed, from linguistics to pragmatics, from semiotics to psycholinguistics, from anthropology to poetics, it is difficult to find a discipline that has not selected—at some point in its history—narrative discourse (or the "story" or the "tale") as its privileged object of analysis.

Three main theoretical frameworks have contributed to our approach to discourse processing.[1] The first of these traditions is that important and innovative way of regarding language phenomena referred to, since the 1970s, as text linguistics. This approach attempts to bring linguistic analysis to the discourse level, that is, to the level of semantic, interpropositional, text-forming relations (e.g., cohesion) and also tries to focus on extralinguistic aspects (e.g., contextual variables) inherent in any communicative act. After its establishment by leading authors such as van Dijk (1972), Kummer (1972), Petöfi and Rieser (1973), Gutwinsky (1976), Halliday and Hasan (1976), and Kiefer (1977), text linguistics rapidly extended beyond the linguistic field and began to exert a decisive influence in the psycholinguistic domain. Simultaneously, text linguistics was itself positively affected by advances in psycholinguistics.

The second theoretical tradition is precisely the result of this productive "scientific co-evolution"—in the sense employed by Churchland (1986)—of psycholinguistic and linguistic theories. It is best represented by the work of Kintsch and van Dijk (1975, 1978) and van Dijk and Kintsch (1983) dealing with the development of a propositional model of text comprehension and memorization, which we briefly review later in this chapter.

Unfortunately, the third and last theoretical framework that has profoundly influenced our work cannot be described in the straightforward manner we have used to present the two preceeding traditions, perhaps because of its more philosophical nature. Indeed, since our work includes the study of discourse processing at both the psycholinguistic and the neurological level, we cannot avoid clarifying our position concerning the famous puzzle of mind-brain relationships, although in a brief manner.[2]

From the outset, we emphasize that the study of the neurological basis of discourse processing is a bona fide example of a most recent field of scientific investigation. Most of the contemporary literature concerning

---

[1] See Guimaraes dos Santos (1992) for a detailed review on this topic.
[2] See Guimaraes dos Santos (1988, 1992) for discussion of this issue.

the neurological basis of language comprehension and memorization in normal subjects—as studied either by imaging techniques (such as PET or SPECT) or by electrophysiological techniques (such as ERP)—deals with this problem almost exclusively at the single word or, at best, at the sentence level (e.g., Goldberg et al., 1989).[3] Data provided by these studies can hardly be useful in the understanding of the neurological mechanisms involved in discourse processing since most of the phenomena pertaining to the discourse level are not only quantitativley but also qualitatively different from phenomena pertaining to the sentence level, not to mention the single-word level.

The key to our epistemological position concerning the mind-brain puzzle is Churchland's co-evolution of scientific theories (Churchland, 1986), which we are willing to adopt with some minor modifications. According to our modified version of this notion, it is obvious that contemporary psycholinguistic theories are not reducible to presently available neurofunctional and neurostructural theories (or vice versa). Yet, one cannot use this current state of affairs to support the inference that, in a perhaps distant future, suitably evolved psycholinguistic theories might not reduce to suitably evolved neurofunctional and neurostructural theories. In other words, whether psycholinguistic theories will ever be reducible to neurofunctional and neurostructural theories is a matter for empirical verification and not a question to be decided by means of a priori reasoning. Accordingly, we have adopted a hybrid heuristic strategy, a "neuropsycholinguistic strategy," in order to approach our object of study discourse processing.

BASIC THEORETICAL STRUCTURE UNDERLYING THE PRESENT WORK

Since the principal aim of this chapter is to discuss some experimental results from a long-range study of the neuropsychological basis of discourse processing by normal subjects, the adoption of a few clearly stated theoretical positions concerning the presumed nature of the neuropsychological structures and mechanisms underlying such processing stands as the necessary first step. After careful consideration of the major available psycholinguistic discourse processing models (Kintsch & van Dijk, 1975, 1978; Mandler, 1978; Mandler & DeForest, 1979; Mandler & Johnson, 1977; Reiser & Black, 1982; Schank & Abelson, 1977),[4] we decided to take one of them, namely that of Kintsch & van Dijk (1975, 1978) and to adapt it to our

---

[3] See Picton and Stuss (1984) for a critical review concerning the use of ERP in the study of language processing. See Hillyard and Kutas (1983) for a general review concerning the electrophysiology of cognitive processing.

[4] See Frederiksen, Bracewell, Breuleux, and Renaud (1990) and Guimaraes dos Santos (1992) for reviews concerning this issue.

own specific theoretical and experimental purposes. Two factors guided our choice. The first one is that, among all the models we examined, only Kintsch and van Dijk's offered both a simple and a detailed account of the fundamental psycholinguistic mechanisms supposedly involved in discourse processing by the normal subject. The second factor, which is more pragmatic in nature, is that this model proved to be easily adaptable to serve our own theoretical and experimental purposes.

Basically, such a process of adaptation implies, among other minor transformations, the elaboration of some explicit statements concerning the possible "hardware" (neurological) representation of the psychological structures and mechanisms that compose Kintsch and van Dijk's model, which is essentially, as we have already mentioned, a psycholinguistic one. Within the context of this chapter, we present only those transformations that are relevant to the interpretation of the results we report in later sections.[5]

For Kintsch and van Dijk (1978), the semantic structure of texts can be fairly adequately described at two basic levels: a *microlevel* and a *macrolevel*. The first one is regarded as being the local level of discourse, that is, the structure of individual propositions and their mutual interrelations. The second level has a more global nature and characterizes discourse as a whole: It can be best understood as being that type of structure that represents the main ideas contained in a text—things such as its theme, gist, or topic. Furthermore, their model proposes that these two levels are related by a set of specific semantic mapping rules, the macrorules (or macro-operators) whose precise function is to reduce the information contained in a text (which consists of a given number of microstructures) to its gist, that is, to its abstract macrostructure.

As far as the psycholinguistic level of analysis is concerned, it has to be emphasized that the research we have undertaken was exclusively concerned with what is called by Kintsch and van Dijk the macrolevel of discourse. The reason for this can be summarized as follows: Since any discourse (whatever its type) is an amazingly complex object of study, it was absolutely crucial for the integrity of our experimental design to choose the level of linguistic structure that should be regarded as the independent variable. Therefore, throughout the development of our study, we tried to keep constant, for all three types of discourse chosen as stimuli, the level of complexity of their microstructural network.

A careful analysis of the distinctive linguistic features that characterize each one of the three types of discourse that were used as stimuli—descriptive without a thematic unit (DD), argumentative (AD), and narrative (ND)—can be useful in clarifying the methodological strategy we have adopted. They can be summarized as follows.

---

[5]See Guimaraes dos Santos (1992) for further discussion.

1. DD-type discourse is defined by (a) concrete referential lexico-semantic content that can be easily conceived of by means of mental images and (b) the absence of any macrostructural network.
2. AD-type discourse is defined by (a) abstract lexico-semantic content that can hardly be conceived of by means of mental images and (b) a well-defined macrostructural network which is, in fact, slightly more complex than the macrostructural network contained in ND-type discourse.
3. ND-type discourse is defined by (a) balanced abstract-concrete lexico-semantic content that is neither predominantly concrete nor predominantly abstract and (b) a well-defined macrostructural network.

SUBJECTS AND METHODS

Sixteen normal, adult, French-speaking volunteers (8 men and 8 women, mean age = 50.3 years ranging from 37 to 66 years, with similar educational backgrounds) were assigned to one of four possible groups (2 men and 2 women each) that corresponded to four different orders of discourse presentation in our auditory comprehension and memorization task: DD-ND-AD, ND-DD-AD, AD-DD-ND, and AD-ND-DD. Subjects' handedness was scored using the Edinburgh Inventory (Oldfield, 1971).

Each type of previously tape-recorded discourse was presented to each subject for 4 minutes, during which the distribution of the regional cerebral blood flow (rCBF) was assessed using a single photon emission tomograph (SPECT) (Tomomatic 64, Medimatic, Copenhägen) and intravenous injection of Xenon 133 (2400 MBeq), which allows the calculation of rCBF on cross-sectional slices of human brain. The rationale underlying the use of rCBF in the mapping of functional activity in the brain is based on the hypothesis that a localized increase in activity in a region of the brain in response to some stimulus results in a local increase in the metabolism in that area, which then causes an increase in the blood flow in the same region.

Data were collected simultaneously from three transverse slices (2-cm thick) parallel and centered at 1 cm (slice 3), 5 cm (slice 2), and 9 cm (slice 1) above the orbitomeatal plane (OM) (see Figure 7–1). The in-plane resolution was 1.7 cm.

During each 4-minute period of SPECT data collection, subjects were kept at rest, with eyes closed, and with headphones in position. Also, pCO_2 was continuously recorded using a cutaneous electrode and a Kontron 634 pCO_2 monitor. For each subject, three measurements corre-

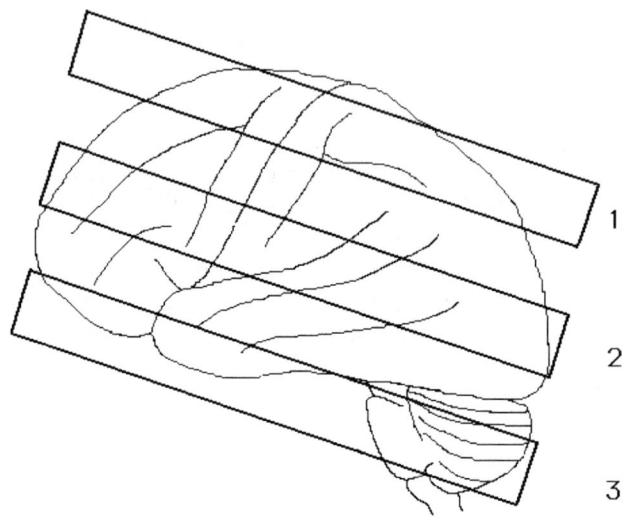

Figure 7–1. Diagram showing the anatomical localization of slices 1, 2, and 3.

sponding to the three types of discourse were performed on the same day, with an interval of 1 hour between each measurement.

Calculation of rCBF was done using a method described by Celsis, Goldman, Henriksen, and Lassen (1981). Mean rCBF values in the whole slices as well as in the regions of interest (ROIs) in slice 2 (OM + 5 cm) (see Figures 7–1 and 7–2) were obtained. The ROIs were determined using predefinite templates and interactive software on a Macintosh II microcomputer with a 256-color display. A homemade image-processing program allowed for corrections necessary to fit templates onto the *flow* pictures of each subject. In addition to absolute values (in ml/100g/min), the differences between homologous interhemispheric regions were considered.

The quality of subjects' performances was evaluated by means of a propositional analysis of each one of the 48 recall protocols obtained after each SPECT data collection session (three for each subject, one for each type of discourse). The difference between the number of correct and the number of incorrect propositions contained in each of the 48 recall protocols proved to be the index that best captured the quality of subjects' performances. This index was defined as follows:

$DDK = NCP_{DD} - NIP_{DD}$ (for DD-type discourse)
$NDK = NCP_{ND} - NIP_{ND}$ (for ND-type discourse)
$ADK = NCP_{AD} - NIP_{AD}$ (for AD-type discourse), where

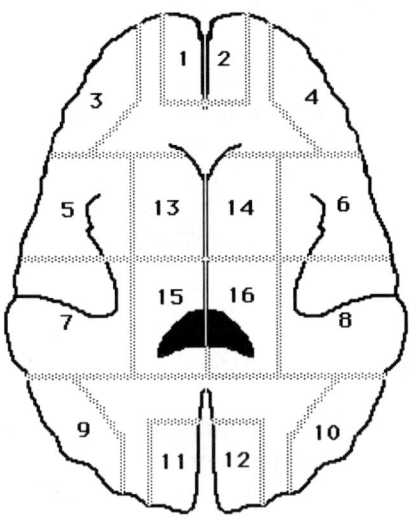

Figure 7–2. Diagram showing the 16 ROIs that have been defined in slice 2.

NCP = number of correct propositions and
NIP = number of incorrect propositions.[6]

Our experimental results do not allow us to draw conclusions that concern exclusively ND-type discourse. All the results obtained using our experimental design must be understood as being *comparative* in the sense that an isolated analysis of the processing of only one type of discourse turns out to be methodologically impossible.

RESULTS

For the sake of simplicity, we shall divide the presentation of our results into three parts.

1. As far as the quality of subjects' performances is concerned, the analysis of the mean values for the variables DDK, NDK, and ADK showed that subjects performed best processing ND-type discourse,

---

[6] See Guimaraes dos Santos (1992) for a full description of the methodology used to evaluate the quality of subjects' performances.

much worse processing ND-type discourse, and worst processing DD-type discourse:

$$DDK = 6.2 < ADK = 7.4 < NDK = 9.8 \ (N = 16, p < .01).$$

2. We also observed a negative correlation between the age variable and the quality of subjects' performances (measured as described above) in processing AD and ND-type discourse (no correlation was found for DD-type discourse):

$$\text{age with ADK: } r = -0.53 \ (N = 16, p < .05)$$
$$\text{age with NDK: } r = -0.58 \ (N = 16, p < .05).$$

These correlations indicate that older subjects gave poorer performances than younger subjects for AD- and ND-type discourse.

3. In addition, we found some corresponding effects in the SPECT data. When rCBF values measured by SPECT during the processing of *only* AD- and ND-type discourse are taken into account, the following relation holds for the anatomical regions indicated in Figure 7–3, which can be considered as being the frontal (medial and lateral), occipital, and posterior temporo-parietal cortical areas:

$$rCBF_{AD} > rCBF_{ND} \ (N = 16, p < .05).$$

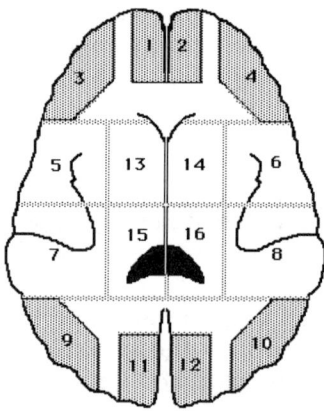

Figure 7–3. Diagram showing the anatomical localization of the cortical regions for which we verified the following relation: **rCBF$_{AD}$ > rCBF$_{ND}$**

DISCUSSION

This discussion is divided into three parts corresponding to those just presented in the Results section.

1. To explain why subjects gave their best performances with ND-type discourse, the poorest with DD-type discourse, and an "intermediate" level with AD-type discourse, we note first that the nonexistence of a well-defined macrostructural network is the only linguistic feature differentiating DD-type discourse both from ND- and AD-type discourses. Next, one can assume the existence of a group of cognitive mechanisms responsible for macrostructural processing, that is, responsible for identifying, "putting together" all the parts that compose a discourse, establishing its coherence, and apprehending the discourse as a "unified whole" (Halliday & Hasan, 1976). Accordingly, it seems quite plausible to us that this particular group of mechanisms would be "overloaded" and engaged in somehow hopeless activity during the processing of DD-type discourse, which does not possess any macrostructural network whatsoever.

Although the hypothesis stated in the preceding paragraph can account for the quality of performances observed during both ND- and DD-type discourse, it is not as useful in explaining the so-called "intermediate" level of performances associated with the processing of AD-type discourse, which is also supposed to present a well-defined macrostructural network (although slightly more complex than the macrostructural network pertaining to ND-type discourse). Interestingly, although both types of discourse (ND and AD) possess a well-defined macrostructural network, *only* the ND-type discourse has a structure based on what has been called since Mandler and Johnson (1977) and Mandler (1978) a *story schema*. It seems to us that this difference could contribute to the better performances associated with ND-type discourse since its processing (and hence its retrieval) could be facilitated or guided by subjects' pre-existing story schema.

An alternative account for the results obtained is based on the opposition between concrete and abstract discourse content that can be used to distinguish among the discourses employed as stimuli. (As stated in the Introduction, DD-type discourse is characterized by concrete referential lexico-semantic content, AD-type discourse by abstract lexico-semantic content, and ND-type discourse by a balance of abstract and concrete lexico-semantic content.) If two discourses present the same level of complexity in their macrostructural networks, as is the case for ND- and AD-type discourses, then processing the one with the more abstract content (AD) will be more difficult and will result in worse recall performance.

In addition to the importance of concreteness when the macrostructural complexity is equivalent, a full explanation of our results also requires consideration of the *relative* importance of macrostructural complexity and concreteness. An auxilliary corollary is that the level of complexity of the macrostructural network of a discourse (i.e., the presence or the absence of a well-defined macrostructural network) seems more crucial than the degree of concreteness or abstractness of its content in determining subjects' facility processing a given discourse (and hence in determining the quality of the memory performance). Such a corollary could explain why the processing of DD-type discourse, which presents a "high imagery" referential content, is more difficult than the processing of the two other types of discourse: In spite of the concreteness of its content, DD-type discourse does not possess any macrostructural network at all.

2. We now turn to the negative correlations observed between age and the quality of performance on AD- and ND-type discourses. As we have already pointed out, these correlations indicate that older subjects gave poorer performances than younger subjects. One reasonable interpretation is that whatever neuropsychological mechanisms are responsible for discourse processing deteriorate with age, as has been well documented for other cognitive functions. (See Habib, Joanette, & Puel, 1991, and van Der Linden & Bruyer,1991, for reviews.) Unfortunately, that view is not able to account for the fact that we did not find a similar correlation for DD-type discourse. We have to confess that, for the moment, we do not have a compelling explanation for this observation. Be that as it may, we could tentatively suppose that the level of difficulty presented by processing DD-type discourse was much higher than the level presented by the two other types of discourse (ND and AD). This extra difficulty may have produced a floor effect which, in turn, restricted the range of subjects' performances which, in turn, would diminish any correlation between age and performance.

3. The findings presented in the third part of the Results section are consistent with the interpretation advanced above. If two discourses present the same level of complexity in their macrostructural networks (as is the case for AD- and ND-type discourses), then processing the one that presents the more abstract content (AD) will be more difficult. Furthermore, the ND-type discourse, in addition to being more concrete, has a second advantage in that it is organized according to a cannonical story schema. Hence, the quality of performances associated with the second tpe of discourse (ND) will be better than those associated with the first (AD) for some combination of these two reasons. Indeed, if we assume that the level of cerebral activity can be fairly evaluated by means of SPECT (i.e., if rCBF can be accepted as a good index of cerebral activity), and if we suppose (as seems reasonable) that more difficult processing is correlated with higher rCBF values, then it becomes easy to explain why rCBF values measured during the processing of AD-type discourse are greater than those measured during the processing of ND-type discourse.

Unfortunately, as was the case for results discussed in paragraph 2, the above rationale cannot explain the rCBF level observed during subjects' processing DD-type discourse. Since the processing of this discourse type is supposed to be the most difficult, it should have produced the highest rCBF values; yet, we did not observe such an effect. The reason for this "unexpected" result (or lack thereof) is not apparent. We must admit that, for the moment, we do not have a satisfying, even tentative explanation.[7]

Finally, as far as the anatomical regions (frontal, medial-lateral, occipital, and posterior temporo-parietal cortical areas) indicated in Figure 7–3 are concerned, their activation during discourse processing was to be expected, particularly for the frontal and posterior temporo-parietal regions. It is not difficult to find in the literature data consistently linking these regions to language processing (e.g., Barbizet, Duizabo, & Flavigny, 1975; Botez, 1987a, 1987b; Caplan, 1987; Geschwind, 1965; Labrecque, 1987).

Even if the results presented above require confirmation in future studies, the questions and hypotheses they suggest can contribute to the organization of this astonishingly complex field of scientific investigation.

ACKNOWLEDGMENT

Dr. Guimaraes dos Santos wishes to thank the CNPq–Conselho Nacional de Desenvolvimento Cientifico e Tecnologico (Brazil) for the grant that allowed him to undertake the research presented in this chapter.

REFERENCES

Barbizet, J., Duizabo, P., & Flavigny, R. (1975). Rôle des lobes frontaux dans le langage: une étude neuro-psychologique expérimentale. *Revue Neurologique (Paris)*, *131*, 525–544.

Botez, M. I. (1987a). Le syndrome pariétal. In M. I. Botez (Ed.), *Neuropsychologie clinique et neurologie du comportement* (pp. 135–154). Montréal: Les Presses de l'Université de Montréal.

Botez, M. I. (1987b). Le syndrome temporal. In M. I. Botez (Ed.), *Neuropsychologie clinique et neurologie du comportement* (pp. 154–167). Montréal: Les Presses de l'Université de Montréal.

Caplan, D. (1987). *Neurolinguistics and linguistic aphasiology*. Cambridge, MA: Cambridge University Press.

Celsis, P., Goldman, T., Henriksen, L., & Lassen, H. A. (1981). A method for calculating regional cerebral blood flow from emission computed tomography of inert gas concentrations. *Journal of Computer Assisted Tomography* , *5*, 641–645.

---

[7] See Guimaraes dos Santos, Nespoulous, Celsis, and Viallard (1991) and Guimaraes dos Santos (1992) for some comments on this problem.

Courtés, J. (1991). *Analyse sémiotique du discours: De l'énoncé à l'énonciation*. Paris: Hachette.

Churchland, P. S. (1986). *Neurophilosophy: Toward a unified science of mind-brain*. Cambridge, MA: M. I. T. Press.

Deschênes, A. -J. (1988). *La compréhension et la production de textes*. Québec: Presses de l'Université du Québec.

Fayol, M. (1985). *Le récit et sa construction: une approche de psychologie cognitive*. Paris: Delachaux & Niestlé.

Frederiksen, C. H., Bracewell, R. J., Breuleux, A., & Renaud, A. (1990). The cognitive representation and processing of discourse: Function and dysfunction. In Y. Joanette and H. H. Brownell (Eds.), *Discourse ability and brain damage: Theoretical and empirical perspectives* (pp. 69–110). New York: Springer-Verlag.

Geschwind, N. (1965). Disconnexion syndromes in animals and man. *Brain, 88*, 237–294, 585–644.

Goldberg, G., Podreka, L., Steiner, M., Willmes, K., Suess, E., & Deecke, L. (1989). Regional cerebral blood flow patterns in visual imagery. *Neuropsychologia, 27*, 641–664.

Guimaraes dos Santos, C. L. N. (1988). *Natureza da diferença existente entre os modos de pensamento pré-verbal, verbal e pos-verbal*. Unpublished master's thesis, Universidade de Sao Paulo, Sao Paulo, Bresil [Brazil].

Guimaraes dos Santos, C. L. N. (1992). *Une étude neuropsycholinguistique du traitement réceptif* (compréhension et mémorisation) du discours par le sujet normal. Unpublished doctoral dissertation, Université de Toulouse-Le Mirail, Toulouse, France.

Guimaraes dos Santos, C. L. N., Nespoulous, J.- L., Celsis, P., & Viallard, G. (1991). Discourse processing and functional inter-hemispheric brain asymmetries. *Journal of Neurolinguistics, 6*, 285–299.

Gutwinsky, W. (1976). *Cohesion in literary texts*. The Hague: Mouton.

Habib, M., Joanette, Y., & Puel, M. (Eds.) (1991). *Démences et syndromes démentiels: approche neuropsychologique*. Paris: Masson.

Halliday, M. A. K., & Hasan, R. (1976). *Cohesion in English*. London: Longman.

Hillyard, S. A., & Kutas, M. (1983). Electrophysiology of cognitive processing. *Annual Review of Psychology 34*, 33–61.

Kiefer, F. (1977). Review of studies in text grammars. *Journal of Pragmatics, 1*, 177–193.

Kintsch, W., & van Dijk, T. A. (1975). Comment on se rappelle et on resume des histoires. *Languages, 10*, 98–116.

Kintsch, W., & van Dijk, T. A. (1978). Toward a model of text comprehension and production. *Psychological Review, 85*, 363–94.

Kummer, W. (1972). Outlines of a model for grammar of discourse. *Poetics, 3*, 29–56.

Labrecque, R. (1987). Le syndrome occipital. In M. I. Botez (Ed.), *Neuropsychologie clinique et neurologie du comportement* (pp. 169–182). Montréal: Les Presses de l'Université de Montréal.

Mandler, J. M. (1978). A code in the node. The use of story schema in retrieval. *Discourse Processes, 1*, 14–35.

Mandler, J. M., & Johnson, N. S. (1977). Remembrance of things parsed: Story structure and recall. *Cognitive Psychology 9*, 111–151.

Mandler, J. M., & De Forest, M. (1979). Is there more than one way to recall a story? *Child Development, 50*, 886–889.

Oldfield, O. D. (1971). The assessement and analysis of handedness: The Edinburgh inventory. *Neuropsychologia, 9*, 97–113.
Petöfi, J., & Rieser, H. (Eds.). (1973). *Studies in text grammar*. Dordrecht, Nederland [Netherlands]: Reidel.
Picton, T. W., & Stuss, D. T. (1984). Event-related potentials in the study of speech and language: A critical review. In D. Caplan, A. R. Lecours, & A. Smith (Eds.), *Biological perspectives on language* (pp. 303–360). Cambridge, MA: M. I. T. Press.
Reiser, B. J., & Black, J. B. (1982). Processing and structural models of comprehension. *Text, 2*, 225–52.
Rondal, J. A., & Thibaut, J. R. (Eds.) (1987). *Problèmes de psycholinguistique*. Bruxelles [Brussels], Belgium: Pierre Mardaga Editeur.
Schank, R. C., & Abelson, R. R. (1977). *Scripts, plans, goals and understanding*. Hillsdale, NJ: Lawrence Erlbaum.
van Der Linden, M., & Bruyer, R. (Eds.) (1991). *Neuropsychologie de la mémoire humaine*. Grenoble, France: Presses Universitaires de Grenoble.
van Dijk, T. A. (1972). *Some aspects of text grammar*. Dordrecht, Nederland [Netherlands]: Reidel.
van Dijk, T. A., & Kintsch, W. (1983). *Strategies of discourse comprehension*. New York: Academic Press.

PART III

Narrative Capacities of Patients with Focal Brain Damage

CHAPTER 8

Comprehension of Narrative Discourse by Aphasic Listeners

ROBERT H. BROOKSHIRE AND
LINDA E. NICHOLAS

Spoken language comprehension in aphasia has been studied since the 1800s. The early work was primarily descriptive, concerned with documenting the presence of comprehension impairments and with demonstrating their relationship to various aphasic syndromes. More recent studies of comprehension in aphasia have followed in the footsteps of research on "normal" language comprehension, which has evolved from studying comprehension of isolated sentences to studying comprehension of information in discourse and gaining an understanding of how the structure of discourse affects comprehension.

A BRIEF HISTORY OF THE STUDY OF NORMAL LANGUAGE COMPREHENSION

From the 1950s to the early 1970s, the focus in studies of normal language comprehension was comprehension of isolated sentences. The sentences tended to be syntactically complex, and they were often unusual, in the sense that normal speakers would rarely produce them in natural environments, as in the following example from Glucksberg and Danks (1975):

The plumber the doctor the nurse met called ate the cheese. (p. 87)

The purpose of studies involving such sentences usually was to test models of language comprehension in which listeners deduced the meaning of a given sentence by means of a sequential series of operations that converted the sentence's "surface structure" into an underlying "deep structure" that had intrinsic meaning. Although those who studied such sentences may have assumed that their experiments represented what listeners do in daily life listening, few attempted to test the assumption. Then, during the late 1960s and early 1970s, the focus shifted from testing models of single-sentence comprehension to appreciating how listeners go about making sense of what they hear in listening situations that more closely resemble daily life.

It became apparent that comprehension was not simply a set of computations by which listeners more or less automatically derived the underlying meaning of sentences or discourse by means of a pre-determined set of mental operations. Rather, the words in the sentences or discourse seemed only to provide a starting point from which listeners set out (often in directions not predicted by the models) to make sense of what they heard. "Bottom-up" models, in which comprehension was seen as a gradual accumulation of meanings from single words to sentences to texts, were replaced by "top-down" models, in which listeners related the linguistic content of the discourse to their general knowledge and to their intuitions concerning the situation, the speaker, and a sense of the speaker's intent.

Numerous models of how discourse comprehension actually transpires have been published (Meyer, 1975; van Dijk & Kintsch, 1983; Winograd, 1977). Most contemporary models assume that discourse comprehension represents an interaction between the linguistic content of the discourse and the listener's strategic use of extralinguistic sources of information to determine the probable meaning of the discourse. Although the terminology differs across models, most agree that listeners go beyond the actual content of what is said to develop presuppositions and expectations, identify the speaker's purpose or intent, decide what is important and what is not, and relate what the speaker says to what the listener already knows. Listeners seem to depend on the lexical and syntactic content of discourse primarily to identify its propositional makeup and to deduce relationships among propositions. They then go on to use their general knowledge, intuitions, and even guessing to arrive at its overall meaning (Caplan & Evans, 1990).

The lexical, syntactic, and propositional analyses can conveniently be called "text-based processes" because they are strongly linked to the actual content of the discourse, in contrast with operations in which the listener invokes general knowledge and intuition to aid in comprehension (knowledge-based or "heuristic" processes). The degree to which listeners engage in lexical, syntactic, and propositional analyses depends, in large part, on the extent to which the meaning of a sample of discourse can be ascertained by means of heuristic processes and intuition. Lexical, propositional, and syntactic analyses usually require more mental effort than heuristic processes. Heuristic processes are said to lessen the processing "load" in comprehension by allowing the listener to deduce general meanings and anticipate the content of upcoming utterances without the need for continuous word-by-word lexical and syntactic analyses. Consequently, normal listeners usually emphasize heuristic processes over text-based ones, and are likely to rely on text-based processes only when forced to do so by the absence of extralinguistic sources of information about the meaning of the discourse, or by arcane vocabulary or complex syntax within the discourse (Carpenter & Just, 1977; Clark, 1977).

EARLY STUDIES OF LANGUAGE COMPREHENSION IN APHASIA

The early studies of language comprehension in aphasia, like early studies of normal comprehension, focused almost exclusively on comprehension of single-sentence utterances. These studies were concerned with how variables such as syntactic complexity, word frequency, sentence length, and speech rate and pauses affected aphasic listeners' comprehension of single-sentence utterances. The general model of comprehension underlying these studies (like the then current conceptualizations of how normal listeners comprehend spoken language) was that comprehension progressed in bottom-up fashion from individual words to the overall meaning of utterances, with heavy reliance on syntactic processes. The results of these studies were important in elucidating the effects of variables such as word frequency, syntactic complexity, sentence length, speech rate, and pauses on aphasic listeners' sentence comprehension, and in identifying differences in the nature and magnitude of comprehension impairments among different "types" of aphasia. However, by the mid-1970s, some began to question whether tests that assess aphasic listeners' comprehension of single-sentence utterances accurately predict their comprehension of multiple-sentence spoken materials (discourse). The first evidence came from studies in which aphasic listeners' comprehension of isolated sentences was compared with their comprehension of short narratives.

RELATIONSHIPS BETWEEN SENTENCE COMPREHENSION AND COMPREHENSION OF DISCOURSE

Stachowiak, Huber, Poeck, and Kerschensteiner (1977) were among the first to evaluate the relationship between brain-damaged listeners' comprehension of single-sentence utterances and their comprehension of narratives. They tested non-brain-damaged, aphasic left-hemisphere-damaged, and nonaphasic right-hemisphere-damaged listeners' comprehension of single-sentence idiomatic expressions placed at the end of five-sentence narratives which set the scene for the idiomatic expressions. They also tested each subject with the Token Test (DeRenzi & Vignolo, 1962).[1] The three groups of subjects did not differ significantly in comprehension of the idiomatic targets. Stachowiak et al. attributed their brain-damaged subjects' good performance on the target sentences to the redundancy afforded by the narratives, which allowed subjects to infer, from context, information about the target sentence, and they attributed their brain-damaged subjects' poor performance on the Token Test to its "strictly nonredundant" nature. They reported generally low correlations (ranging from .17 to .31) between Token Test scores and text comprehension scores for brain-damaged subjects. They concluded that linguistic context facilitates comprehension for both aphasic and right-hemisphere-damaged listeners and that Token Test scores do not predict their text comprehension performance.

Pashek and Brookshire (1982) subsequently compared aphasic adults' comprehension of information from spoken expository paragraphs with their Token Test performance. For subjects who performed well on the Token Test, the correlation between Token Test and paragraph comprehension scores was $r = .76$, and for those who performed poorly on the Token Test it was $r = .26$, suggesting that single-sentence tests of comprehension might predict discourse comprehension better for aphasic listeners with relatively good single-sentence comprehension than for those whose single-sentence comprehension is relatively poor.[2]

Brookshire and Nicholas (1984) tested aphasic adults' comprehension of stated and implied main ideas and details from spoken stories. They also administered the Token Test to each subject. They reported generally

---

[1] The Token Test requires subjects to touch or manipulate large and small colored circles and squares in response to single-sentence commands of various lengths and syntactic structures.

[2] Our subsequent work, and that of others, suggests that the correlation of .76 may have been affected by sampling anomalies or some other artifact. Our subsequent work has not replicated this relatively high correlation, and we know of no one else who has reported a correlation of this magnitude.

low correlations (Pearson correlation coefficients ranged from .20 to .27) between Token Test scores and narrative comprehension performance.

Caplan and Evans (1990) reported somewhat higher correlations between aphasic and non-brain-damaged adults' comprehension of isolated sentences (representing seven syntactic structures) and their comprehension of short narratives. Spearman rank-order correlation coefficients between subjects' narrative comprehension scores and their sentence comprehension scores ranged from .32 to .52. Caplan and Evans concluded that sentence comprehension and discourse comprehension represent, at least in part, different processes and that discourse comprehension can occur without syntactic analysis of the sentences in the discourse.

The evidence from these studies indicates that aphasic and right-hemisphere-damaged listeners' performance on single-sentences tests of comprehension does not predict their discourse comprehension. Correlations between scores on sentence comprehension tests and scores on discourse comprehension tests generally range from the .20s to the .30s, with Caplan and Evans (1990) reporting correlations ranging from the low .30s to about .50. Although these correlations may be statistically significant (meaning that there is *some* relationship between the two), they are not large enough to permit accurate prediction of discourse comprehension from sentence comprehension test scores.[3] Consequently, it seems clear that if we are to predict brain-damaged listeners' comprehension of discourse, then we must test their comprehension of discourse. We cannot infer their comprehension of discourse from their comprehension of isolated sentences.

The weak relationship between brain-damaged listeners' comprehension of isolated sentences and their comprehension of discourse, and the fact that their discourse comprehension usually is better than one would expect from their sentence comprehension performance suggest that brain-damaged listeners, like normal listeners, use sources of information beyond the sentence to facilitate their com-prehension of discourse. Studies of aphasic and right-hemisphere-damaged listeners' discourse comprehension suggest that brain-damaged listeners do, in fact, call on extrasentential sources of information to facilitate their comprehension of spoken discourse. The first of these sources to receive extensive study was *linguistic context*.

---

[3] The statistic that best captures the *strength* of the relationship expressed by a correlation coefficient is called the *coefficient of determination*, represented by r^2. The coefficient of determination for a correlation of .17 (the lowest reported) is approximately .03, which means that less than 5% of a group's variability in discourse comprehension scores is related to their sentence comprehension performance. The coefficient of determination for a correlation of .30 (approximately the average of the reported correlations) equals .09, which means that less than 10% of a group's variability in discourse comprehension scores is related to their sentence comprehension performance.

THE EFFECTS OF LINGUISTIC CONTEXT ON APHASIC LISTENERS' COMPREHENSION

Stachowiak et al. (1977), were interested in assessing whether providing linguistic context facilitated aphasic and right-hemisphere-damaged listeners' comprehension of idiomatic statements. As mentioned previously, they placed idiomatic statements near the end of short contextual passages, as in:

Werner and his wife meet with friends every Friday. This time the men want to play poker. Because Werner plays riskily, he soon loses all of his money. *The others strip him right down to his shirt.* His wife gets quite annoyed.

Stachowiak et al. concluded that the contextual passages facilitated brain-damaged listeners' comprehension of the idioms, based on their good performance on the contextualized idiomatic sentences and their poor performance on the Token Test. However, they apparently did not verify that their subjects could not comprehend the idiomatic sentences in isolation. Consequently, they did not directly test the effects of context on comprehension of the sentences, which would have been possible had they tested comprehension of the idiomatic sentences in isolation.

There followed numerous studies in which others examined the relationship between aphasic (and sometimes right-hemisphere-damaged) listeners' comprehension of isolated sentences and comprehension of sentences that came at the end (usually) of short contextual passages. Nicholas and Brookshire (1983) compared aphasic adults' comprehension of comparative and embedded-clause reversible sentences presented in isolation with their comprehension of the same sentences presented at the end of short narratives that set the scene for the final sentences, as in the following example.

A man was standing at the bus stop reading a newspaper. A woman was waiting for the same bus. The woman quietly stepped over behind the man and began to read the newspaper over his shoulder. She could read the paper easily. *The woman was taller than the man.*

Nicholas and Brookshire reported that most (but not all) aphasic listeners comprehended target sentences in context better than they comprehended the same sentences in isolation. Pierce and his associates (Cannito, Jarecki, & Pierce, 1986; Hough, Pierce, & Cannito, 1989; Pierce, 1988; Pierce & Beekman, 1985; Pierce & Wagner, 1985) also reported several studies of aphasic adults' comprehension of sentences presented in isolation and following context provided by single sentences or short narratives. Their subjects consistently comprehended sentences in context better than they comprehended the same sentences in isolation.

For some time it was not clear whether context actually facilitated aphasic listeners' comprehension of target sentences, or simply made them superfluous, by providing all the information contained in the target sentences (Boyle & Canter, 1986). However, the results of studies by Cannito et al. (1986), Pierce (1988), and Hough et al. (1989), in which contexts were structured so that they provided no information about the syntactic relationships depicted in the target sentences, indicate that context does, in fact, facilitate comprehension of syntactically complex sentences and that this facilitation is not explainable by the effects of simple redundancy.

The foregoing studies show that aphasic listeners can use linguistic context to facilitate their comprehension of target sentences that come at the end of the linguistic context. Waller and Darley (1978), took a somewhat different approach, and measured the effects of prior linguistic or pictorial context on comprehension of information located throughout short narratives, rather than on target sentences at the end of the narratives. They evaluated aphasic listeners' comprehension of short narratives in three conditions. In *verbal prestimulation condition*, two or three sentences providing general information about the theme of each paragraph were read to subjects before each paragraph was read. In *visual prestimulation condition*, colored pictures representing the theme of each paragraph were shown to subjects before each paragraph was read. In *verbal plus visual prestimulation condition*, visual and verbal prestimulation were presented together before each narrative. First they tested the effects of these conditions on comprehension of highly cohesive paragraphs. Then they tested the effects of verbal pre-stimulation alone on less cohesive paragraphs. They reported that combined prestimulation facilitated aphasic listeners' comprehension of highly cohesive paragraphs, and that visual prestimulation caused their performance to deteriorate, though the effects were not statistically significant. There was a significant positive effect of verbal prestimulation on aphasic listeners' comprehension of less cohesive paragraphs. Waller and Darley concluded that prior verbal context "may" facilitate aphasic listeners' comprehension of certain kinds of spoken narratives.

In most studies of the effects of context on comprehension, the investigators were interested in the extent to which aphasic listeners' impairments in comprehension of syntactically complex sentences might be mitigated by providing them with supportive context. Caplan and Evans (1990) approached this relationship from the other direction. They designed a study to determine if aphasic listeners' impairments in syntactic analysis affected their comprehension of information from discourse. They tested aphasic and non-brain- damaged listeners' comprehension of syntactically simple and syntactically complex folk tales and narratives. They found that aphasic listeners did significantly less well overall than non-brain-damaged listeners. However, there was no significant effect of syntactic complexity on the discourse comprehension performance of either group. The authors reached the following conclusion.

> In common discourse structures containing semantically and discourse-constrained sentences, the syntactic complexity of the sentences in the discourse does not have an independent effect upon aphasic patients' abilities to answer questions about the content of a passage, regardless of a patient's ability to comprehend sentences by a syntactic route. (p. 224)

However, they noted that their subjects reported subjective feelings of greater difficulty with the syntactically complex stories than with the syntactically simple ones. They also commented that making the task more difficult by requiring recall, rather than recognition of information from the passages, or making more of the sentences in the passages semantically reversible and not easily predicted from the previous discourse may have made the role of syntactic variables more prominent. Nevertheless, Caplan and Evans's results clearly show that aphasic listeners are capable of using information from the context provided by discourse to facilitate their comprehension of syntactically complex sentences within that discourse—a conclusion that is consistent with the results of the studies that preceded theirs.

MENTAL REPRESENTATIONS AS A SOURCE OF CONTEXT IN DISCOURSE COMPREHENSION

In addition to making use of the context inherent in discourse itself, normal listeners often draw on their general knowledge to construct a mental representation of the situation or events portrayed by discourse. This mental representation may function as a context or frame of reference for the discourse.[4] For example, if the speaker is describing what transpired at a party the previous night, the listener may call on his or her knowledge

---

[4] The labels applied to these mental representations differ across studies. Some have called them "schemata" (Rumelhart, 1975); others have called them "scripts" (Schank & Ableson, 1977); and others have called them "frames" (van Dijk, 1980). Although there are subtle differences in the exact definitions of these terms, they all refer to mental representations that organize information in memory. We use the label "script" herein.

of what typically transpires at parties to construct a set of expectations regarding what most likely took place. Thus, once the listener establishes the topic as "party," he or she can predict much of the likely content of the discourse from a mental "script" of a typical party scenario:

- That a number of other people were there.
- That food and drink were served.
- That there was a host or hostess.
- That the party was at the host or hostess's home.
- That social conversations took place.

Numerous studies of normal discourse comprehension support the idea that listeners invoke such mental representations to organize information from discourse and to make predictions and construct expectations about the likely meaning of discourse (Adams & Collins, 1979; Bower, Black, & Turner, 1979; and others). Such mental representations no doubt also help listeners separate "new" information from that which is already known, thereby diminishing the amount of processing resources needed by allowing listeners to focus processing on the "new" information.

Armus, Brookshire, and Nicholas (1989) have shown that aphasic adults' script knowledge is apparently well preserved. They had aphasic and non-brain-damaged adults *discriminate* phrases identifying test scripts from phrases identifying foil scripts, *identify the central events* in test scripts, and *sequence* the central events in test scripts in the order in which they would occur in real life. Neither aphasic nor non-brain-damaged subjects made many errors in any of the three tasks, and the two groups did not differ in discriminating script events or identifying the central events in scripts. Aphasic subjects were significantly poorer than non-brain-damaged subjects at sequencing script events, but the actual difference was so small that it seems clinically unimportant (a mean difference of 0.17 points of a possible 5 points). The authors concluded that "the script knowledge of aphasic adults is relatively well preserved for scripts of this level of complexity, at least when aphasia is mild or moderate" (p. 526). They also suggested that preserved script knowledge might help to account for aphasic listeners' good comprehension of discourse relative to their comprehension of single sentences.

Roman, Brownell, Potter, Siebold, and Gardner (1987) reported similar findings for adults with right-hemisphere brain damage. They had young normal, older normal, and (older) right-hemisphere-damaged adults produce scripts for common situations, as well as identifying the important elements of scripts and putting the elements of scripts in temporal order. They found that older normal and right-hemisphere-damaged subjects performed somewhat less well on all tasks than the younger normal subjects, but they concluded that these deficiencies did not represent impaired knowledge of scripts or impaired use of scripts in discourse comprehension. Rather, they concluded that the older normal and right- hemisphere-damaged subjects "fell prey to general cognitive abnormalities, that from time to time disrupt their use of script knowledge under various task demands" (p. 161).

EFFECTS OF DISCOURSE STRUCTURE ON BRAIN-DAMAGED LISTENERS' COMPREHENSION

The foregoing studies show that brain-damaged listeners can use linguistic context and mental scripts to facilitate their comprehension of discourse. Other studies of brain-damaged listeners' discourse comprehension provide insights into how the structure of discourse itself affects their comprehension of information in the discourse. These studies have investigated listeners' sensitivity to the salience of information in discourse. **Salience** refers to how important certain information is to the essential meaning of the discourse. By means of devices such as repetition, paraphrase, elaboration, and cohesive ties, speakers emphasize some information (the main ideas) while other information (the details) receives less emphasis and remains peripheral to the essential meaning of the discourse. Normal listeners customarily comprehend and remember the main ideas from discourse better than the details (Meyer, 1975; Meyer and McConkie, 1973; Kintsch, 1974; and others).

In most of the studies of the effects of salience on brain-damaged listeners' discourse comprehension, the **directness** of certain information (i.e., whether information was directly stated or implied) was also manipulated to determine if aphasic listeners have unusual difficulty with constructing inferences from information in discourse. The studies of directness were motivated by previous literature showing that normal speakers do not always specify all the information needed for listeners to comprehend the meaning and intent of the speaker's utterances (Clark & Haviland, 1977), but often leave informational gaps in what they are saying. They expect the listener to fill these gaps by drawing on their existing knowledge. For example, in a narrative fragment such as "The body lay on the floor. *The knife lay nearby.*" it is left to the listener to infer the connection between the knife and the body. Listeners fill these inferential gaps by constructing "implicatures" (Clark & Haviland, 1977) or "connecting propositions" (Kintsch, 1974). There is little doubt that normal listeners routinely engage in such gap filling, usually without conscious attention, although older listeners may have difficulty constructing inferences when discourse is spoken at a fast rate (Cohen, 1979).

Because they have been studied together, we will discuss the evidence regarding listeners' sensitivity to discourse structure and their ability to construct inferences suggested by discourse together, even though they most likely represent different processes. We will review the evidence regarding aphasic listeners' appreciation of discourse structure first and then discuss the evidence regarding inference.

The studies of the effects of salience and directness on listeners' discourse comprehension have generally followed a similar format. Non-brain-damaged adults, aphasic adults, and sometimes right-hemisphere damaged adults listen to short (100-word to 200-word) narratives and subsequently answer yes-no questions about the narratives. Half of the questions assess comprehension and retention of main ideas and half assess comprehension and retention of details. Half of the main idea questions and half of the detail questions assess information that is directly stated in the narratives. The other half of each type assess information that must be inferred from statements in the discourse. The following example of a narrative and its questions is from Nicholas and Brookshire (1986) (MI = main idea; DT = detail; S = stated; I = implied).

One day last Fall, several women on Willow Street decided to have a garage sale. They gathered odds and ends from all over the neighborhood. Then they spent an entire day putting prices on the things that they had collected. On the first day of the sale they put up signs at both ends of the block and another one at a nearby shopping center. Next they made a batch of iced tea and sat down in a shady spot beside the Anderson's garage to wait for their first customer. Soon a man drove up in an old truck. He looked around and finally stopped by a lumpy old mattress that was leaning against the wall. He gestured to it and asked how much they wanted for it. Mrs. Anderson told him that it wasn't for sale. Then she added that they were going to put it out for the trash collectors the next day. The man asked if he could have it. Mrs. Anderson said that he could. Then she asked, "Why do you want such a terrible mattress?" "Well," he said, "My no-good father-in-law is coming to visit next week and I don't want him to get too comfortable."

QUESTIONS

1. Did several women *have a party*? (No) [MI-S]
2. Were there a *large number of things* at the garage sale? (Yes) [MI-I]
3. Did the women put up a sign *at a shopping center*? (Yes) [DT-S]
4. Was it *cold* the day of the garage sale? (No) [DT-I]
5. Was the man driving *a car*? (No) [DT-S]
6. Was the mattress *in terrible condition*? (Yes) [MI-S]
7. Was the man *married*? (Yes) [DT-I]
8. Was the man *fond of his father-in-law*? (No) [MI-I]

Studies by Brookshire and Nicholas (1984), Nicholas and Brookshire (1986), and Brookshire and Nicholas (1993) used this general format and consistently found that non-brain-damaged and brain-damaged listeners (aphasic left-hemisphere-damaged and nonaphasic right-hemisphere-damaged) comprehended and remembered main ideas significantly better than details, with brain-damaged listeners' showing a larger effect than non-brain-damaged listeners. As a general rule, brain-damaged listeners were nearly as good at comprehending main ideas as non-brain-damaged listeners. Non-brain-damaged listeners made almost no errors on items which tested main ideas, and brain-damaged listeners typically missed less than 10% of main idea test items. Similar results were reported by Wegner, Brookshire, and Nicholas (1984) who evaluated the effects of salience, but not directness, on non-brain-damaged and aphasic listeners' comprehension of coherent and noncoherent narratives and by Katsuki-Nakamura, Brookshire, and Nicholas (1988) for non-brain-damaged and aphasic listeners' comprehension of main ideas and details from monologues and two-person dialogues. Figure 8–1 summarizes results from Brookshire and Nicholas (1993) who tested 40 non-brain-damaged, 20 aphasic, and 20 right-hemisphere-damaged listeners' comprehension of main ideas and details in 200-word narratives like the garage sale story provided previously. These results are representative of the

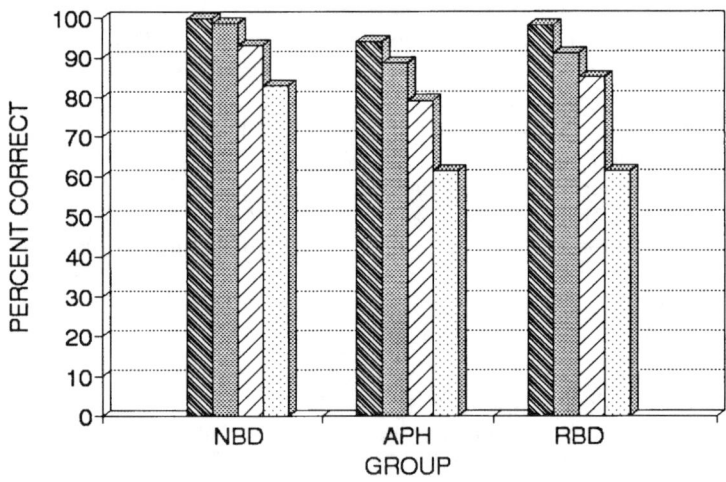

Figure 8–1. Non-brained-damaged (NBD) aphasic (APH) and right-hemisphere-damaged (RBD) subjects' performance on items that tested stated main ideas (MIS), implied main ideas (MII), stated details (DTS) and implied details (DTI), as reported by Brookshire and Nicholas (1993).

general results of the other studies of non-brain-damaged and brain-damaged listeners' comprehension of main ideas and details reviewed herein.

In contrast with the consistent effects of salience across studies, the effects of directness have been less predictable. Brookshire and Nicholas (1984) and Katsuki-Nakamura et al. (1988) found no significant effects of directness on either non-brain-damaged or brain-damaged listeners' comprehension of main ideas or details, whereas Nicholas and Brookshire (1986) and Brookshire and Nicholas (1993) found that directness significantly affected both non-brain-damaged and brain-damaged subjects' comprehension of details (stated details were comprehended and remembered better than implied details), but did not affect their comprehension of main ideas.[5] Figure 8–1 summarizes the results from Brookshire and Nicholas (1993) for subjects' comprehension of stated and implied main ideas and details.

This inconsistency in results across studies appears at least partially explainable by differences in the difficulty of the inferences required. In Brookshire and Nicholas (1984) and Katsuki-Nakamura et al. (1988) many of the items testing implied information merely paraphrased information stated in the narratives and did not actually require subjects to construct bridging assumptions. The following example, from Brookshire and Nicholas (1984), exemplifies the issue.

One night Joe and his friend Sam were having a few beers down at the local bar. They were laughing and talking and then, suddenly, they got into an argument and Joe punched Sam. Right away, the bartender called the cops and Joe wound up spending the night in jail. When Sam showed up in court the next morning, he had a bruise on his cheek and a real beauty of a shiner. The judge asked Sam if he wanted to press charges. He thought for a minute and then smiled and patted his friend on the back. "Nope," he said, "after all, a guy needs a good drinking buddy."

Here are three items that tested implied information. Subjects responded "yes" or "no" to the truth of pairs of statements, presented once in true form and once in false form. The words which falsified the statement are given in parentheses:

1. One of the men (the bartender) was arrested.
2. One of the men got a black eye (broken arm).
3. The two men remained friends (enemies).

---

[5]However, directness had a small but statistically significant effect on comprehension of main ideas by right-hemisphere-damaged subjects in Brookshire and Nicholas (1993). They comprehended stated main ideas significantly better than implied main ideas. However, the actual difference between means was 1.4 points of a possible 20, which yielded a 7% difference between means (Figure 8–1). Whether this statistically significant difference is clinically meaningful appears questionable.

Item 1 can be deduced easily from "Joe spent the night in jail". Item 2 is represented in the narrative by the paraphrase "real beauty of a shiner." Only item 3 requires the listener to use his or her general knowledge to form bridging assumptions between items of information in the narrative.

In contrast, the questions testing implied information from the garage sale narrative (p. 13) all require the listener to use his or her general knowledge to construct relationships that are not stated in the narrative. The information tested by question 2 does not appear in the text in any form. It is only recoverable by inferring that if the women spent an entire day putting prices on things, there must have been a large number of them. Likewise for question 3 which depends on establishing a logical connection between sitting in the shade and drinking iced tea with the probable temperature on the day of the sale. Question 7 requires the listener to make a logical connection between having a father-in-law and being married. Question 8 is recoverable from the phrase "no-good father-in-law," and from the implication that the man doesn't want his father-in-law to stay very long.

At this time we feel that the inconsistent effects of directness on brain-damaged listeners' comprehension across studies is explainable by differences in the difficulty of the inferences required. Systematic study of the relationship between the difficulty of inferences and brain-damaged listeners' ability to construct them would be an appropriate direction for further study.

In summary, the results of studies of brain-damaged adults' discourse comprehension suggest that the salience of information has strong effects on discourse comprehension for both non-brain-damaged and brain-damaged listeners. Even when main ideas are implied, rather than stated, both non-brain-damaged and brain-damaged listeners are likely to comprehend them. Details, on the other hand, generally are comprehended less well than main ideas and are more strongly affected by whether they are stated or implied. Because the main ideas in discourse, taken together, best represent the overall meaning of the discourse, missing main ideas, whether stated or implied, seem likely to leave relatively obvious gaps in the overall sense of the discourse. Missing details, however, would be less noticeable, because their absence is less likely to seriously affect the overall meaning of the discourse. Consequently, when main ideas are not stated, but only suggested by discourse, listeners are likely to construct the associated inferences. When details are only suggested, listeners may or may not construct the associated inferences.

Whether listeners construct inferences may depend on how hard they are working at comprehending a particular sample of discourse. Cohen (1979) suggested that normal older listeners' ability to construct inferences may deteriorate as processing demands increase. Cohen studied the effects of speech rate on young and old non-brain-damaged listeners' comprehension of short narratives. The listeners were further subdivided into high-education and low-education groups. (The results for the young listeners will not be reported or discussed here.) The narratives were spoken at either 120 words per minute (wpm) or 200 wpm. Subjects answered both *verbatim questions* and *inference questions* about the narratives. Verbatim questions required subjects to reproduce or para-phrase facts from the narratives, whereas inference questions required subjects to draw inferences based on information that was stated in the narratives. Older high-education subjects correctly answered significantly fewer inference questions when narratives were spoken at 200 wpm than when they were spoken at 120 wpm, but their performance on verbatim questions was not affected by speech rate. Speech rate did not affect older low-education subjects' comprehension of either verbatim questions or inferential questions—probably because they were performing at near chance levels on inferential questions in both speech rate conditions. Cohen concluded that making inferences "is a vulnerable stage of pro-cessing which tends to drop out when total processing demands exceed capacity" (p. 419).

EFFECTS OF SPEECH RATE ON BRAIN-DAMAGED LISTENERS' DISCOURSE COMPREHENSION

Speech rate also appears to affect brain-damaged listeners' comprehension of information from spoken discourse. Brain damage, like normal aging, seems to diminish the rate at which the brain can process information. The concept of processing capacity has received considerable attention in the comprehension literature in recent years, particularly in "resource allocation" models of comprehension. In such models, comprehension, like other cognitive activities, is said to be served by a limited-capacity system with a finite pool of processing resources (McNeil & Kimelman, 1986). This finite pool of resources is drawn on for all cognitive operations, and investing resources in one comprehension process (e.g., syntactic analysis) means that fewer resources are available for other comprehension processes (e.g., drawing inferences).[6] When the demands for processing resources exceed the available pool, performance deteriorates.

Pashek and Brookshire (1982) had aphasic and non-brain-damaged subjects listen to and answer questions about 12 expository paragraphs. Six were read at slow rate (120 wpm) and 6 were read at fast rate (150 wpm).

---

[6]Likewise, investing resources in cognitive processes other than comprehension (e.g., formulating a verbal response) diminishes the amount of resources available for comprehension.

(They also manipulated the emphatic stress placed on important information in the paragraphs, but that is not of concern herein.) Aphasic listeners answered significantly more questions correctly when paragraphs were spoken at slow rate than when they were spoken at fast rate, regardless of the severity of their sentence comprehension impairments, as measured by a short version of the Token Test (DeRenzi & Vignolo, 1962).

Nicholas and Brookshire (1986), in a more extensive study, found that the rate at which discourse is spoken, listeners' familiarity with the discourse, and the severity of aphasic listeners' comprehension impairments all may interact with the effects of salience and directness to affect comprehension. They had non-brain-damaged, aphasic, and right-hemisphere-damaged adults listen to 10 stories and then answer questions that tested stated and implied main ideas and stated and implied details. Each subject heard 5 stories at slow speech rate (110–130 wpm) and 5 stories at fast speech rate (190–210 wpm). To assess the effects of familiarity with the materials on comprehension, the brain-damaged subjects were tested twice, with 7 to 10 days intervening between Session 1 and Session 2.

Non-brain-damaged subjects made almost no errors on main ideas, whether stated or implied, and speech rate did not significantly affect their performance on main ideas. Non-brain-damaged subjects comprehended main ideas better than details in both fast rate and slow rate condition. However, fast speech rate had significant negative effects on their comprehension of implied details. Their comprehension of implied details was significantly worse than their comprehension of stated details in fast rate condition, but when stories were read at slow rate, there was essentially no difference between their comprehension of stated and implied details.

Both aphasic and right-hemisphere-damaged subjects comprehended main ideas better than details, regardless of the rate at which the stories were read. Familiarity with the stories did not change this relationship— the difference between main ideas and details was significant both in Session 1 and Session 2. Directness had no significant effect on brain-damaged subjects' comprehension of main ideas—their comprehension of stated main ideas did not differ from their comprehension of implied main ideas in either session. However, directness significantly affected brain-damaged subjects' comprehension of details—they comprehended stated details significantly better than they comprehended implied details in both sessions. The rate at which stories were read affected comprehension of main ideas only for a subgroup of 7 aphasic patients with Boston Diagnostic Aphasia Examination (BDAE) (Goodglass & Kaplan, 1983) auditory comprehension subtest percentiles below 80. These subjects comprehended main ideas significantly better in slow rate condition than in fast rate condition. In contrast, rate significantly affected both aphasic and right-hemisphere- damaged subjects comprehension of details in unfamiliar stories—they comprehended details better in slow rate condition than in fast rate condition in Session 1. However, familiarity with the stories reduced the rate effect. In Session 2 there was no significant effect of rate on comprehension of details for any brain-damaged group.

These results suggest that resource allocation models may appropriately be applied to aphasic listeners' comprehension of discourse. Comprehension of main ideas appears less vulnerable to shortages in processing resources than comprehension of details (perhaps because comprehension of main ideas requires fewer resources). Although aphasic listeners may have an overall reduction in the resources available for comprehension, they perform almost as well as non-brain-damaged listeners in comprehension of main ideas. Furthermore, the effects of fast speech rate (which hypothetically increases processing demands) on comprehension of the main ideas in discourse appear to be minimal, unless the available processing resources are substantially diminished by aphasia. Comprehension of the details in discourse appears more vulnerable to shortages in processing resources than comprehension of main ideas—brain-damaged listeners' comprehension of details usually suffers when discourse is spoken at a fast rate. As Cohen (1979) has suggested, making inferences seems to be particularly vulnerable to shortages in processing resources—brain-damaged listeners' comprehension of implied details is significantly worse than their comprehension of stated details, even at slow rate.

The results of these studies also suggest that one can lighten the processing load for listeners in several ways. The most dependable way to make information in discourse easier to comprehend and retain is to increase its salience through redundancy and elaboration. Directly stating information, rather than requiring listeners to construct inferences, also is likely to improve its comprehension and retention. Slowing the rate at which the discourse is spoken also may have positive effects on compre-hension, especially for new information that does not have strong contex-tual support.

CONCLUSION

The studies reviewed in this chapter demonstrate that sentence comprehension and discourse comprehension, at least in part, call on different processes and that performance on one does not predict performance on the other. These studies also demonstrate that brain-damaged (aphasic and right-hemisphere-damaged) listeners, like normal listeners, rely more on knowledge-based processes than on text-based processes when comprehending spoken discourse that deals with familiar topics. They comprehend and retain the main ideas from discourse better than the details and stated information better than implied information.

However, numerous questions remain unanswered. We do not know how (or if) the overall severity of comprehension impairment influences brain-damaged listeners' use of knowledge-based and text-based processes, because studies of brain-damaged listeners' discourse comprehension have included mostly persons whose comprehension impairment is mild to moderate. We do not know whether the similarities between aphasic and non-brain-damaged persons' discourse comprehension reported in the literature would persist if their comprehension were tested with recall tasks rather than the recognition tasks that have been the norm to date. We also do not know to what extent the difficulties aphasic listeners have on inferential questions result from problems in constructing inferences per se or result from problems in retrieving the relevant information from memory to construct the inferences.

Nevertheless, what we know about aphasic listeners' discourse comprehension is encouraging. It suggests that most aphasic listeners probably do better at comprehending discourse in daily life than traditional sentence-level tests of comprehension suggest that they should. It suggests that aphasic listeners usually are quite good at getting the main ideas from spoken discourse, even though they may miss some of the details. It suggests that aphasic listeners can deduce at least some of the inferences that normal speakers expect their listeners to construct and that providing information at a slower rate may help them to make inferences that they might otherwise miss, especially when the information is complex or unfamiliar.

Finally, what we know about aphasic listeners' discourse comprehension poses a challenge for clinicians, because it suggests that treatment programs for auditory comprehension impairments in aphasia should move away from drill on single-sentence messages toward comprehension of materials that provide the structure and contextual support that resemble more closely what the aphasic listener is likely to encounter in daily life. Along with changes in how we treat auditory comprehension impairments in aphasia must come standardized instruments for measuring both the extent and the nature of their deficiencies in comprehension of spoken discourse.

ACKNOWLEDGMENTS

Preparation of this chapter was supported by the Medical Research Service, Department of Veterans Affairs and by the Research Service, Minneapolis Veterans Affairs Medical Center.

REFERENCES

Adams, M. J., & Collins, A. (1979). A schema-theoretic view of reading. In R. O. Freedle (Ed.), *New directions in discourse processing*. Norwood, NJ: Ablex.

Armus, S. R., Brookshire, R. H., & Nicholas, L. E. (1989). Aphasic and non-brain-damaged adults' knowledge of scripts for common situations. *Brain and Language, 36*, 518–528.

Bower, G. H., Black, J. B., & Turner, T. J. (1979). Scripts in memory for text. *Cognitive Psychology, 11*, 177–220.

Boyle, M., & Canter, G. J. (1986). Verbal context and comprehension of difficult sentences by aphasic adults: A methodological problem. In R. H. Brookshire (Ed.), *Clinical aphasiology: Conference proceedings, 1986*. Minneapolis, MN: BRK Publishers.

Brookshire, R. H., & Nicholas, L. E. (1984). Comprehension of directly and indirectly stated main ideas and details in discourse by brain-damaged and non-brain-damaged listeners. *Brain and Language, 21*, 21–36.

Brookshire, R. H., & Nicholas, L. E. (1993). *The Discourse Comprehension Test*. Tucson, AZ: Communication Skill Builders.

Cannito, M., Jarecki, J., & Pierce, R. S. (1986). Effects of thematic structure on syntactic comprehension in aphasia. *Brain and Language, 27*, 38–49.

Caplan, D., & Evans, K. L. (1990). The effects of syntactic structure on discourse comprehension in patients with parsing impairments. *Brain and Language, 39*, 206–234.

Carpenter, P. A., & Just, M. A. (1977). Integrative processes in comprehension. In D. LaBerge & S. J. Samuels (Eds.), *Basic processes in reading: Perception and comprehension* (pp. 217–242). Hillsdale, NJ: Lawrence Erlbaum.

Clark, H. H. (1977). Inferences in comprehension. In D. LaBerge & S. J. Samuels (Eds.), *Basic processes in reading: Perception and comprehension*. Hillsdale, NJ: Lawrence Erlbaum.

Clark, H. H., & Haviland, S. E. (1977). Comprehension and the given-new contract. In R. O. Freedle (Ed.), *Discourse comprehension and production*. Norwood, NJ: Ablex.

Cohen, G. (1979). Language comprehension in old age. *Cognitive Psychology, 11*, 412–429.

DeRenzi, E., & Vignolo, L. (1962). The Token Test: A sensitive test to detect receptive disturbances in aphasics. *Cortex, 85*, 655–678.

Glucksberg, S., & Danks, J. H. (1975). *Experimental psycholinguistics: An introduction*. Hillsdale, NJ: Lawrence Erlbaum.

Goodglass, H., & Kaplan, E. (1983). *The Boston Diagnostic Aphasia Examination*. Boston: Lea & Febiger.

Hough, M. S., Pierce, R. S., & Cannito, M. P. (1989). Contextual influences in aphasia: Effects of predictive versus nonpredictive narratives. *Brain and Language, 36*, 325–334.

Katsuki-Nakamura, J., Brookshire, R. H., & Nicholas, L. E. (1988). Comprehension of monologues and dialogues by aphasic listeners. *Journal of Speech and Hearing Disorders, 53*, 408–415.

Kintsch, W. (1974). *The representation of meaning in memory*. Hillsdale, NJ: Lawrence Erlbaum.

McNeil, M. R., & Kimelman, M. D. Z. (1986). Toward an integrative information-processing structure of auditory comprehension and processing in adult aphasia. In L.L. LaPointe (Ed.), Aphasia: Nature and assessment. *Seminars in Speech and Language, 7*, 123–146.

Meyer, B. J. F. (1975). *The organization of prose and its effect on memory*. Amsterdam: North Holland.

Meyer, B. J. F., & McConkie, G. W. (1973). What is recalled after hearing a passage? *Journal of Educational Psychology, 65,* 109–117.

Nicholas, L. E., & Brookshire, R. H. (1983). Syntactic simplification and context: Effects on sentence comprehension by aphasic adults. In R. H. Brookshire (Ed.), *Clinical aphasiology: Conference proceedings, 1983*. Minneapolis, MN: BRK Publishers.

Nicholas, L. E., & Brookshire, R. H. (1986). Consistency of the effects of rate of speech on brain-damaged adults' comprehension of narrative discourse. *Journal of Speech and Hearing Research, 29,* 462, 470.

Pashek, G. V., & Brookshire, R. H. (1982). Effects of rate of speech and linguistic stress on auditory paragraph comprehension. *Journal of Speech and Hearing Research, 25,* 377–382.

Pierce, R. S. (1988). Influence of prior and subsequent context on comprehension in aphasia. *Aphasiology, 2,* 577–582.

Pierce, R. S., & Beekman, L. (1985). Effects of linguistic and extralinguistic context on semantic and syntactic processing in aphasia. *Journal of Speech and Hearing Research, 28,* 250–254.

Pierce, R. S., & Wagner, C. (1985). The role of context in facilitating syntactic decoding in aphasia. *Journal of Communication Disorders, 18,* 203–214.

Roman, M., Brownell, H. H., Potter, H. H., Seibold, M. S., & Gardner, H. (1987). Script knowledge in right-hemisphere-damaged and in normal elderly adults. *Brain and Language, 31,* 151–170.

Rumelhart, D. E. (1975). Notes on a schema for stories. In D. G. Bobrow & A. Collins (Eds.), *Representation and understanding* (pp. 211–236). New York: Academic Press.

Schank, R. C., & Abelson, R. P. (1977). *Scripts, plans, goals, and understanding*. New York: Lawrence Erlbaum.

Stachowiak, F., Huber, W., Poeck, K., & Kerschensteiner, M. (1977). Text comprehension in aphasia. *Brain and Language, 4,* 177–195.

van Dijk, T. A. (1980). *Macrostructures*. Hillsdale, NJ: Lawrence Erlbaum.

van Dijk, T. A., & Kintsch, W. (1983). *Strategies of discourse comprehension*. New York: Academic Press.

Waller, M. R., & Darley, F. L. (1978). The influence of context on the auditory comprehension of paragraphs by aphasic subjects. *Journal of Speech and Hearing Research, 21,* 732–745.

Wegner, M. L., Brookshire, R. H., & Nicholas, L. E. (1984). Comprehension of main ideas and details in coherent and noncoherent discourse by aphasic and nonaphasic listeners. *Brain and Language, 21,* 37–51.

Winograd, T. (1977). A framework for understanding discourse. In M. A. Just & P. A. Carpenter (Eds.), *Cognitive processes in comprehension*. Hillsdale, NJ: Lawrence Erlbaum.

CHAPTER 9

Selected Aspects of Narratives in Polish-Speaking Aphasics as Illustrated by Aesop's Fables

HANNA K. ULATOWSKA, MARIA SADOWSKA,
JAN KORDYS, AND DANUTA KADZIELAWA

SOCIAL FUNCTION OF FABLES

The use of fables in neurolinguistic investigations of discourse in aphasia can be justified in terms of the model character of this class of texts. In nonliterate societies, folk tales, the category described in the classic book by Propp (1968), function as a specific model of cohesive text which members of society use to form other texts. The basis of cohesion in the fables of ancient folklore consists of strict adherence to action sequences which lead to a given result, making a fable similar to a game. This feature, together with other features described below, makes it possible to treat texts of fables as cognitive representations of certain complex situations and behaviors similar to those that readers of a fable may have encountered in their lives.

In the past, peasant families told fables at a specific developmental stage of child rearing, namely, after the child learned to solve riddles. If a riddle is considered a task of looking for a concrete solution, then a fable represents the next stage of acquiring semiotic and cognitive structures by utilizing language as a means of transmitting and preserving tradition. Understanding fables involves grasping the meaning and keeping in memory sequences of actions. It does not solely depend on the actual actions, but on modeling an imagined solution which allows one to adopt the perspective of the main character in the narrative (Revzin, 1975).

The function of modeling actions is one of the most important tasks of the mythology of illiterate cultures. Mythology creates a model of the world for a given collective group. The model is realized through various semiotic systems (i.e., myths, rituals, kinship systems) which act either on a conscious level or on the unconscious aspects of the psyche. A model of the world conceived as a program for action for an individual and a collective group defines a set of rules and motivations for acting on the world and for regulating the life of the collective group (Ivanov & Toporov, 1965). This type of model ensures the stability of a society because it preserves in a constant form the basic agreed standards. Hence, the model allows for consistency and predictability of actions and for formulating institutional methods for resolving conflicts and achieving goals useful to a given community.

The modeling of situations and actions inherent in the structure of a fable is one of its most important characteristics. Functionally, a fable resembles a myth. A fable reveals the order of reality and provides a model for actions. Thus, the assumed temporal space of a fable becomes a model of the world in that fables' events are repeated ad infinitum following the same principles, which are conventionally prescribed. A fable represents a general model that contains scenarios dealing with specific aspects of peoples' lives and describing specific situations (Abramowska, 1991).

However, some fables contain tasks and goals outside of the conventional rules, which entail high risks or require unconventional methods and individual characteristics. The hero who undertakes such tasks represents a different model than the model described above in that this latter model presupposes the use of methods contrary to conventional schemes. In literary texts and myths, the activities of such "tricksters" and mythological cheaters are regarded by ordinary people as paradoxical violations of the norm, completely unjustifiable by common sense. The importance of this trickster's success is derived not only from its information value (low probability) and emotional value (everybody can be defeated, but only an exceptional person such as a trickster can win), but also from its cognitive value. Taking a risk and being victorious shows the importance of searching for unconventional solutions, which enrich the traditional repertoire. According to Toporov, this type of cognitive activity characterizes not only every tradition and collective group but also the mental structure of every individual (Levi-Strauss, 1991; Toporov, 1987). The duality of cognitive mechanisms relying on conventional norms and on the actions falling outside these norms has also been discussed by Minsky (1985) in his book *The Society of Mind*. Minsky notes that storing all of these mechanisms in one's memory would require an enormous memory capacity. Therefore, a more convenient solution would be to partially transfer these mechanisms to a collective level and preserve them in the form of texts.

STRUCTURAL FEATURES OF FABLES

Fables are particularly useful in investigations of narrative competence due to certain structural features. The first feature is a paradigmatic set of characters (the actants in a fable) who are unambiguously classified and who possess capabilities for performing specific actions. The choice of animals as main characters (possessing a human way of thinking, feeling, and acting) enables a specific interplay between the general and particular since the name of an animal can be associated with a specific animal or an entire species. This feature enables one to perform a reverse operation in the construction of a moral, namely, transforming an animal character into a human character. All characteristics of the fable's actants (assigned conventionally to specific animals and also used to describe human characteristics) are carefully selected and appropriately matched to allow a high predictability of outcome (Abramowska, 1991). Note that the character's mental structure is considered not as a dynamic structure but as a sum of these characteristics. The plot of a fable consists of a sequence of simple functions (actions of a given character) that are ordered according to four links: exposition, motivation to act, action itself and, unexpected outcome. This schema, when filled, does not undergo any changes to achieve an artistic form of a text. In that sense, Aesop's fables exist only at the level of deep structure and not at the surface structure level (Paduceva, 1984). Thus, the primary purpose of a fable is to transmit the main point or semantic meaning rather than to express its literary form through the surface structure. This feature is of special importance in investigating responses of various populations in experimental studies of fables. This specific structure is reflected in the reduction of all temporal-spatial references, generalization, and ellipticity of the world that is represented. The primary function is to make the comprehender of a fable focus on the narrative structure itself. Thus, fables do not represent only a concrete text with specific linguistic and narrative organization; they represent a metatext with universal principles of organization both at the level of plot and at the level of represented interactions.

TYPES OF FABLES ACCORDING TO METIS

In fables involving a trickster or mythological character, the basic task for the comprehender of a fable is to grasp the "fabular knot," that is, the structure of the deceit or trick which the hero uses. The texts of fables allow an investigation of this type of comprehension. In some Aesop's fables, the plots refer to archaic mythological concepts and related cognitive categories which organize the structure of the texts (Gasparov, 1971). In Greek mythology, the actions characteristic of the trickster are associated with a specific type of practical intelligence called "metis." The hero utilizing metis chooses an unconventional means of deceit or trick. The art of metis involves a specific time and space and is used in an unstable situation when complex actions are applied based on adapting to changing circumstances, on foreseeing the unforeseen, and on perceptiveness and smartness (Detienne & Vernant, 1974).

The Aesop's fables selected for the investigation described later in the chapter exhibit the operation of different types of metis; one type of metis is achieved by concealing and camouflaging one's true nature (Raven and Pigeons) or by pretending and creating illusions. In another category of fables, metis is exhibited through the use of language: enticement through speech (Raven and Fox) or through literal and metaphoric uses of speech resulting in a complex interplay between words and actions (Old Woman and Doctor). This interrelationship between speech and action was described by Detienne (1967). As a result of this interplay, the seemingly weaker actant succeeds by utilizing metis in a more efficient way.

Utilization of metis can lead to success or failure in terms of fulfilling the goal of the protagonist. For example, in the fables Raven and Fox and Old Woman and Doctor, the basic theme is "triumphant metis," that is, achieving a goal such as getting food or exposing the dishonest doctor; whereas in the fables Raven and Pigeons and Two Donkeys, metis leads to failure (see Appendix for the fables). Moreover, in fables, the goals of different protagonists produce a double perspective. For example, from the perspective of the fox in Raven and Fox, the action unfolds according to the following scheme: A fox saw a raven with a piece of cheese; he decided to get the cheese; he used flattery; he achieved his goal. The scheme from the perspective of the raven has the following form: A raven saw a fox; he listened to his flattery; he decided to show off his voice; he lost the cheese. In listening to the fable, the listener's attention shifts from the fox to the raven, a feature which Gasparov (1968) finds rather unusual for this type of fable.

TEXT TRANSFORMATION TASKS

There are various ways to transform the information contained in a fable to reveal levels of understanding of the various aspects of meaning. These transformations are governed by rules of macrostructure which manipulate information (van Dijk, 1980).

RETELLING AND SUMMARY

Retelling a fable constitutes the simplest task cognitively and, provided that a fable is short and simple, can be reproduced either verbatim or with minimal transformations of information, primarily through deletion.

Summarizing a fable, however, is cognitively more complex than retelling a fable. Summarizing, if done properly, involves not only deletion of information, in its simplest form, but also construction of new structures often produced by generalization. It is easier to see whether a reader understands the meaning of a fable in a summary than in retelling since, ideally, only essential or core information should be included in the summary. Therefore, the process of selection of information is of great importance in producing a summary.

IDENTIFICATION AND JUSTIFICATION OF THE MAIN CHARACTER

There are two components in the task of identifying the main character. The first is the selection of one character from a set of characters occurring in the fable, and the second is justifying one's choice of the character. At a surface level, one can state one's choice on the basis of the shear frequency of occurrence of a character, or on intuitive grounds based on his perceptual saliency, or on the level of deep meaning based on his contributions to the primary function of the fable, its didactic function, that is, moral. The main character can be either a winner who should be praised or a loser who should be admonished. In the latter case, the choice depends on the type of metis, that is, whether the trickster operates through camouflage and illusion or through speech and metaphoric use of language.

Consequently, a correct identification of the fable's main character with an appropriate justification requires proper assessment of whether a given character is the center of action, whether he is the instigator of the events, or whether a moral or a lesson can be derived from his actions. These tasks involve metalinguistic processes and, therefore, are cognitively complex. Although an identification of the main hero in simple fables with a small number of characters may be quite simple and may require only a surface level of comprehension, the task of justification often requires deeper processing of both the content of the fable and knowledge about the real world.

GIST AND MORAL

Grasping the gist or main idea can be regarded as a process of selection based on knowledge and hypotheses that the reader possesses, of information contained in the text which the reader considers the most essential, and of the underlying structure of a given text (Sperber & Wilson, 1986). When deriving a gist, a person is concerned less with the structure of the message than with the person's preferences that reveal individual ways of organizing experience.

Understanding the moral of a fable, on the other hand, should be regarded as a different cognitive process than that of formulating a gist, although sometimes the products may be similar or the same. Whereas the gist is more subjective, the moral is governed by rules similar to those governing the formation of a fable in that the moral is based on collective rules and wisdom familiar to all members of a given group.

Morals have specific semantic quantifiers and semantic and syntactic forms. The predicate of a moral is usually expressed in the present tense, which is unmarked as to time reference, and is often modified by "usually" and "always." Often, predicates have an imperative form or occur in an impersonal form. Similarly, persons and items occurring in morals are often modified by the quantifiers "every" or "all" to refer to the producer and the receiver of a moral. This lack of specificity of the basic grammatical categories is relevant to the interpretation and use of morals. Avoiding communicative precision facilitates achieving a didactic effect. Hence, this low specificity and vagueness is a testimony to the tendency to educate an individual by a collective experience and by demonstrating the principles that govern society (Nikolaeva, 1990).

The cognitive aspect of Aesop's fables is related to metis and is often didactic in nature: The narrator is teaching and the receiver of the fable is learning. This didactic function of fables, usually external to the text, is achieved by the speaking and acting characters. The heroes personify different values and opinions that undergo verification in the course of the action. Some of the values are ridiculed and rejected. Those that remain constitute the didactic program of a fable. The first stage of the program requires grasping the general principle. The next stage in the didactic program involves transformation from the world of animals to the world of humans. Finally, the listener must match the general principle against analogous situations found in personal experience (Abramowska, 1991).

The receiver of a fable, however, can use different cognitive strategies in the process of forming a moral. One can either interpret a fable in the light of similar cases from one's own experience or one can compare the actions of animals to those of a specific individual or a group of individuals. One can also focus on the model itself, that is, on metis in the action schema or on metis in the use of language. However, it is essential to grasp the use of language to derive the moral. In the Old Woman and Doctor fable, the woman's utterances contain a play on words that constitutes the finale of the fable. This play on words requires simultaneous comprehension of both literal and metaphoric meaning. Moreover, it is necessary for one to get to a metatextual level in order to reach an interpretation of a fable. In formulating a gist and a moral, one can adopt the perspective of one character in a fable, for example, a victor, or one can also shift perspective in that the gist can be formulated from the perspective of a victor and a moral from the perspective of a victim or vice versa.

AN INVESTIGATION USING FABLES IN APHASIA

PURPOSE OF THE STUDY

Investigations of Aesop's fables in aphasia are of particular importance since the fables constitute texts in which retrieving the deep meaning of the fable is possible only when both linguistic and experiential information is taken into account. The processing of this type of text may reveal strategies that aphasics utilize in their manipulation of these two different types of information in the process of comprehending and producing discourse. In this section, an investigation is described which focused on the cognitive strategies used by aphasic subjects in interpreting Aesop's fables. The analyses described pertain primarily to the semantic and pragmatic aspects of the responses. The semantic aspect consists of operations, that is, the text transformations, performed on the meaning components of the original texts in formulating the main idea or gist, the moral, and the identification and justification of the choice of the main character in the derived texts. The semantic operations involve recovering the "deep" meaning of a fable that includes various types of social interactions expressed through a limited number of combinations of simple actions of the characters in the fable. The pragmatic aspect of the analysis is revealed in both the external relationship between the subject and the text, that is, the cognitive strategies the reader uses to understand the text, and also in the internal organization of the moral he provides that determines the rules of interpersonal behavior. The analyses presented here are preliminary and descriptive.

EXPERIMENTAL STIMULI

The ability to transform texts of Aesop's fables was examined using the subjects' responses to the following tasks: (1) retelling, (2) summarizing, (3) identification of the main character, (4) formulating the gist, and (5) formulating a moral. Four fables were selected for the present investigation based on specific criteria. Fables with clarity of content, potential ease of formulating a moral and suitable length, not exceeding 20 propositions, were selected. When necessary, fables were simplified in conceptual and linguistic form and freed of archaic terms. The fables consisted of the following: Raven and Fox (18 propositions), Raven and Pigeons (13 propositions), Two Donkeys (15 propositions), and Old Woman and Doctor (15 propositions) (see Appendix).

The selected fables can be subdivided by type according to the following criteria: (a) more (Raven and Fox) or less (Two Donkeys) conventional structure; (b) type of metis of the main hero performing specific actions or using language, especially metaphoric language (Old Woman and Doctor); (c) effect of the actions of hero in victory (Raven or Fox) or in defeat (Raven and Pigeons); and (d) presence or absence of elements of humor. For the discussion presented in this chapter, the first three criteria are the most important because they provide insight into whether the structure of a text has an effect on an aphasic patient's ability to transform it.

The experiment was performed in a written modality. In this way, the subjects performed under optimal conditions, that is, unlimited time for the execution of the tasks. The subjects could read each fable several times, but they had to generate their responses without looking at the stimulus fables. They were allowed to use dictionaries. Before starting the tasks, care was taken to ensure that the subjects understood the requirements of the tasks.

SUBJECTS

The subjects selected for this study included 18 aphasic patients, (8 women and 10 men) ranging in age from 25 to 70 years. All were speakers of Polish who were seen for therapy in the outpatient clinic of the Medical School in Warsaw. Ten aphasics had a high school education, and 8 had a college education. All subjects suffered a single cerebrovascular accident (CVA) and were right handed. The etiology was occlusion in 10 cases, aneurysm in 5, post-traumatic hematoma in 2, and viral meningitis in 1. Nine subjects exhibited anterior lesions and the other 9 exhibited posterior lesions in the left hemisphere. Severity of aphasia ranged from 2.5 to 5 as measured by the Severity Scale of the Boston Diagnostic Aphasia Examination (Goodglass & Kaplan, 1983). On cognitive tests, aphasic subjects scored a mean of 22.6 (range 14–23) on the Ravens Coloured Progressive Matrices Test, a mean of 11.0 (range 6–15) on the Picture Arrangement Subtest of the Wechsler Adult Intelligence Scale-Revised (WAIS-R), and a mean of 11.4 (range 6–19) on the Similarities Subtest (WAIS-R). Subjects were selected for the experiment on the basis of clinical assessment of suitability for this study. The subjects were assessed on their ability to produce discourse and on tasks of naming, comprehension of spoken and written language, that is, all abilities considered important for performing the experimental tasks. All selected subjects had good comprehension of spoken and written language. None of the subjects had any emotional problems or depression, and all were willing to participate in the study. The control group consisted of 18 subjects, ranging in age from 23 to 70 years. There were 9 women and 9 men. Five had a high school education and 13 had a college degree.

RESULTS

In this section, the global findings of the investigation are discussed first, followed by more specific results pertaining to the three tasks of identifying and justifying the choice of the main character, giving the gist, and giving the moral. Special emphasis is given to the qualitative aspect of the analysis, that is, the types of responses given with exemplifications. First, the basic terms used in the following section are defined. **Superstructures** are schemata for conventional text forms such as stories, procedures or scientific articles. Knowledge of these forms facilitates generating, remembering and reproducing information. **Macrostructure** of a text is a theoretical construct accounting for the global meaning of a text which may be expressed as the gist or the topic of a text. The macrostructure is generated by the application of the macrorules of deletion, construction, and generalization. The function of these rules is organizational. They delete redundant or irrelevant information or replace entailed or specific information with more general or abstract information (van Dijk, 1980).

The findings indicate that the separate tasks revealed different levels of difficulty despite the same experimental conditions, that is, written form and unlimited time. This was seen in both the results of the tasks and also in the reports given by the subjects when asked which task was the most difficult.

The easiest task was retelling the fable, followed in order by summarizing the fable, identifying the main character, giving the gist, and finally producing a moral. These tasks required, in varying degrees, utilization of the structure of the original stimulus fable. Thus, the highest degree of adherence to the stimulus was required in reconstructing the content of the story and the lowest degree of adherence to the stimulus was required in formulating the moral. The results of the investigation indicated that the degree of difficulty of the task was inversely related to its closeness to the stimulus fable. This finding is understandable since reconstructing the content requires manipulation of the superstructure of the text which, as previous studies have shown (Ulatowska & Sadowska, 1992), is relatively well preserved in the narrative competence of aphasic subjects. This reconstruction of text involves relatively simple processes of memory and language. In contrast, the tasks of producing the gist and moral entail manipulation of the macrostructure of the text, which involves complex cognitive processes of selection, generalization, and analogy.

RETELLING TASKS

The majority of the aphasic subjects retold the stimulus fables by retaining most of the essential information and preserving the superstructure and sequence of the actions of the fable. Aphasic subjects, especially those with more pronounced language deficits, produced simplified and reduced versions. Additionally, their fables were characterized by diminished coherence, for example, "Two mules carried bags on their shoulder. One had salt and one had sponge. The mule with salt cross the rivers and he lessened his burden. The other one also wanted to do the same and got into the water. However his burden was heavier" (Two Donkeys). The retellings could be differentiated primarily by the degree of cohesion they displayed. The aphasic subjects with mild language impairment produced the most cohesive texts.

SUMMARY TASKS

The data on the summary tasks are preliminary at this time because only a subset of the subjects was given the summarizing task. On the whole, the aphasic subjects had difficulty with this task in that their summaries showed minimal or no reduction and contained unnecessary details. Moreover, the strategies utilized on this task were different for aphasic patients as compared to the control subjects. Aphasic subjects primarily used the macrorule of deletion; whereas normal control subjects used the macrorule of generalization in producing summaries.

IDENTIFICATION OF THE MAIN CHARACTER

All aphasic subjects identified a main character in the fables; however, their choices were not always correct. In their choice of the main character, they showed a tendency toward identifying the concept of the main character with an actant who has a plan, reaches his goal, and becomes a winner. Consequently, the most appropriate responses were found for the fables where the main character was both the winner and the one who fulfilled his goal (e.g., Raven and Fox). The most frequent departures from the correct identification of the main character were in the fables Two Donkeys and Old Woman and Doctor. In the fable Two Donkeys, where paradoxically the main character is the one that suffers a defeat, correct identification of the main character is possible only through proper utilization of the macrostructure and grasping the deep meaning. Only two aphasic subjects (exhibiting mild aphasia) made the right choice with the appropriate identification, for example, "The main character is the donkey carrying on his back a bag with sponge. The animal did not think about the consequences of crossing the river by a donkey carrying on his back a bag of salt and of his crossing while carrying a bag full of sponge." Several aphasic subjects identified both donkeys as the main characters and could not give any justification for the choice or would give a justification in terms of specific actions performed by the animals and not in terms of the deep meaning of the whole fable, for example, "Two donkeys. One had salt and got out of the water and the other one had sponge and drowned." There also were responses identifying the main character as the winner as opposed to the victim around whom the main gist of the fable revolves, for example, "The first donkey because he carried salt and the bag became lighter," or "The first one because he was thinking what he was doing."

Difficulties with identifying the main character in the fable of the Old Woman and Doctor were presumably influenced by the patients' inabilities to understand metaphoric language and the humor contained in it. This problem is evident in the aphasic subjects' justifications of the choice of the main character, given in terms of specific actions and not in the metaphoric language used, for example, "The old woman—she could not see her possessions and refused to pay the doctor." There also were cases of identifying both characters instead of one, for example, "The old woman and the doctor, help to patients." Finally, cases of wrongly identifying the main character were found in aphasic subjects, for example, "The main character is the mean doctor who, not considering professional ethics and the poverty of the old woman, deprived her of all her possessions."

The most revealing aspect of the task of justifying the choice of the main character was the types of transformations of information contained in the original fable performed by the aphasic subjects. At one end of the continuum, aphasic subjects' responses with justifications utilized information explicitly stated in the fable in the form of a summary (the strictest adherence to the original stimulus), or a specific action or state related to setting or outcome, for example, "A raven—he painted his feathers white" (setting) "A fox because he got the cheese" (outcome). At the other end of the continuum, there were aphasic subjects' responses with justifications containing information characterized by certain amounts of inference or evaluation based on the information contained in the stimulus fable, for example, "The main character is the raven because he wanted to change his group but he did not succeed" (Raven and Pigeons).

Metatextual responses that reflect the overall structure and content of the stimulus fable belong to the inferential end of the continuum and were produced primarily by the control subjects. "The main character is a raven because his actions constitute the content of the story and his unfortunate experience" (Raven and Pigeons). It is important to note that it is the inferential responses that are related to the deep meaning of the fable and its didactic nature.

Although the aphasic subjects produced some justifications of the inferential and the metalinguistic types, they showed a clear tendency to give justifications formulated in terms of explicitly stated information (i.e., showing a minimal amount of transformation). This was especially evident in aphasic subjects with more severe language impairments. Only a few control subjects had difficulty identifying the main characters appropriately and giving appropriate justifications. The difficulties were observed predominately in the most difficult fables, Two Donkeys and Old Woman and Doctor. None of the control subjects gave justifications in the form of summaries or setting actions, although some justified their choice of the main character by the outcome action. Interestingly, some of the control subjects cited two main characters, justifying their choice in terms of the relationship and the interaction between them from which the gist of the fable could be derived, for example, "The main characters are fox and raven. The first one had an ingenious idea, the other one was defeated through his vanity" (Raven and Fox); "The main characters are two donkeys since their actions are the basis for teaching the lesson" (Two Donkeys). These types of responses were not found in the aphasic subjects. Thus, the findings of the analysis indicated that the performance of the aphasic subjects and normal controls varied along an intratextual and extratextual response continuum.

CONSTRUCTIONS OF GIST AND MORAL

The findings of the analysis of gists and morals are discussed together because of the relationship between them. Inability to give a gist or moral or the giving of inappropriate gists and morals occurred only in aphasic subjects. Two aphasic subjects were unable to give gists and seven aphasic subjects were unable to give the morals of different fables. As it was in the task of identifying the main character, the structure of the stimulus fable was an important factor in the success rate on these tasks. The fables with stereotypic situations such as a proverbially sly fox outwitting a less intelligent animal were the easiest (Raven and Fox); whereas fables with more complex plots (Two Donkeys) or with metaphorical language (Old Woman and Doctor) were the most difficult for both producing a gist and a moral. Although the fables do also differ along a dimension of familiarity, that is, Raven and Fox being more familiar and Two Donkeys being less familiar, familiarity was not explored in this study. It is important to note that all aphasic subjects who produced responses had a notion of what a gist and moral were even if their responses were different than those of the normal subjects.

Only aphasic subjects produced gists and morals that utilized only information explicitly stated in the stimulus fable. Surprisingly, this was particularly apparent in one aphasic subject with an anterior lesion and with a relatively mild level of language impairment, for example, "The gist is about fox and raven. He had cheese in his beak. The cheese fell to the ground, the fox grabbed it." Note that the essential component of flattery is missing from the response. Gists in the form of explicitly stated components such as setting were characteristic only of aphasic subjects, for example, "The old woman suffered of a disease of the eyes." Similarly, both gists and morals consisted of resolution components of the stimulus fables only in aphasic subjects, for example, "The raven lost his own kind by painting his feathers white." Both aphasic subjects and controls produced gists in the form of a theme, especially in the fables with stereotypic content or with a transparent message such as stealing (Raven and Fox; Old Woman and Doctor). It is important to note that the metis of a trickster is often identified as the gist of a fable by both populations, but especially in the aphasics as a form of didactic theme, for example, "cunning of fox," "flattery," "a trick of the raven," "lie," (Raven and Fox) which in more elaborate responses become lessons in the few aphasic subjects with only mild language impairments, for example, "Do not dress in somebody's else feathers" (Raven and Pigeons), "The compliments are not always true" (Raven and Fox).

Another type of response in gist formulation attesting to aphasics' sensitivity to didactic messages in fables was nongeneralized advice with close adherence to the explicitly stated information (e.g., "You should not paint yourself in the future" [Raven and Pigeons]). These types of responses are characteristic of aphasic types of morals, for example, "Do not behave like a donkey with a sponge because you will end up like him" (Two Donkeys). "If you have cheese in your mouth, keep your mouth shut" (Fox and Raven). The nongeneralized morals did not occur in control subjects. They produced primarily generalized morals often of the proverbial type. Only two aphasic subjects with mild language problems produced proverbial morals, for example, "Stolen things will not fatten you up," and "A smart man will always outfox a stupid man" (Fox and Raven). However, some aphasic subjects produced a reduced form of a moral in a proverbial saying pertaining to the features of the main character, for example, "Sly as a fox" (Fox and Raven) and "Stupid as a donkey" (Two Donkeys) as both gists and morals.

RECOVERING METIS

The findings reported in the above sections described the responses from the point of view of transformations of information contained in the stimulus fables in relation to that given on specific experimental tasks. The part that follows briefly describes the basic findings of semantic analysis to assess patients' success in recovering metis of the fables.

Nearly all aphasic subjects and all control subjects were able to correctly identify the concept of metis as a specific cognitive activity. The identification of metis was recovered from the analysis of responses in the justification of the main character and the formulations of gist and moral, for example, "The main character is a fox. Not being able to get food in an honest way he uses a *trick*. In a story the fox utilized weakness for flattery" (Raven and Fox); or "The main gist is the idea of a trick to get the cheese from the raven" (Raven and Fox); or "The moral is that one should not listen to flattery" (Raven and Fox).

The identification of metis was much easier in the fables where metis leads to victory of the main character and where the structure of the fable is relatively easy as in Raven and Fox. In the two fables where metis leads to failure, the recognition of metis was more difficult due to the additional complexities of the fable's plot. In both fables, metis consists of thoughtless imitation of the actions of somebody else (Two Donkeys) or camouflage (Raven and Pigeons). The recognition of metis emphasized the negative consequences of thoughtless imitation, for example, "The main gist is imitation" (Two Donkeys); "[Moral] Think twice before you do something" (Two Donkeys). The responses displayed different levels of abstraction, some of them being rather concrete or evaluative in nature, for example, "The main gist is that the donkey is stupid" (Two Donkeys). In the fable of Raven and Pigeons, most of the subjects grasped the idea of metis, although the responses varied again in the level of generalization; the aphasic subjects tended to produce concrete responses, for example, "The main gist is the *trick* of the raven"; [Moral] "Deceit will be uncovered sooner or later and one has to answer for one's actions"; [Gist] "If you are a raven you should not pretend to be a pigeon." It was clear from many responses that included contextual elements that the aspect of camouflage could have facilitated recovery of metis. This aspect was especially salient for the Polish subjects in view of the sociopolitical history of the country since under the Communist regime people were often forced to conceal their political and religious beliefs.

Finally, in the fable Old Woman and Doctor, metis is expressed through the language that provides the argumentation of the Old Woman in court and leads to her vindication. Only 2 aphasic subjects, in contrast with 13 control subjects, recognized the metaphorically expressed metis. One aphasic subject commented on humor resulting from the use of language in giving the gist of the fable, for example, "The hero—the old woman is great, even her disease did not defeat her and did not deprive her of her sense of humor." Several of the control subjects signaled the grasping of metis of the literal and metaphoric use of the verb "see" by putting it in quotation marks while formulating the gist of the fable. Some of the other responses of the control subjects were: "[The moral is] intelligence, sense of humor, creative problem solving is a way to live and overcome difficulties." Since the structure of the fable consists of two parallel planes, the plane of action of the dishonest doctor and his patient, the old woman, and the plane of verbal exchange containing metis, the subjects who did not grasp metis interpreted the fable in terms of the action plane, the script knowledge of the doctor-patient relationship, and their own experiential knowledge, for example, "One should not trust doctors in every aspect."

In summary, the above findings indicate that on the whole the aphasic and control subjects could recover the meaning of the metis in the fables; however, the aphasic subjects displayed a higher incidence of failures, especially on the fables with more complex structures which used metaphoric language and/or consisted of two parallel planes.

SINGLE VERSUS DOUBLE PERSPECTIVE

In reproducing any narrative text, one can adopt two perspectives: one that is associated with the objective of recounting the events from the perspective of an outside observer or one that represents a subjective point of view of a protagonist allowing one to reconstruct the psychological plans, motivations, and emotional states (Uspenskij, 1970). The tasks of this present experiment allowed the subject to change perspectives from an objective reconstruction of events in the fables to individualized and evaluative formulations of the gist and moral which required simultaneous outside perspectives and evaluations.

The findings indicated that both aphasic and control subjects were utilizing two different cognitive strategies in formulating gists and morals. One cognitive strategy was applied to the fables with metis leading to success where the same perspective was maintained in identifying main character and in formulating gist and moral, for example, "The main character is fox because he wants to get raven's cheese"; "The gist is the deceit of the fox"; "The moral is that the smart one always wins and the stupid one loses" (Raven and Fox). This strategy is referred to as a "single perspective." The occurrence of this "single perspective" was rare for either population. The other cognitive strategy, referred to as a "double perspective," occurred more often in both subject populations. A change of perspective was utilized when a moral was derived as a lesson for a victim from his own mistakes with a simultaneous negative evaluation of the victor in the gist, for example, "Gist is deceiving a raven by a smart fox in order to achieve something"; "A moral is one should not boast because one can lose everything."

In fables with the metis leading to defeat, both groups usually adopted a single perspective where both gist and moral referred to the fiasco of the actions of the main character, for example, "The gist of the fable is that the raven changed its color to look like pigeons"; The moral is that change of appearance for gains not always pays" (Raven and Pigeons). It is important to note, however, that although both populations of subjects displayed both single and double perspective in their gists and morals, their responses differed in the level of generalization, that is, in the degree to which they used intratextual as opposed to extratextual information.

CONCLUSION

The analysis of text transformations in this investigation revealed several important findings regarding the level of semantic processing in these aphasic patients. First, it appears that both aphasic subjects and control subjects were able to discover the deep meaning of the fables as manifested by: (a) their identification of a trickster and metis through proper interpretation of the roles of actors and the relations between actions and actors; (b) their recovery of a didactic component in their formulations of gists and morals; and (c) their ability to manipulate single and double perspective in their interpretations of actions.

Second, the aphasic subjects were sensitive to the structure of the fables. Their performance on discovering deep meaning depended upon the complexity of the stimulus fable. The easiest fable was the one with a stereotypic trickster whose metis led to a successful outcome, and the most difficult fable was the one which used metaphoric language. The same response tendency was observed in the control subjects.

Finally, analysis of text transformations at a pragmatic level revealed that aphasic subjects exhibited a strong and consistent tendency to utilize information contained in the stimulus fables (i.e., intratextual responses) in formulating gists and morals at a concrete level, often reducing the fable to the form of a single component taken from it. The control subjects tended to generalize the information contained in the stimulus fable to a much broader class of texts utilizing information derived from world knowledge, experiential knowledge, and conventionalized sets of values (extratextual responses). Although there was a quantitative difference in responses, both types of responses were found in the two populations, they differed primarily in the level of abstraction.

It is important to note that there was a tendency to resort to script knowledge and experiential knowledge in interpreting gists and morals in those fables with more complex structures, especially in the aphasic subjects. No clear difference was found in the performance of the aphasic subjects with anterior as compared to posterior lesions although concrete intratextual responses were characteristic of aphasic subjects with more severe language impairment. Concrete responses were produced also by aphasic subjects with only mild language impairments.

One of the aphasic subjects with a mild language impairment who volunteered for an in-depth 1-year study utilizing tasks of text transformation made an insightful comment about her experience with the tasks: "Summarizing is a real nightmare for me, a real pain. I do not know whether I will ever be able to break the text into segments and *abstract* the information contained in the main plots. As far as I remember I was quite good at abstracting, but I do not remember how I reduced information in the process of abstracting and generalizing the main points." However, the patient *did* improve in her ability to summarize texts and to abstract in the course of the study, so it is believed that the approach to narrative studies reported here may become useful if extended and applied to clinical practice.

REFERENCES

Abramowska, J. (1991). *Polska bajka ezopowa*. Poznan:Wydawnictwo Naukowe Uniwersytetu im. Adama Mickiewicza.

Detienne, M. (1967). *Les maitres de verite dans la Grece archaique*. Paris: Maspero.

Detienne, M., & Vernant, J. P. (1974). *Les ruses de l'intelligence. La metis des Grecs*. Paris: Flammarion.

Gasparov, M. L. (1968). "Sjuzet i ideologija v ezopovskix basnjax." *Vestnik drevnej istorii*, 2, 116–127.

Gasparov, M. L. (1971). *Anticnaja literaturnaja basnja* (Fedr i Babrij). Moskva: Izd. Nauka.

Goodglass, H., & Kaplan, E. (1982). *The assessment of aphasia and related disorders* (2nd ed.). Philadelphia: Lea and Febiger (Adapted and translated into Polish by Ulatowska, H. K., Sandowska, M., Grotecki, S. and Kaczmarek, B. 1984.)

Ivanov V. V., & Toporov, V. N. (1965). *Slavjanskie jazykovye modelirujuscie semioticeskie sistemy*. (*Drevnij period*). Moskva: Izd. Nauka.

Levi-Strauss, C. (1991). *Histoire de lynx*. Paris: Plon.
Minsky, M. (1985). *The society of mind*. New York: Simon and Schuster.
Nikolaeva, T. M. (1990). O principe "nekooperacii" i/ili okategorijax sociolingvisticeskogo vozdejstvija. In N. D. Arutjunova (Ed.), *Logiceskij analiz jazyka. Protivorecivost i anomal'nost' teksta* (pp. 225–235). Moskva: Izd. Nauka.
Paduceva, E. V. (1984). O semanticeskix svjazjax mezdu basnej i eo moralju (na materiale basen Ezopa). In G. L. Permyakov (Ed.), *Paremiologiceskie issledovanija* (pp. 223–251). Moskva: Izd. Nauka.
Propp, V. (1968). *Morphology of the folk-tale*. Austin and London: University of Texas Press.
Revzin, I. I. (1975). K obscesemioticeskomu istolkovaniju trex postulatov Proppa (analiz skazki i teorija svjaznosti teksta). In E. M. Meletinsky & S. Ju. Nekludov (Eds.), *Tipologiceskie issledovanija po fol'kloru. Sbornik statej pamjati V. J. Proppa (1895–1970)* (pp. 77–91). Moskva: Izd. Nauka.
Sperber D., & Wilson, D. (1986). *Relevance, communication and cognition*. Oxford: Basil Blackwell.
Toporov, V. N. (1987). Obraz trikstera v enisejskoj tradicii. In I. N. Gemujev & A. M. Sagalaev (Eds.), *Tradicionnye verovanja i byt narodov Sibiri XIX—nacalo XX veka* (pp. 5–27). Novosibirsk: Izd. Nauka.
Ulatowska, H. K., & Sadowska, M. (1992). Some observations on aphasic texts. In S. J. Hwang & W. R. Merrifield (Eds.), *Language in context: Essays for Robert E. Longacre* (pp. 51–66). Arlington: The Summer Institute of Linguistics and The University of Texas at Arlington.
Uspenskij, B. A. (1970). *Poetika kompozicii. Struktura xudozestvennogo teksta i tipologija kompozicionnoj formy*. Moskva: Izd. Iskusstvo.
van Dijk, T. A. (1980). *Macrostructures*. Hillside, NJ: Lawrence Erlbaum.

APPENDIX

FABLE WITH TRIUMPHANT METIS

RAVEN AND FOX

A raven was sitting on a tree holding a piece of cheese in his beak. A fox saw him and decided he wanted the cheese. He stood under the tree and began to praise the raven. He told the raven that he was a very beautiful bird and that he should become a king. The fox said that he would like to hear the raven's voice to be sure that the raven could give orders. Then the raven decided to show off his voice. He opened his beak and the cheese fell out onto the ground. The fox grabbed the cheese and ran away.

FABLES WITH METIS LEADING TO FAILURE

RAVEN AND PIGEONS

A hungry raven saw that pigeons in the pigeon coop had a lot of food. He painted his feathers white to look like them. But when he started to crow, they realized that he was a raven and chased him away. So he returned to his own kind. But the other ravens did not recognize him because he had his feathers painted white, so they chased him away.

TWO DONKEYS

Two donkeys were carrying heavy bags. One was carrying a bag of salt and the other was carrying a bag of sponges. They came to a river and wanted to get to the other side. The donkey carrying the salt got into the water first. When he got out of the water his bags were lighter because some of the salt dissolved. The other donkey also wanted to make his bundle lighter so he got into even deeper water. But his bags became much heavier because the sponges filled with water and the donkey drowned.

FABLE WITH METAPHORIC LANGUAGE

OLD WOMAN AND DOCTOR

A certain old woman suffered from a disease of the eyes. She called a doctor. The doctor came every day and rubbed some ointment on her eyes. When the old woman had her eyes closed, the doctor secretly carried her belongings out of her house. When he finished his treatment, he demanded a payment. The old woman refused. The doctor took her to court. In court, the old woman said that her vision was worse because before the treatment, she saw all of her belongings. But after the treatment, she could not see any of them. That is why she refused to pay.

CHAPTER 10

Discourse Production Patterns in Neurologically Impaired and Aged Populations
GUILA GLOSSER

All approaches to the study of natural discourse share the idea that it may be analyzed at multiple levels of structure, organization, and meaning. Implicit in this idea is the further notion that the different levels of analysis and representation of discourse correspond to different cognitive operations or abilities of speakers and listeners. To the extent that discourse analysis is assumed to yield structures and relations that are "psychologically real," it must also be assumed that these structures and representations correspond in some fashion to cognitive processes that are activated during actual discourse comprehension and production.

Because of its multilevel structure and the complexity of organizational relations in discourse, production and comprehension of discourse can be expected to involve the activation of many different linguistic and nonlinguistic cognitive processes. Analysis of discourse production and comprehension reveals the operation of these different cognitive processes (Fredriksen, Bracewell, Breuleux, & Renaud, 1990).

This chapter deals with two broad kinds of cognitive functions that are assumed to be involved in discourse processing: **Microlinguistic** functions refer to language-specific procedures for processing phonological and syntactic aspects of single words and sentences. These are procedures specialized for processing linguistic units in a relatively decontextualized manner. **Macrolinguistic** functions involve cognitive procedures for integrating linguistic and nonlinguistic knowledge for the purposes of maintaining the conceptual, semantic, and pragmatic organization of discourse. In general, microlinguistic processes are performed on smaller structural units at the level of the word or sentence, whereas macrolinguistic processes deal with larger suprasentential discourse units. The more critical distinction between micro- and macrolinguistic processes, however, is whether linguistic units are analyzed only with respect to an abstract system of context-independent rules dictating relationships among language forms or whether the language units are analyzed as contextual events in relation to other types of nonlinguistic textual and extratextual knowledge.

It has been claimed in some cognitive models of discourse processing that the mental computations necessary for microlinguistic processing of individual words and sentences do not overlap completely with those required for macrolinguistic processing of suprasentential units (van Dijk, 1980). Macrolinguistic processing is not viewed as a mere elaboration of microlinguistic processing, but rather these are considered to entail independent cognitive functions.

Studies of the discourse abilities of subjects with compromised brain functioning offer a means for testing the proposed distinctions and relationships among component cognitive processes hypothesized to be involved in the comprehension and production of discourse. Demonstrations of dissociable impairments in various component discourse abilities in patients with different types of brain damage provide evidence supportive of claims that these abilities reflect cognitive procedures that are not only psychologically distinct, but are also represented independently in the nervous system. In the studies reported below, data from subjects with focal and multifocal cerebral disorders were analyzed to explore the neuropsychological bases of microlinguistic and macrolinguistic cognitive abilities.

STUDY METHODS

To enable comparisons of discourse abilities among subjects with different kinds of compromised brain functioning who present with diverse profiles of cognitive and behavioral deficits, an informal discourse production task was developed. Subjects were asked to describe events of personal relevance in an informal interview format where there was minimal structuring or input from the interviewer. This method of assessment has the advantage that performance on a single task, descriptive discourse, can be used to simultaneously assess different aspects of language processing, involving both micro- and macrolinguistic functions. Measures were derived from conversational behavior, which constitutes a generally nonthreatening, familiar, high-frequency activity for all subjects. Unlike other methods of eliciting discourse, which are reliant on retelling stories or describing presented pictures, the language production deficits elicited in discourse descriptive of personal experiences are less confounded by cognitive impairments in other domains such as auditory comprehension, verbal memory, or visuospatial functions. Using naturally occurring verbal behaviors as the corpus for analysis facilitates direct comparisons among groups of neuropsychologically impaired subjects who may otherwise vary in their capacity to engage in formal test procedures.

The same methods of eliciting and analyzing discourse productions were used in all the studies reported below. Subjects were interviewed individually for about 10–20 minutes, during which time they were asked to describe family and work experiences. These two content areas were chosen to sample different types of descriptive discourse (Glosser, Wiener, & Kaplan, 1988). Description of one's family tends to be structured according to a fairly standard format or schema. This type of discourse usually is comprised of less complex linguistic forms (e.g., less complex syntax and more familiar vocabulary), and it contains relatively few linguistic and speech errors. Describing one's work in detail, however, is a less practiced task that results in new formulations of relatively more complex linguistic structures, but it also contains more linguistic errors and speech disruptions.

Audiotapes of subject interviews were transcribed and subsequently segmented into sentence-like units (Loban, 1963). Protocols were scored independently by two raters. Interrater agreement for blind scoring of protocols was generally acceptable and ranged from 79–98% agreement for various measures. In all cases of disagreement between raters, a compromise score was arrived at through discussion prior to data analyses. On average, there were about 500 total words for analysis for each subject. There were no differences among any of the subject groups participating in the studies reported below in terms of either discourse length (total words produced) or mean length of utterance.

The following measures were derived from the discourse samples to assess various aspects of intrasentential (microlinguistic) and suprasentential (macrolinguistic) discourse abilities.

1. Microlinguistic abilities are reflected in the complexity and adequacy of intrasentential syntactic organization. The complexity of sentence combining syntactic transformations is estimated by a **Weighted Index of Subordination** (Loban, 1963). This scoring system assigns greater weight to sentence units containing recursively embedded subordinate structures.

Two additional measures of the adequacy of intrasentential syntactic organization were also computed: the proportion of all verbalizations that were **syntactically complete** and that contained no syntactic errors and the rate of errors of **omission** of required morphosyntactic units.

2. Single word production measures provide additional indexes of microlinguistic discourse abilities. Different types of lexical errors reflect disturbance in different aspects of word production. **Literal paraphasias**, defined as uncorrected omissions or substitutions of phonemes in a recognizable English word, reflect problems in phonemic realization. **Verbal paraphasias** represent referential errors and are comprised of uncorrected substitutions of one English word by another. Nonspecific, **indefinite** nouns and pronouns that make ambiguous or general reference and are substituted for substantive words are scored to represent failures in semantic specification at the lexical level.

3. Coherence is a term that has been used to characterize the suprasentential conceptual organization of discourse, and thus, it reflects macrolinguistic abilities. The coherence of a text or discourse depends, at least in part, on the speaker's ability to maintain thematic unity (Agar & Hobbs, 1982). Thematic unity is achieved by the integration of textual units that form a coherent representation because they denote conditionally related "real world" events and facts (Keenan, Baillet, & Brown, 1984; van Dijk, 1977).

Several models of discourse analysis distinguish between "global" and "local" coherence relations (Agar & Hobbs, 1982; Kintsch & van Dijk, 1978; Mross, 1990). **Global coherence** refers to the manner in which discourse is organized with respect to an overall goal, plan, theme or topic. It reflects unity in the themes and topics underlying the semantic macrostructure of the text or discourse as a whole. **Local coherence**, by contrast, refers to the maintenance of meaningful conceptual links between individual sentences or propositions in a text or discourse. Local coherence is reflected in contents and meanings shared between contiguous propositional units at the microstructural level of discourse organization.

A five-point scale was used to separately rate the global and local coherence of each verbalization in the discourse. A higher global coherence rating is assigned to verbalizations that provide substantive information directly related to the designated topic of discourse. Ratings of local coherence reflect judgments of the relatedness between the content of a verbalization and the content or meaning of the immediately preceding utterance in the conversational exchange. Higher ratings of local coherence are assigned to verbalizations that continue, repeat, elaborate, or coordinate with the topic in the immediately preceding discourse.

4. Another component of macrolinguistic abilities is reflected in discourse cohesion. This refers to linguistic devices that are employed in the surface structure of texts to index interconnections between various

segments of discourse. These interconnections typically span across sentences and larger discourse units. Cohesive linguistic devices share the property that interpretation of one linguistic element, such as a pronoun, depends on or presupposes another linguistic element, such as a preceding noun (Halliday & Hasan, 1976). Cohesive devices such as co-reference and anaphora are linguistic means through which thematic unity or coherence may be sustained. Though cohesion contributes to maintaining the coherence of a text or discourse, it is neither necessary nor sufficient for achieving thematic unity (Brown & Yule, 1983), and, thus, it is considered to be separate from coherence.

Of the four major types of cohesive devices outlined by Halliday and Hasan (1976), referential and lexical types of cohesion are recognized to be the most commonly occurring in natural discourse (Patry & Nespoulous, 1990). **Referential cohesion** is indexed by the appropriate use of personal pronouns, demonstrative pronouns, and definite articles that have an unambiguous lexical referent in the preceding discourse. **Lexical cohesion** is indexed by the production of nouns that are exact repetitions, synonyms, superodinate designates, or subordinate exemplars of a referent linguistically indexed in the preceding discourse. **Incomplete cohesion** is a measure of discourse cohesion errors consisting of the inappropriate use of personal pronouns, demonstrative pronouns, and definite articles that do not have an unambiguous lexical referent in the preceding discourse.

A sample transcript presented in Table 10–1 includes all of the subject's linguistic output that has been segmented into sentence-like units. Segmentation of the discourse into scorable units was guided principally by syntactic criteria, but prosodic and/or semantic features were used sometimes when the syntactic form was grossly distorted, incomplete, or ambiguous. The underlined text portions, hereafter termed verbalizations, represent the best or most complete syntactic units that could be identified in the stream of discourse. Syntactic errors, syntactic complexity and lexical errors were scored after the grammatically most complete verbalization was extracted. All the false starts, repetitions, and self corrections (the nonunderlined portions of the transcript) were excluded first, so that only the best-formed linguistic segments were used when scoring for the correctness of syntactic and lexical microlinguistic structures. By contrast, when deriving macrolinguistic measures of coherence and cohesion, *all* of the available linguistic material was used, regardless of its grammatical or lexical well-formedness. Since it is assumed that even the most poorly formed speech can potentially convey appropriate meaning, all of the information available in the linguistic context was considered when rating the conceptual-linguistic integrity and unity of the discourse. These distinctions in the types of information used for

Table 10–1. Sample discourse protocol scored for syntactic and lexical errors and global and local thematic coherence

Coherence			
Global	Local		
5	5		I had my father my mother and two and three brothers three brothers.
3	3	**	Good family good family.
5	3		One brother's still in the one one one in the service.
5	3		and another brother he quit he died.
3	3	**	Very nice fally we got.

** syntactic omission   ⁀ literal paraphasia
See text for discussion of scoring methods

scoring micro- and macrolinguistic aspects of discourse are based on the notion that whereas the correctness of syntactic, phonological, and lexical characteristics of language output can be evaluated with respect to a set of formal, context insensitive invariant rules specifying the well-formedness of language, the acceptability of textual organization cannot be defined in reference to a set of universal rules. Rather, textual coherence and cohesion can only be evaluated with regard to the total social-linguistic context of the particular discourse event (de Beaugrande, 1985).

FACTOR ANALYSIS OF DISCOURSE PRODUCTION MEASURES

The results of a factor analysis of the discourse measures described above are reviewed as a prelude to the ensuing discussion of patterns of disrupted discourse abilities in neurologically compromised subjects. This factor analysis was conducted to determine if separate factors that might correspond to hypothesized component micro- and macrolinguistic cognitive processing abilities could indeed be identified empirically. Eight discourse measures from 68 healthy and brain-damaged subjects who participated in the studies described below were submitted to a principal components factor analysis with varimax rotation. Three factors emerged that together accounted for 70% of the total variance (Table 10–2).

The first factor that was extracted is termed "coherence-cohesion" because it includes high loadings from the ratings of both global and local thematic coherence. The measure of appropriate cohesion, which is the sum of the all appropriate occurrences of referential and lexical cohesive

Table 10–2. Factor analysis of discourse measures

	Factor 1	Factor 2	Factor 3
	Coherence-Cohesion	Lexical	Syntax
Global coherence	**.787**	−.108	.217
Local coherence	**.855**	−.129	.284
Appropriate cohesion	**.721**	−.118	−.168
Incomplete cohesion	−.122	**.787**	−.356
Verbal paraphasia	−.041	**.715**	−.387
Indefinite terms	−.212	**.796**	.185
Index of subordination	−.036	−.163	**.814**
Syntactic errors	−.382	.109	**−.714**

ties, also loads highly on this coherence-cohesion factor. This first factor seems to represent a composite of what have been identified as macrolinguistic components of discourse. Note that despite the emergence in this analysis of a single factor encompassing all the macrolinguistic measures, data are presented in the ensuing discussion that suggest that this factor may be parsed further into more discrete components.

The second factor that was extracted is termed "lexical." It consists of traditional measures of impaired lexical retrieval or naming. Verbal paraphasias and the use of indefinite, nonspecific or semantically empty terms load highly on this factor. Incomplete cohesion also loaded highly on this lexical factor. In this subject sample, which included many aphasic patients, it was not surprising to find that the production of cohesive markers in the surface text that did not have an antecedent lexical text referent was closely related to other errors in word retrieval. Because textual cohesion is realized in part through the grammatical system and in part through the lexical system, some cohesion errors may be expected with concurrent microlinguistic lexical-grammatical processing deficits. The second factor extracted in the analysis, therefore, seems to reflect a lexical microlinguistic component of discourse.

The third factor is composed of measures of syntactic errors and syntactic complexity. This factor, termed "syntax," appears to capture another separate microlinguistic component of discourse.

The results of the factor analysis provide empirical support for the conceptual groupings of the different measures employed in the studies reported below. This analysis also confirms the distinctions between micro- and macrolinguistic processes outlined above, as these were captured as statistically independent factors. The analysis reveals the well-recognized subdivision of microlinguistic abilities into separate lexical and syntactic components of intrasentential organization. Macrolinguistic abilities were represented in the factor analysis by combined measures of thematic coherence and appropriate cohesion. Additional analyses of discourse production performances of patients with neuropsychological disorders described below, however, suggest that coherence and cohesion may be distinct subcomponents of macrolinguistic abilities.

DISCOURSE PATTERNS IN THE CONTEXT OF FLUENT LANGUAGE DISORDERS

Glosser and Deser (1990) compared discourse productions of three groups of brain-damaged adult patients, all of whom presented with acquired fluent language disorders. At least superficially, the three groups displayed equally severe impairments in their abilities to produce meaningful linguistic communications. The groups were matched on the overall Boston Diagnostic Aphasia Examination (Goodglass & Kaplan, 1983) severity rating and performance on a visual confrontation naming test (Glosser & Kaplan, 1989). Despite apparent similarities in the superficial manifestations of their language disorder, the three groups differed in terms of the profile of accompanying nonlinguistic cognitive deficits and the neuropathology underlying the cognitive and linguistic disturbances. These groups were chosen because disparities in their neuropsychological dysfunction were expected to impact on and disrupt different aspects of discourse production.

The first group consisted of nine right-handed patients who displayed a fluent aphasia (FA) as a result of a single cerebrovascular lesion in the posterior region of the left hemisphere. Based on previous research, it was expected that the FA patients would demonstrate disturbances in microlinguistic phonological, lexical, and syntactic aspects of language production (Blumstein, 1981; Caramazza & Berndt, 1978). Based on other work (Stachowiak, Huber, Poeck, & Kerschensteiner, 1977; Ulatowska, Allard, & Chapman, 1990), these same patients were expected to show preserved macrolinguistic skills for conveying meanings at the suprasentential level of discourse.

The second group consisted of nine patients with mild and moderate dementia with the clinical diagnosis of probable Alzheimer's disease (AD). These patients' language disorder evolved in the context of generalized cognitive loss that is assumed to be the result of multifocal cerebral disease. Although AD patients have well-recognized impairments in naming (Huff, Corkin, & Growden, 1986), they have been reported to show relatively preserved phonological and syntactic processing at the single word and sentence levels (Glosser & Kaplan, 1989; Kempler, Curtiss, & Jackson, 1987; Schwartz, Marin, & Saffran, 1979). Impairments in the conceptual and pragmatic aspects of language comprehension and production are characteristic of AD patients (Bayles & Kaszniak, 1987). Such impairments were expected to impact most directly on macrolinguistic abilities for maintaining organization at the suprasentential level of discourse.

The third brain-damaged group consisted of nine patients who developed a fluent type of aphasia as the result of a severe closed head injury (CHI). Because closed head injuries result in both focal and multifocal brain injuries (Levin, Benton, & Grossman, 1982), such patients tend to have impairments in both domain specific (e.g., linguistic) cognitive functions, as well as in the more diffusely organized cognitive processes of attention, memory, and executive control. It was expected that these CHI patients with disproportionately severe disorders in language (possibly as a consequence of focal trauma to the left hemisphere) would be similar to the FA group in showing impaired microlinguistic abilities, and like the AD group with multifocal cerebral disease, CHI patients were also expected to show impaired macrolinguistic abilities.

Thus, it was hypothesized that relative to healthy controls ($n = 17$), the FA group would be impaired in microlinguistic aspects of discourse production; the AD group was expected to be selectively impaired in the macrolinguistic aspects of discourse production; and the CHI group was expected to show impairments on *both* micro- and macrolinguistic measures of discourse production.

As predicted, on the two sets of measures of microlinguistic abilities the patients with focal left hemisphere dysfunction, the FA and CHI patients, were impaired relative to normal controls, whereas the AD patients were unimpaired. In terms of the adequacy of the syntactic structure of discourse, FA subjects were impaired relative to normals on measures of the completeness of the syntactic form, syntactic errors, and syntactic complexity. The CHI subjects produced proportionately fewer syntactically complete verbalizations and made more syntactic errors than normals, but they did not differ from normals in syntactic complexity. The AD patients, by contrast, did not differ from normals on any of the syntactic measures.

All three groups differed from normals in terms of the overall lexical error rate. This was not unexpected, since the subjects were chosen for inclusion in the study because of their naming problems. More detailed linguistic analyses, however, revealed qualitatively different lexical error types among the three groups of brain-damaged patients: The FA subjects produced significantly more verbal paraphasias and indefinite terms than normals, and they also produced some uncorrected phonemic errors (literal paraphasias). Like the FA group, the CHI group produced more verbal paraphasias than normals, and they also produced a few literal paraphasias. Compared to normals, the AD subjects produced significantly more semantically nonspecific indefinite terms, but they made no more uncorrected verbal paraphasias and they did not make any phonemic errors.

The results of analyses of macrolinguistic measures of discourse coherence contrast sharply with the findings on microlinguistic measures. The

AD patients who seemed to produce speech that was generally correct in terms of intrasentential linguistic forms were significantly impaired relative to normals in terms of the thematic coherence of their discourse. AD subjects were significantly impaired on ratings of global coherence, but they did not differ from normals on ratings of local coherence. The AD subjects were much more likely to lose the main topic of the discourse or to produce utterances that were only tangentially related to the discourse topic than were normals, though they generally maintained conceptual relationships locally between immediately contiguous verbalizations. CHI subjects were even more profoundly impaired relative to normals on coherence measures. They showed significant deficits on rating of *both* local and global thematic organization.

The FA subjects did not differ from normals in either global or local thematic coherence ratings. Despite numerous errors and simplifications in the production and organization of intrasentential forms, these patients managed to convey coherent intersentential meaning relationships in their discourse. It should be emphasized that the ratings of thematic coherence were based strictly on transcribed data. Neither paralinguistic nor nonlinguistic behaviors contributed to ratings of thematic coherence. The findings suggest that the FA patients were able to convey successfully suprasentential discourse meanings through oral language, even when they could not produce linguistically correct single words and sentences.

Measures of appropriate discourse cohesion did not discriminate between any of the subject groups. It is especially significant that the AD and CHI subjects obtained normal discourse cohesion scores despite disturbed discourse coherence, suggesting that cohesion and coherence are dissociable components of discourse processing. Although FA subjects evidenced normal rates of production of appropriate referential and lexical cohesion terms, at times there was no unambiguous and proximal antecedent linguistic referent for the coreferential terms produced. As discussed earlier, the higher rates of incomplete cohesion for FA subjects are most likely related to the higher incidence of verbal paraphasic errors produced by these subjects, not to a specific deficit in the ability to maintain intratextual cohesive relations.

The group findings discussed above are illustrated by selected protocols of individual subjects. Table 10-3 presents the discourse of a 49-year-old male who was recovering from a Wernicke's aphasia following an infarct in the region of the left temporal-parietal junction that extended deep to the body of the lateral ventricle. Although the patient produced many gross syntactic and lexical errors, the thematic coherence ratings for this discourse are relatively intact in comparison to age-matched normals who obtained mean global coherence ratings of 4.21 (SD = .41) and mean local coherence ratings of 4.13 (SD = .34). Overall, this FA subject produced surprisingly informative and well-organized discourse, even though the discourse contains many linguistic errors.

Table 10–4 presents the discourse of a moderately demented (Mini Mental State [Folstein, Folstein, & McHugh, 1975] = 11) 78-year-old former executive who had carried the diagnosis of probable AD for about 4 years. This speech sample reveals no linguistic or paraphasic errors per se, but many vague nonspecific terms are produced, and these seem to contribute to the overall impression of semantically empty noninformative speech. Table 10–4 also presents discourse of a mildly demented (Mini Mental State = 20) recently diagnosed 82-year-old male AD patient. Again, there are no apparent lexical or syntactic errors in the

Table 10–3. Discourse about work from a patient recovering from Wernicke's Aphasia following a left hemisphere stroke

Coherence			
Global	Local		
5	5		I was in the service.
5	3		Then I became a truck driver.
5	5	**	Drove every*place.
3	5	**	The big trucks.
5	5	**	G$\overset{+}{e}$t em all over the country.
3	3	**	Very good job.

** syntactic omission   * indefinite term   + verbal paraphasia

Table 10–4. Discourse from two patients with the diagnosis of probable Alzheimer's Disease. The first excerpt is discourse about work, and the second is about family

Coherence		
Global	Local	
3	3	I did quite a lot of thi*ngs.
3	3	I graduated as I told you from Williams.
3	3	And then I did a number of different thi*ngs.
4	3	And finally I* thought I might do some*thing in a certain field of food or some*thing like that, but it never worked out.
5	5	Two of my boys are in selling.
5	5	And they do pretty well.
5	3	And one other is in chemical engineering in a laboratory.
1	3	I used to do that.
1	5	I didn't like it, but I did it.
1	3	And I'd rather be selling, too.
1	5	And that's what I did do.

* indefinite term

discourse, intrasentential organization is adequate, and the patient appropriately maintained thematic relationships between contiguous sentences (local coherence). Midway through the interview, however, he shifted from the given topic of discourse about his family, and he began to describe his own work, a topic that had not yet been introduced into the interview. The patient continued the idiosyncratic topic excursion and never returned to the designated topic.

An excerpt from the discourse of a 25-year-old male who sustained a severe CHI in a motor vehicle accident 7 months prior to the interview is presented in Table 10–5. This protocol illustrates breakdown in both the local thematic organization of contiguous verbalizations and in the global thematic organization of discourse.

The comparisons among the three brain-damaged groups provide evidence consistent with the postulated independent neuropsychological organization of micro- and macrolinguistic discourse abilities. The comparisons between the FA and AD patients indicate that impairments in macrolinguistic discourse organization may occur without any impairments in microlinguistic operations and that macrolinguistic organization can be adequately maintained despite very impaired syntax and word finding. When taken together, these results indicate a type of double dissociation (Teuber, 1955). Since the two sets of cognitive operations appear to be independently disrupted by different types of brain damage, then it might be inferred that these operations are subserved by different brain systems.

Table 10–5. Discourse about work from a patient recovering from a severe closed head injury

Coherence		
Global	Local	
5	5	I worked in eight plȧces.*
5	5	The last one was Playboy.
3	3	The last Playboy was in New York which I remember, but I don't** exactly where it is.
1	1	Mrs. White let me use her car to drive.
1	5	And I used her car.
1	3	She drove.
1	3	I drove.
1	4	And I drove the o~t~her car.
1	1	And I never had any problems.
2	1	~It~ was in New York.

** syntactic omission   * indefinite term   ~~ incomplete cohesion

The observed patterns of disrupted discourse production in the three patient groups are also relevant to understanding how the broader category of macrolinguistic cognitive functions may be parsed into dissociable components. The data suggest that discourse cohesion and discourse coherence are separable. The performance patterns for the AD and CHI patients suggest that intact cohesion in the surface structure of the text does not guarantee coherence in the underlying conceptual semantic organization of discourse. Production of cohesive linguistic devices, unlike discourse coherence, may be more driven by automatized linguistic processes, rather than by higher order conceptual processes. The findings of preserved thematic coherence for the FA group, despite increased production of cohesion errors, further suggest that linguistic cohesive devices are not prerequisites for establishing and maintaining thematic conceptual coherence. These results support hypothesized distinctions between discourse cohesion and discourse coherence (Halliday & Hasan, 1976; Keenan, Baillet, & Brown, 1984).

Finally, the analyses of thematic coherence suggest that different cognitive processes may underlie local and global discourse organization. Both the AD and CHI patients showed apparently greater impairments in maintaining global coherence compared to local coherence. The disordered discourse of the AD patients, in particular, seemed to stem less from a disruption in relationships of meaning between contiguous concepts and more from impaired macro-organizational abilities. This apparent difference in the degree of disruption in local and global coherence following brain damage would be consistent with the view of some investigators that local and global coherence represent different sets of underlying cognitive procedures (Kintsch & van Dijk, 1978; Tracy, 1984).

MICROLINGUISTIC AND MACROLINGUISTIC ASPECTS OF DISCOURSE PRODUCTION IN NORMAL AGING

The observed dissociations among component macrolinguistic abilities were explored further in a study of age-related changes in the discourse productions of healthy adults (Glosser & Deser, 1992). Changes in the quantity, precision, cohesion and organization of the language productions of the elderly have long been noted (Critchley, 1984; Obler, 1989). One interpretation of these changes is that they result from age-related declines in processes of attention, memory, and executive control functions (Au, Obler, & Albert, 1991; Kemper, 1988). Such declines in higher-level cognitive processes would be expected to selectively disrupt macrolinguistic aspects of discourse production, while sparing more automatized and modularized microlinguistic cognitive processes.

Discourse samples from 14 middle-aged (mean age = 51.9) and 13 elderly (mean age = 76.2) healthy subjects were compared on the measures described above to assess for age-related declines in micro- and macrolinguistic abilities.

It was found that although elderly subjects' absolute scores on microlinguistic measures of syntactic integrity, syntactic errors, and syntactic complexity were less adequate than those of middle-aged subjects, there were no statistically significant group differences on any of these measures. The groups also did not differ significantly on either of the two lexical error measures of verbal paraphasias and indefinite terms. As expected, there were no apparent deficits in phonological, lexical, and syntactic aspects of language production for the elderly subjects.

As in the study of brain-damaged subjects, there were no age-related differences in rates of production of appropriate referential and lexical cohesive ties, nor did groups differ in terms of incomplete cohesion errors.

Analyses of thematic coherence ratings revealed a specific deficit for the elderly group. Compared to middle-aged subjects the elderly subjects obtained significantly lower ratings on global thematic coherence, although groups did not differ on local coherence ratings. Elderly subjects not only obtained significantly lower mean global coherence ratings than middle-aged subjects, but they also produced a significantly higher proportion of verbalizations that were totally unrelated to the designated topic of discourse.

The pattern of disruption, though not the absolute level of impairment, in discourse production seen in healthy subjects of advanced age closely matches that found in AD patients. Both groups evidence disproportionate disruption in certain macrolinguistic abilities for organizing discourse to maintain a coherent overall theme or topic, whereas they maintain meaning relationships at the microstructural level of discourse organization relatively well. The similarities in the discourse patterns of AD patients and healthy subjects of advanced age are not unexpected as these groups share many features in terms of their pattern of cognitive and linguistic performances (Bayles & Kaszniak, 1987; Light & Burke, 1988) and neuropathological abnormalities (Berg, 1985).

The finding that normal aging differentially affects macro- but not microlinguistic processes reinforces the conclusions of the study of patients with fluent language disorders supporting the idea that micro- and macrolinguistic processes are organized separately psychologically and also neurologically. Unfortunately the exact neurobiological substrates of these different cognitive functions are not completely known. One hundred years of research of the anatomy of various aphasic disorders leaves little question that microlinguistic syntactic, phonological, and lexical abilities depend primarily on the integrity of function in focal neural systems within the left cerebral hemisphere. Macrolinguistic processing abilities, however, are less obviously localized neuroanatomically. One suggestion that had been put forth is that at least certain macrolinguistic processes are dependent on the integrity of the right cerebral hemisphere.

DISCOURSE PRODUCTION FOLLOWING RIGHT HEMISPHERE DAMAGE

It is now well-recognized that damage in the right cerebral hemisphere can disrupt certain higher-order linguistic functions. Patients with right hemisphere damage (RHD), for example, have been shown to be impaired in comprehending verbal information in connected texts, in appreciating intentions and attitudes conveyed indirectly in speech, and in comprehending metaphoric and connotative word meanings (see Joanette, Goulet, & Hannequin, 1990, for a comprehensive review). RHD patients' impairments on complex linguistic tasks may be understood as reflecting failures to integrate linguistic information with its surrounding context to achieve coherent meanings (Weylman, Brownell, & Gardner, 1988). RHD patients manipulate individual linguistic units without difficulty, but they are specifically impaired when required to deal with multiple linguistic units in an organized, contextually bound fashion. Unlike left-hemisphere-damaged aphasic patients who have selectively impaired microlinguistic abilities for processing phonological, syntactic, and semantic aspects of individual words and sentences, the impairment for nonaphasic RHD patients seems to lie in macrolinguistic abilities for maintaining conceptual and pragmatic organization at the suprasentential level (Joanette, Goulet, & Hannequin, 1990; Molloy, Brownell, & Gardner, 1990).

The differential contribution of the right cerebral hemisphere to microlinguistic and macrolinguistic discourse processes was evaluated in a study of the discourse productions of a small group of patients who had suffered a single cerebrovascular accident in the right hemisphere (Glosser, Deser, & Weisstein, 1992). Seven right-handed RHD patients (mean age = 57.9) were compared to seven healthy controls matched individually to each patient in terms of age and educational background.

Using the methods of analyses described above, *no* group differences were found on any of the measures taken to reflect microlinguistic abilities (Table 10–6), including measures of the completeness and complexity of syntactic structure and lexical error measures.

Significant group differences were obtained, however, in analyses of measures of certain macrolinguistic abilities (Table 10–7). Analyses of

Table 10–6. Microlinguistic measures of discourse production in right hemisphere damaged patients and normal controls

	Right Hemisphere	Normal Control
	Mean (SD)	Mean (SD)
Lexical Errors[1]		
Verbal paraphasias	.005 (.001)	.005 (.001)
Indefinite terms	.011 (.003)	.010 (.002)
Syntax		
Syntactically complete[2]	.81 (.08)	.77 (.05)
Syntactic omissions[3]	.02 (.01)	.01 (.01)
Index of subordination[4]	.63 (.22)	.39 (.27)

[1] Scores are computed as a proportion of total spoken words.
[2] Proportions of all verbalizations that are syntactically complete.
[3] Omissions are computed as proportions of total spoken words.
[4] Mean score for all verbalizations.

Table 10–7. Macrolinguistic measures of discourse production in right hemisphere damaged patients and normal controls

	Right Hemisphere	Normal Control	
	Mean (SD)	Mean (SD)	
Discourse Cohesion[1]			
Appropriate cohesion	.13 (.02)	.12 (.01)	
Incomplete cohesion	.03 (.01)	.01 (.01)	**
Thematic Coherence Mean Rating[2]			
Global coherence	3.7 (.63)	4.2 (.48)	
Local coherence	3.9 (.22)	4.2 (.32)	
Proportion Thematically Incoherent Verbalizations[3]			
Global incoherence	.18 (.17)	.09 (.11)	
Local incoherence	.06 (.03)	.02 (.04)	**

** Significant group difference ($p < .05$)
[1] Cohesion scores were computed as proportions of total spoken words.
[2] Higher ratings indicate greater thematic coherence (range = 1–5).
[3] Proportion of all verbalizations rated "1" on the 5-point scale.

discourse cohesion measures revealed that compared to normals RHD patients used significantly more cohesive ties that did not have a clear antecedent linguistic referent in the discourse (incomplete cohesion).

There were no differences between groups in the rate of production of appropriate lexical and referential cohesive ties, but they made more referential cohesion errors. Since they made no more of the other kinds of lexical errors, the cohesion errors of the RHD patients may be taken to reflect specific impairment in the capacity to maintain textual unity lexically. RHD patients were also more likely than normals to produce utterances that were incoherent with respect to the local, but not the global, thematic context within the discourse. These utterance were totally unrelated to the content of the immediately preceding utterance (reflected in a measure of the proportion of locally "incoherent" verbalizations). It is important to note, however, that groups did not differ on the overall mean ratings of local, as well as global, coherence.

Unlike left-hemisphere-damaged patients who show selectively impaired microlinguistic discourse abilities for producing correct lexical and syntactic forms in discourse, RHD patients were found to be impaired only on measures of certain macrolinguistic abilities. They maintained the overall (global) thematic coherence of discourse appropriately, but they made errors that intermittently disrupted thematic coherence and cohesion at the local level of intersentential organization.

The disruption in macrolinguistic discourse abilities seen in RHD patients differs qualitatively from that documented for patients with multifocal CNS disorders such as Alzheimer's disease and closed head injury and for healthy elderly subjects. Patients in the latter groups were found to be impaired principally in their ability to maintain macrostructural or global thematic organization. In contrast, RHD patients were found to be impaired in the ability to clearly specify co-referential and shared thematic relationships between more proximal linguistic units. Together these findings support the claim that different cognitive procedures underlie local and global discourse organization as different types of damage in the nervous system can disrupt these different component macrolinguistic abilities.

The contribution of the right cerebral hemisphere to what have been defined in this discussion as macrolinguistic abilities is a specific one. It seems to involve appropriate coordination of contiguous thematic and referential units, but it spares the overall macrostructural organization of discourse. Furthermore, the disruption of referential coherence and cohesion at the local level of discourse organization seen in RHD patients is intermittent. In a stream of otherwise normally structured discourse, RHD patients sporadically produced verbalizations that are totally unrelated to the immediately surrounding context. This is not dissimilar to RHD patients' performance on a word association task where they sometimes produced idiosyncratic and bizarre word associations that bore no relationship at all to the presented stimulus words (Glosser & Goodglass, 1991). An attentional disorder was suggested to explain this occasional disruption in language use that was documented in the context of otherwise normal linguistic performance. Coslett, Bowers, and Heilman (1987), among others, have argued that reduced attention or arousal underlie the cognitive and linguistic deficits seen following RHD. Such an inability to maintain activation or attention may also account for intermittently disrupted local coherence and cohesion in these patients' descriptive discourse.

CONCLUSION

These studies of discourse production patterns in neurologically impaired and aged populations are informative about the ways in which discourse abilities may be parsed into component cognitive processes. The distinctions proposed between the two broad categories of macrolinguistic and microlinguistic cognitive functions have been supported by findings of dissociations in these functions among patients with different types of neurological disorders. The data suggest further refinements within the general category of macrolinguistic functions. Just as there are accepted distinctions among component phonological, lexical-semantic and syntactic processes subsumed under the category of microlinguistic processes, interesting distinctions have emerged within the broad category of macrolinguistic processes. The performance patterns of different neurologically compromised subject groups indicate dissociations between the macrolinguistic procedures required for sustaining cohesion in the surface structure of texts and conceptual coherence in the deeper semantic structure and also dissociations between local and global levels of textual thematic organization.

The neurological bases of the component cognitive operations entailed in discourse processing are also revealed by these types of studies. Consistent with the expectation that microlinguistic abilities for phonological, syntactic and certain aspects of lexical processing are critically dependent on the integrity of functioning in the left cerebral hemisphere, selective deficits in these processes were documented for aphasic stroke and CHI patients with insults in the left hemisphere. Also consistent with previous research suggesting that the right cerebral hemisphere is critical for the adequate expression of higher-level communication abilities, RHD patients evidenced impairments in certain macrolinguistic abilities. The observed disturbance in these patients' ability to maintain coherence and cohesion at the local level of discourse organization seemed to be intermittent, not absolute, suggesting that the failure lies in accessing the requisite cognitive operations rather than in the operations themselves.

The neurological bases for the abilities to organize the macrostructure of discourse remain elusive. Though selective deficits in these abilities were found in normally aging subjects and mildly to moderately demented AD patients, it is not possible to determine what, if any, single aspect of these individuals' neurological dysfunction accounts for the impairment in processing the global organization of discourse. One possibility that may be considered is that the multifocal nature of the neurological dysfunction in these populations, rather than disruption in any focal neurological region, accounts for the observed disturbance in macrostructural discourse organization. This proposal follows from distinctions that have been made in neuropsychology between cognitive operations that can be decomposed into discrete modules having focal regions of representation in the nervous system and central cognitive functions that are represented in more widely distributed neuronal networks (Fodor, 1983). The hypothesis that the cognitive operations underlying the organization of the macrostructure of discourse, in contrast to other aspects of discourse processing, rely primarily on central, nonfocally represented neuropsychological processes and are globally disrupted with multifocal types of neurological disorders awaits further investigation.

REFERENCES

Agar, M., & Hobbs, J. R. (1982) Interpreting discourse: Coherence and the analysis of ethnographic interview. *Discourse Processes, 5*, 1–32

Au, R., Obler, L. K., & Albert, M. L. (1991). Language in aging and dementia. In M. T. Sarno (Ed.), *Acquired aphasia* (2nd ed., pp. 405–424). San Diego: Academic Press.

Bayles, K. A., & Kaszniak, A. W. (1987). *Communication and cognition in normal aging and dementia.* Boston: Little, Brown.

Berg, L. (1985). Does Alzheimer's Disease represent an exaggeration of normal aging? *Archives of Neurology, 42*, 737–739.

Blumstein, S. E. (1991). Phonological aspects of aphasia. In M. T. Sarno (Ed.), *Acquired aphasia* (2nd ed., pp. 151–174). San Diego: Academic Press.

Brown, G., & Yule, G. (1983). *Discourse analysis.* Cambridge, England: Cambridge University Press.

Caramazza, A., & Berndt, R. S. (1978). Semantic and syntactic processes in aphasia: A review of the literature. *Psychological Bulletin, 85*, 898–918.

Coslett, H. B., Bowers, D., & Heilman, K. M. (1987). Reduction in cerebral activation after right hemisphere stroke. *Neurology, 37*, 957–962.

Critchley, M. (1984). And all the daughters of musick shall be brought low. *Archives of Neurology, 41*, 1135–1139.

de Beaugrande, R. (1985). Text linguistics in discourse studies. In T. A. van Dijk (Ed.), *Handbook of discourse analysis*, (vol. 1, pp. 41–70). New York: Academic Press.

Fodor, J. (1983). *The modularity of mind.* Cambridge, MA: MIT Press.

Folstein, M. F., Folstein, S. E., & McHugh, P. R. (1975). "Mini Mental State": A practical method for grading the cognitive state of patients for the clinician. *Journal of Psychiatric Research, 12*, 189–198.

Fredriksen, C. H., Bracewell, R. J., Breuleux, A., & Renaud, A. (1990). The cognitive representation and processing of discourse: Function and dysfunction. In Y. Joanette & H. H. Brownell (Eds.), *Discourse ability and brain damage: Theoretical and empirical perspectives* (pp. 69–110). New York: Springer-Verlag.

Glosser, G., & Deser, T. (1990). Patterns of discourse production among neurological patients with fluent language disorders. *Brain and Language, 40,* 67–88.

Glosser, G., & Deser, T. (1992). Aging changes in microlinguistic and macrolinguistic aspects of discourse production. *Journal of Gerontology: Psychological Sciences, 47,* 266–272.

Glosser, G., Deser, T., & Weisstein, C. (1992). Structural organization of discourse production following right hemisphere damage. *Journal of Clinical and Experimental Neuropsychology, 14,* 40.

Glosser, G., & Goodglass, H. (1991). Idiosyncratic word associations following right hemisphere damage. *Journal of Clinical and Experimental Neuropsychology, 13,* 703–710.

Glosser, G., & Kaplan, E. (1989). Linguistic and non-linguistic impairments in writing: A comparison of patients with focal and multifocal CNS disorders. *Brain and Language, 37,* 357–380.

Glosser, G., Wiener, M., & Kaplan, E. (1988). Variations in aphasic language behaviors. *Journal of Speech and Hearing Disorders, 53,* 115–124.

Goodglass, H., & Kaplan, E. (1983). *The assessment of aphasia and related disorders.* Philadelphia: Lea and Febiger.

Halliday, M. A. K., & Hasan, R. (1976). *Cohesion in English.* London: Longman.

Huff, F. J., Corkin, S., & Growden, J. H. (1986). Semantic impairment and anomia in Alzheimer's Disease. *Brain and Language, 28,* 235–249.

Joanette, Y, Goulet, P., & Hannequin, D. (1990). *Right hemisphere and verbal communication.* New York: Springer-Verlag.

Keenan, J. M., Baillet, S. D., & Brown, P. (1984). The effects of causal cohesion on comprehension and memory. *Journal of Verbal Learning and Verbal Behavior, 23,* 115–126.

Kemper, S. (1988) Geriatric psycholinguistics: Syntactic limitations of oral and written language. In L. L. Light & D. M. Burke (Eds.), *Language, memory, and aging* (pp. 58–76). New York: Cambridge University Press.

Kempler, D., Curtiss, S., & Jackson, C. (1987). Syntactic preservation in Alzheimer's Disease. *Journal of Speech and Hearing Research, 30,* 343–350.

Kintsch, W., & van Dijk, T. A. (1978). Toward a model of text comprehension and production. *Psychological Review, 85,* 363–394.

Levin, H. S., Benton, A. L. & Grossman, R. G. (1982). *Neurobehavioral consequences of closed head injury.* New York: Oxford University Press.

Light, L. L. & Burke, D. M. (1988). Patterns of language and memory in old age. In L. L. Light & D. M. Burke (Eds.), *Language, memory and aging* (pp. 244–271). New York: Cambridge University Press.

Loban, W. D. (1963). *The language of elementary school children.* Champaign, IL: National Council of Teachers of English.

Molloy, R., Brownell, H. H., & Gardner, H. (1990). Discourse comprehension by right hemisphere stroke patients: Deficits of prediction and revision. In Y. Joanette & H. H. Brownell (Eds.), *Discourse ability and brain damage: Theoretical and empirical perspectives* (pp. 113–130). New York: Springer-Verlag.

Mross, E. F. (1990). Text analysis: Macro- and microstructural aspects of discourse processing. In Y. Joanette & H. H. Brownell (Eds.), *Discourse ability and brain damage: Theoretical and Empirical Perspectives* (pp. 50–68). New York: Springer-Verlag.

Obler, L. K. (1989). Language beyond childhood. In J. Berko Gleason (Ed.), *The development of language*. Columbus, OH: Merrill Publishing.

Patry, R., & Nespoulous, J.-L. (1990). Discourse analysis in linguistics: Historical and theoretical background. In Y. Joanette & H. H. Brownell (Eds.), *Discourse ability and brain damage* (pp. 3–27). New York: Springer-Verlag.

Schwartz, M. F., Marin, O. S. M., & Saffran, E. M. (1979). Dissociations of language function in dementia: A case study. *Brain and Language, 7*, 277–306.

Stachowiak, F. J., Huber, W., Poeck, K., & Kerschensteiner, M. (1977). Text comprehension in aphasia. *Brain and Language, 4*, 177–195.

Teuber, H. L. (1955). Physiological psychology. *Annual Review of Psychology, 9*, 267–296.

Tracy, K. (1984). Staying on topic: An explication of conversational relevance. *Discourse Processes, 7*, 447–464.

Ulatowska, H. K., Allard, L., & Chapman, S. B. (1990). Narrative and procedural discourse in aphasia. In Y. Joanette & H. H. Brownell (Eds.), *Discourse ability and brain damage* (pp. 180–192). New York: Springer-Verlag.

van Dijk, T. A. (1977). *Text and context*. London: Longman.

van Dijk, T. A. (1980). *Macrostructures: An interdisciplinary study of global structures in discourse, interaction, and cognition*. Hillsdale, NJ: Lawrence Erlbaum.

Weylman, S. T., Brownell, H. H., & Gardner, H. (1988). "It's what you mean, not what you say": Pragmatic language use in brain-damaged patients. In F. Plum (Ed.), *Language communication and the brain* (pp. 229–243). New York: Raven Press.

CHAPTER 11

Contextual and Thematic Influences on Narrative Comprehension of Left and Right Hemisphere Brain-Damaged Adults

MONICA STRAUSS HOUGH AND ROBERT S. PIERCE

The study of discourse comprehension has been spurred by recent concern in understanding how individuals comprehend and interpret information in more naturalistic contexts. This has been of particular interest in various brain-damaged populations. The comprehension of one type of discourse, narratives, has been examined most frequently, possibly because of the greater ease of investigating this genre as well as the general importance of narratives in normal communication. Narratives are oriented around characters and events with their primary function providing specific sequential information to the listener. Furthermore, narratives have a relatively conventional superstructure; that is, there is consistency in the elements that comprise the narrative. Typically, elements include a setting, complicating action, and resolution (Ulatowska, Allard, & Chapman, 1990).

During narrative comprehension, normal listeners construct a representation of the situations described in the narrative. They combine their linguistic knowledge with knowledge of the objects and actions that are being described (Morrow, Bower, & Greenspan, 1989; Morrow, Bower,

& Greenspan, 1990; van Dijk & Kintsch, 1983). Listeners gradually construct a "model" of the described situations by integrating information from each sentence of the narrative into the model. Therefore, this situation model of the narrative is dependent on the individual's general world knowledge and pragmatic reasoning. In addition, the listener identifies a sequence of causal links that connect a narrative's opening to its final outcome (Fletcher & Bloom, 1988). To do this, the listener also must develop a text base of the propositions of the narrative. These propositions represent the meaning conveyed by the text, that is, the topic level information (Kintsch & van Dijk, 1978; Morrow, Bower, & Greenspan, 1989; Speelman & Kirsner, 1990). Therefore, people understand narratives by constructing a model of the situation as well as a representation of the text meaning (Morrow, Greenspan, & Bower, 1987; Mross, 1990; van Dijk & Kintsch, 1983).

Although there has been a current surge of investigations examining the narrative comprehension abilities of adults with left and right hemisphere brain damage, minimal information has been acquired from these studies regarding the variables which influence and/or contribute to comprehension. In this chapter, we discuss the comprehension of short narratives by adults with left and right hemisphere brain damage as a result of cerebrovascular accident. The first part of the chapter addresses influences of context on the narrative comprehension of aphasic adults. Specifically, the effect of contextual predictiveness on the comprehension of syntactically complex sentences and predictive-nonpredictive narratives in fluent and nonfluent aphasic adults is discussed. The second part of the chapter is devoted to how organization of the theme of a narrative may influence comprehension in right and left hemisphere brain-damaged adults. The focus here is on the effect that organizational manipulation of the central theme of the narrative has on comprehension for these two populations. Possible variables that influence and/or contribute to the comprehension of narratives in regard to contextual and thematic information is discussed from a neuropsychological perspective.

CONTEXTUAL INFLUENCES ON NARRATIVE COMPREHENSION

Listening is an active process. World knowledge possessed by the listener is applied to information contained in the verbal input to form an integrated meaning representation. This is seen clearly in syntactically complex sentences presented in isolation. Those that are semantically and/or pragmatically constrained are easier for aphasic patients to comprehend than those without such constraints (Caramazza & Zurif, 1976; Deloche &

Seron, 1981; Heilman, Scholes, & Watson, 1976; Kudo, 1984; Sherman & Schweickert, 1989). This finding has been extended to the narrative level by Caplan and Evans (1990). These authors found that stories containing complex syntactic structures, that were all semantically or pragmatically constrained, were comprehended as accurately by aphasic subjects as were comparable stories containing only simple grammatical constructions.

However, not all contextually supportive information comes from world knowledge. Much of it derives from the surrounding linguistic and extralinguistic environment, that is, from the narrative itself. The purpose of this section of the chapter is to explore these more local, microstructural effects in adults with aphasia, to see how information contained in a narrative impacts on the comprehension of other information within the narrative. Two primary sources of context, prediction and redundancy, are discussed as they impact on the processing of syntactic and semantic target information.

CONTEXTUAL INFLUENCES ON SYNTACTIC PROCESSING

Prediction

Prediction refers to the notion that some specific information predicts the occurrence of other information. For example, in the semantically reversible sentence "The boy was hit by the girl," the listener must rely on syntactic-based decoding strategies because there is no other information that would predict which person served as the agent of the sentence. However, Pierce and Wagner (1985) found that aphasic subjects comprehended this type of sentence more accurately when it was preceded by a contextual sentence that predicted which person would act as the agent (e.g., The boy had a black eye. The boy was hit by the girl.). In contrast, comprehension was not significantly enhanced by information that did not predict the forthcoming subject-object relationship (e.g., The boy and girl were playing. The boy was hit by the girl.). Accordingly, the aphasic subjects benefitted from prior contextual information that predicted the forthcoming agent-object relationship. Presumably, the predictive context created a pragmatic environment that influenced comprehension of the reversible passive target sentence in a manner similar to the plausibility factor generated by world knowledge (Deloche & Seron, 1981). Provided the fact that the boy had a black eye, it was more plausible that he received the action rather than giving it (although not essential).

This result was replicated by Pierce and Beekman (1985) who also extended the finding to include extralinguistic contextual information. In this study, a picture was substituted for the contextual sentence (e.g., a picture of a boy with a black eye in the previous example). The picture was shown to the aphasic subjects and then removed before the reversible passive target sentence was provided. As in the contextual sentence condition, comprehension was significantly enhanced by the presence of the contextual picture. The aphasic subjects were able to derive knowledge from the picture that predicted the subsequent subject-object relationship.

An important aspect of these two studies is that the significant contextual effects were found only for those subjects with poorer comprehension skills. This is consistent with Sherman and Schweickert (1989) who found that subjects with Broca's aphasia could perform some syntactic analyses but resorted to the use of semantic and pragmatic strategies when the syntax became more complex. It also partially explains the negative results of Waller and Darley (1979) whose aphasic subjects did not benefit from prior contextual sentences. Their subjects' comprehension of the target syntactic structures without the context was quite good (approximately 76% accuracy). The other problem with this study was that the contextual sentences were very general in nature and not predictive. In contrast to the influence of comprehension level on the extent of contextual benefit, aphasia type based on fluency does not influence performance. Both fluent and nonfluent aphasic subjects benefit from context in a similar manner (Hough, Pierce, & Cannito, 1989; Pierce & Beekman, 1985).

Obviously, the research paradigm used in these studies is tapping comprehension at the level of an integrated meaning representation (compared to some on-line or priming paradigms). Accordingly, it was questioned whether the order of presentation of target and contextual information would affect performance. Pierce (1988) presented predictive contextual sentences either before or after reversible passive target sentences and found that both formats generated significantly more accurate comprehension than presenting the target sentence in isolation. As long as aphasic subjects can process and integrate both target and contextual information prior to responding, then the order of presentation does not seem to matter (at least for these two sentence combinations). Pierce also found that simply repeating the reversible passive target sentence once did not lead to significantly enhanced comprehension. This result further supports the notion that pragmatic prediction contributes to the contextual effect apart from merely repeating the nouns and verbs.

The positive effect of predictive context on the comprehension of syntactic structures has been expanded to include five-sentence narrative contexts for listening (Hough, Pierce, & Cannito, 1989) and reading (Germani & Pierce, 1992). That is, aphasic subjects' comprehension of reversible passive sentences was more accurate when they were preceded by five-sentence narratives that predicted the subject-object relationship than when they were presented alone. However, it has been questioned whether the predictive narrative contexts actually facilitate the comprehension of the subsequent reversible passive sentences or whether they simply allow these sentences to be ignored (Brookshire, 1987; Huber, 1990). These authors argued that the subjects may be responding based only on the information contained in the narrative contexts. Germani and Pierce (1992) tested this notion by comparing aphasic subjects' comprehension in three conditions: reversible passive sentences in isolation, reversible passive sentences preceded by five-sentence narrative contexts, and the narratives in isolation (i.e., without the target reversible passive sentences). The subjects comprehended the narratives alone as accurately as they did the reversible passive sentences alone. However, comprehension of the two together was significantly more accurate than either alone. Accordingly, it appears that predictive context exerts its influence by interacting with the target information, not by replacing it.

Redundancy

Not all linguistic context is predictive in nature. Sometimes it introduces the key lexical items (e.g., nouns) and may lead to expectations about possible actions but does not predict thematic roles. Accordingly, a reversible passive sentence following a nonpredictive context remains just as reversible as it is in isolation. In contrast to the finding mentioned earlier (Pierce & Wagner, 1985) that single sentence nonpredictive contexts do not enhance comprehension of reversible passive sentences, nonpredictive five-sentence narratives improve comprehension as much as predictive narratives do (Cannito, Jarecki, & Pierce, 1986; Germani & Pierce, 1992; Hough, Pierce, & Cannito, 1989). Examples of the narratives are presented in Table 11-1.

The reasons for this effect are not obvious, but a possible explanation relates to the allocation of processing resources as a function of information redundancy. As the subjects hear (or read) the narrative, they become familiar with the main characters and events that are happening. By the time they reach the target sentence, the key lexical items are no longer "new" information and, thus, require less processing attention. Accordingly, more processing attention can be devoted to determining the thematic roles. In contrast, when a reversible passive sentence is encountered in isolation, processing resources must be divided among identifying the primary lexical items, decoding morphosyntactic elements, and determining thematic roles. Thematic role identification is often the most difficult task (Caramazza & Miceli, 1991) and can suffer when processing resources are divided. The notion of dividing processing resources is consistent with concepts of working memory (Baddeley, 1986; Moscovitch & Umilta, 1990) and has been shown to occur in other tasks attempted by aphasic subjects (Arvedson & McNeil, 1988; McNeil & Kimelman, 1986).

Recall that comprehension of reversible passive sentences was not significantly enhanced by either single sentence nonpredictive contexts (Pierce & Wagner, 1985) or target sentence repetition (Pierce, 1988). It is possible that these single sentence contexts did not provide sufficient

Table 11–1. Examples of predictive and nonpredictive narrative contexts

Predictive Narrative

A cat is attempting to eat its food. A dog walks by the cat. The cat begins to hiss at the dog. The dog tries to eat some of the cat's food. The cat arches its back as the dog begins to run. The dog is chased by the cat.

Nonpredictive Narrative

A cat is eating its dinner. A dog walks over to the cat. The cat hisses at the dog. The dog growls at the cat. They both begin to run. The dog is chased by the cat.

---

exposure to the key lexical items to alleviate processing demands during the forthcoming target sentence.

Even though both redundancy and prediction can contribute to enhanced comprehension, the data so far indicate that these effects are not additive. Both predictive and nonpredictive narrative contexts improved comprehension to the same extent (Germani & Pierce, 1992; Hough, Pierce, & Cannito, 1989). However, since the predictive contexts also contained the factor of redundancy, it is possible that redundancy rather than prediction generated the effect associated with the predictive narratives. There are several reasons to believe that prediction and redundancy are separate factors. First, the effects of each one are dissociable. A group of aphasic subjects tested by Cannito, Vogel, and Pierce (1991) demonstrated significantly better comprehension of reversible passive sentences following predictive but not nonpredictive narrative contexts. Further analysis (Cannito, Vogel, Pierce, & Hough, 1991) revealed that those aphasic subjects who did not benefit from the nonpredictive contexts (redundancy factor alone) had significantly shorter times post-onset of insult and significantly poorer auditory comprehension skills than those subjects who did benefit from the nonpredictive narrative contexts. This suggests that the contextual feature of prediction is usable at an earlier stage of recovery from aphasia than is redundancy. This dissociation between predictive and nonpredictive contexts also was found at the level of single sentence contexts (Pierce & Wagner, 1985). Second, aphasic subjects performed above chance level (66% accuracy) when the predictive narrative contexts were provided without the subsequent reversible passive target sentences (Germani & Pierce, 1992). In this case, redundancy could not occur, so the subjects had to rely on prediction.

CONTEXTUAL INFLUENCES ON SEMANTIC PROCESSING

All of the research reviewed in the previous section used reversible passive sentences as the target information. This was done to maintain uniformity across studies and to focus on a difficult syntactic construction for aphasic subjects to understand in isolation. However, linguistic and extralinguistic context can also influence the comprehension of semantic information, which is usually easier for aphasic individuals to process. Pierce and Beekman (1985) found that aphasic subjects' comprehension of a specific noun was better when preceded by a contextual sentence (or picture) that predicted the target noun. For example, the stimulus "The woman went to the movies. Where did she go? (dentist or movies)" was more accurately comprehended when preceded by the sentence "The woman has popcorn." Placing the contextual sentence after the target information also generated significantly enhanced comprehension (Pierce, 1988). In contrast, comprehension was not significantly improved when the contextual information was presented alone (Clark & Flowers, 1987) or the target sentence was simply repeated once (Pierce, 1988).

Despite these results, which mirrored those found for syntactic targets discussed previously, narrative context does not always improve comprehension of semantic information; it can cause performance to deteriorate. For example, Pierce and DeStefano (1987) tested aphasic subjects' comprehension of target nouns placed in the middle of three-sentence narratives. The narratives varied in the extent to which they predicted the target nouns. The subjects responded to a question about these target nouns by selecting from four printed words with the following characteristics: the correct word, a word that logically fit in the narrative but differed from the target noun in its initial phonemes, a word that shared the same initial phonemes as the target but did not logically fit in the narrative, and an unrelated word. An example is presented in Table 11–2. When the narrative only loosely predicted the target word (weak context condition), the subjects performed quite accurately. However, when the narratives predicted the target noun more strongly, performance deteriorated significantly. This deterioration was completely accounted for by erroneous selection of the word foil that logically fit in the narrative. One implication of these results is that aphasic subjects, at times, may be more responsive to contextual influences than they are to what is actually presented. If the subjects had been able to block out the stronger contextual information, then they should have performed as well as they did in the weak context condition.

The process of comprehension usually entails the integration of what is heard (or read) with what is known (either based on world knowledge or from the surrounding context) (Morrow, Bower, & Greenspan, 1990; Mross, 1990; van Dijk & Kintsch, 1983). This integration, while enhancing comprehension, can make it difficult to determine whether the comprehended message reflects what was heard or what the listeners thought they heard as colored by their prior knowledge. For example, Rosenthal and Bisiacchi (1992) found evidence for the tacit integration, through the automatic application of causal inferences, of what aphasic

Table 11–2. Example of a predictive narrative

> There is too much noise in here.
> Please turn down the TV.
> We do not want the neighbors to complain.
>
> What needs to be turned down?
>
> (a) TV
> (b) radio
> (c) teapot
> (d) window

subjects read with what they knew. Specifically, subjects were presented sentences that had compelling tacit implications (e.g., "The ball hit the window" and "The woman slips on the stairs"). They were then asked to select the picture that represented the sentence from a set of three: the correct picture, one that showed the compelling pragmatic implication of the event, and a distractor that contained the same characters but in a different action. The aphasic subjects selected the foil representing the compelling implication of the event significantly more often than did either young or elderly non-brain-damaged normals. Accordingly, the strong application of knowledge measurably influences comprehension, but this can generate an integrated message that may differ from what was actually presented.

An issue that relates to prediction is expectation (Schwanenflugel & Shoben, 1985). Despite the extent to which context predicts a set of possible words, certain words are usually more expected than others. For example, "car" is a highly expected completion for the utterance "I drive a _____" However, "tractor" and "lorry," among others, are also possible completions. The predictive stimuli in the studies described were high on both the predictive and expectation dimension. Puskaric and Pierce (1991) investigated the interaction between prediction and expectation in a reading comprehension task with aphasic subjects. When sentences were strongly predictive (eliciting a small set of possible word completions), expected and unexpected words were equally well comprehended. However, when the sentences were weakly predictive (eliciting a larger set of possible word completions), highly expected words were comprehended more accurately than unexpected words. According to a model in the normal literature (Schwanenflugel & LaCount, 1988; Schwanenflugel & Shoben, 1985; Simpson, Peterson, Casteel, & Burgess, 1989), strongly predictive sentence stems generate a large number of specified features that activate a small set of possible word completions. Because of the small number of words and the large set of features, each word becomes highly activated. Accordingly for aphasic subjects, the additional impact of expectation may be negligible.

In contrast, weakly predictive sentence stems generate a limited number of features that are consistent with a large number of word possibilities. Each word is activated to a much smaller extent, thus leaving an opportunity for the (additive) impact of expectation to affect performance.

THE NARRATIVE OF DAILY LIFE

This section of the chapter has been concerned with the nature of contextual influences that exist within narratives. Two primary factors, prediction and redundancy, have been discussed. However, in one sense, the function of narratives is to provide continuous information with which additional information can be integrated. The same can be said for the events of daily life, and the mechanisms of contextual influence could be as prevalent in daily events as they are in narratives. For example, if one hears the utterance "John was hit by Bill," it is usually accompanied by some event such as John crying or having a large bruise. Those events would certainly predict the subject-object relationship of the utterance. Conversely, one may know both John and Bill, who are playing, and then hear a loud smack. On asking what happened, one is told that "John was hit by Bill." Certainly, most of one's processing resources could be devoted to determining the thematic roles within the sentence because the other information is already known.

Contextual influences are prevalent throughout the natural linguistic and extralinguistic environment. Advances in our understanding of these influences will help improve both our treatment procedures for patients with aphasia (Pierce, 1989) and our understanding of how language is normally processed.

NARRATIVE PROCESSING IN RIGHT AND LEFT HEMISPHERE BRAIN-DAMAGED ADULTS

This section addresses both right and left hemisphere brain-damaged adults' use of macrostructure in comprehending narratives. Research with individuals with right hemisphere brain damage has revealed difficulties in the integration of linguistic information into coherent wholes (Gardner, Brownell, Wapner, & Michelow, 1983; Millar & Whitaker, 1983; Myers, 1984, 1986, 1990). These adults have been observed to miss the intended meaning of narrative level materials, such as stories (Huber, 1990; Huber & Gleber, 1982; Myers & Linebaugh, 1981; Rehak et al., 1992; Wapner, Hamby, & Gardner, 1981), dialogs and conversational remarks (Gardner et al., 1983; Kaplan, Brownell, Jacobs, & Gardner, 1990; Myers, 1984; Rehak, Kaplan, & Gardner, 1992), indirect requests (Foldi, 1987; Hirst, LeDoux, & Stein, 1984; Weylman, Brownell, Roman, & Gardner, 1989), jokes (Bihrle, Brownell,

Powelson, & Gardner, 1986; Brownell, Michel, Powelson, & Gardner, 1983), and inferences (Brownell, Potter, Bihrle, & Gardner, 1986; Joanette, Goulet, Ska, & Nespoulous, 1986; Myers, 1990; McDonald & Wales, 1986).

Some research has shown that right hemisphere brain-damaged adults do not differ from non-brain-damaged and/or left hemisphere brain-damaged aphasic individuals in narrative comprehension. Brookshire and Nicholas (1984) found that aphasic, right hemisphere brain-damaged, and normal adults all exhibited a similar pattern of better comprehension for main ideas than for details. Furthermore, main idea comprehension was not influenced by narrative coherency for any of these populations (Wegner, Brookshire, & Nicholas, 1984). Stachowiak, Huber, Poeck, and Kerschensteiner (1977) found no differences between left and right hemisphere brain-damaged and non-brain-damaged individuals in text comprehension. Tompkins and Mateer (1984) observed similar performance between right hemisphere and normal subjects in comprehending highly redundant short narratives. Delis, Wapner, Gardner, and Moses (1983), however, observed that redundancy did not influence the poor performance of right hemisphere brain-damaged adults on a task requiring sentence arrangement in paragraphs. These inconsistent findings may be the result of differences in contextual redundancy.

A few investigations have revealed narrative comprehension differences in left and right hemisphere brain-damaged subgroups. Brookshire and Nicholas (1984) found that fluent but not disfluent aphasic adults had significantly worse comprehension than non-brain-damaged adults for main ideas and details. Wapner et al. (1981) observed that fluent aphasic adults were less accurate than nonfluent adults in the integration and comprehension of narratives. Low, but not high, comprehending aphasic adults performed significantly poorer than non-brain-damaged adults in the comprehension of both monologues and dialogues (Katsuki-Nakamura, Brookshire, & Nicholas, 1988). Grossman (1982) found that adults with anterior right hemisphere brain-damage displayed greater difficulty in interpreting linguistic materials presented in noncanonical form than other adults with brain-damage.

THEMATIC INFLUENCES ON NARRATIVE COMPREHENSION

DEFINITION OF THEMES AND THEME PROCESSING

To comprehend a narrative, normal adults rely on an abstract underlying structure, frequently termed a macrostructure. This construct is an abstract semantic description of the total content of any type of discourse, including narratives (Kintsch & van Dijk, 1978; Mross, 1990). The macrostructure is part of the base of the narrative that represents or includes the main idea(s) (Bransford & Johnson, 1972) or theme (Dooling & Lachman, 1971; Thorndyke, 1977) of a text. The *theme* is the topic or gist of a narrative (Mross, 1990). The theme enables a person to extract meaning from individual sentences and integrate that meaning into the context supplied by other sentences in the narrative. Successful comprehension is dependent on this theme integration process. At times, however, the process may be more difficult because semantic links between sentences are not explicitly stated or theme organization is unexpected. Normal adults show no difference in comprehending narratives that have the expected organization of a theme at the beginning of the passage and those that have the presentation of the theme delayed until the end of the text. Normal adults have been observed, however, to display a deterioration in comprehension when narratives have no theme (Thorndyke, 1977).

Normal and aphasic adults have been found to synthesize all semantic information available to them prior to determining the meaning for a target sentence. More importantly, the order of presentation of this information has been found to have no influence on comprehension of the material. As mentioned previously, Pierce (1988) found that supportive or contextual information, regardless of whether it was presented before or after the target information to be understood, was observed to aid comprehension of aphasic adults. In a normal discourse (e.g., conversation), supportive information may be presented after other related information particularly when a speaker wants to clarify an issue already stated. This clarification may enhance previously heard statements (i.e., redundancy) or may actually promote comprehension of information by providing the central theme of the discourse. The latter occurrence is observed frequently in normal conversation. That is, the central theme of a discourse may not always be presented at the beginning and may, in fact, be presented at the end of a discourse.

In this section, we report on a study (Hough, 1990) that looked at the effects of delayed presentation of theme on narrative comprehension[1] in adults with left and right hemisphere brain-damage and non-brain-damaged individuals. Specific subgroups of right (anterior vs. posterior) and left (nonfluent vs. fluent) hemisphere groups also were examined. Narratives were used because it is easier to control manipulation of the central theme in regard to organization of the narrative and they can be visually represented in the form of a picture. Specifically, we were interested in whether individuals with brain damage were able to retain information without the aid of a central theme and subsequently organize and

---

[1] The original study investigated the delayed theme effect on narrative comprehension as well as interpretation-production of narratives. Only the comprehension findings are reported here.

comprehend this information when the theme was presented at the end of the narrative. Performance of the right hemisphere subjects was of particular interest because of these individuals' reported difficulties in integrating information in a coherent and holistic manner, especially when information is presented in noncanonical form (Delis et al., 1983; Gardner et al., 1983; Grossman, 1982; Hough, 1990; Myers, 1986, 1990).

STUDY METHODS

We analyzed the narrative comprehension of 30 native adult speakers of English. Twenty of the adults had suffered single unilateral cerebrovascular accidents, 10 of which suffered left hemisphere brain damage and 10 suffered right hemisphere brain damage. All brain-damaged subjects were right-handed by self-report. The other 10 participants were neurologically intact control subjects. There were no significant differences between groups on age and education level.

For the right hemisphere subjects, five had anterior lesions limited to prerolandic areas and five had posterior lesions limited to postrolandic regions. For the left hemisphere subjects, five displayed fluent aphasia and five exhibited nonfluent aphasia. Behavioral data were used to identify these subgroups because of incomplete lesion localization information.

The stimuli were 32 paragraphs, a sample of which is presented in Table 11–3. All paragraphs were equivalent in regard to the number of: (a) sentences, (b) words per sentence, (c) independent clauses per paragraph, (d) dependent clauses per paragraph, and (e) amount of information conveyed regarding propositions. This last factor aided the reduction of information redundancy in the narratives. All paragraphs, which were developed by the first author (Hough, 1990), were at or below a sixth-grade reading level (Dale & Chall, 1948). Paragraph main ideas as well as the primary main idea or central theme of each paragraph were empirically derived from a study with non-brain-damaged middle-aged adults. The central theme was manipulated in regard to the organization of each narrative.

Thirty-two black and white line drawings were generated, each one depicting the central theme of a particular narrative. This was utilized to provide subjects with an extralinguistic context of the central theme. The picture that accompanies the sample narrative is presented in Figure 11–1.

Subjects were presented with four multiple-choice questions per narrative. The questions corresponded to each of the four most salient narrative main ideas.[2] For each question, subjects pointed to one of four

---

[2] For half of the narratives (16), subjects were presented with a multiple-choice format (4 questions per narrative, yielding a total of 64 questions); for the other narratives, subjects were required to produce verbal responses regarding the most salient main ideas. As mentioned, production data is not reported.

Table 11–3. Sample stimuli

Narrative 1

Normal Theme Organization

Susan was sitting at her desk in her office. She was unhappy because she had not received any candy, flowers, or cards for Valentine's Day. She thought that her fiance would send her something but it was getting close to five o'clock. Just before five, there was a knock at her door. Her secretary walked in with two huge baskets of roses. She was followed by a handsome man who also was carrying flowers. Susan jumped up and ran over to kiss Paul, her fiance. Susan was sorry that she ever doubted him on Valentine's Day.

Delayed Theme Organization

Susan was sitting at her desk in her office. She thought that her fiance would send her something but it was getting close to five o'clock. Just before five, there was a knock at her door. Her secretary walked in with two huge baskets of roses. She was followed by a handsome man who also was carrying flowers. Susan jumped up and ran over to kiss Paul, her fiance. Susan was sorry that she ever doubted him on Valentine's Day. She had been unhappy because she had not received any candy, flowers, or cards for Valentine's Day.

Sample Multiple Response Choices

Question: "Why was Susan unhappy?"

Correct response	"had not received any gifts"
Unrelated plausible response	"fighting with her boyfriend"
Related implausible response	"secretary walked in her office"
Unrelated nonsensical response	"stealing gifts"

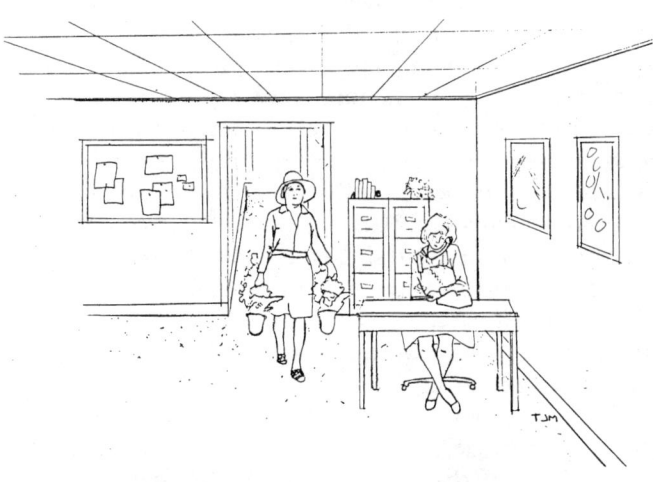

Figure 11–1. Stimulus picture depicting the central theme of Narrative 1.

foils, each foil consisting of words and phrases. The foils included: (a) the correct response, (b) an unrelated but plausible incorrect response, (c) an implausible but related incorrect response in that it contained information mentioned in the narrative, and (d) a nonsensical response unrelated to the narrative context.

Subjects were informed that they would hear a short story and would be asked questions about it. For each subject, half the narratives were presented with the central theme at the beginning and half were presented with the central theme delayed until the end of the narrative. Half of the narratives were accompanied by the central theme picture and half were presented without the picture. All narratives were presented auditorily via live voice. After a paragraph was read aloud to a subject, the subject was engaged in a 5-minute conversation with the examiner on topics unrelated to the preceding narrative context. The conversational delay was used to reduce the possibility of rehearsal and eliminate the recency effect (Glanzer, 1972; Glanzer & Cunitz, 1966). After the delay, narrative comprehension was ascertained through the multiple-choice task.

RESULTS

The first analysis addressed overall accuracy on the multiple-choice questions about the narratives. As can be seen in Table 11-4, the right hemisphere group performed significantly poorer when central theme to presentation was delayed compared to normal theme organization. There were no differences between theme conditions for the aphasic and non-brain-damaged groups. The non-brain-damaged subjects were significantly more accurate than both brain-damaged groups, regardless of theme condition. However, the aphasic group was significantly more accurate than the right hemisphere brain-damaged group only for the delayed theme condition. The central theme picture did not influence performance of any group.

Table 11-5 is a display of the overall accuracy for the left and right hemisphere brain-damaged subgroups. For the subgroup analyses, comparisons were made only between the particular hemisphere subgroups and the non-brain-damaged group. For the aphasic groups, theme organization or presence of the central theme picture did not appear to have an influence on the performance of either group. The non-brain-damaged and nonfluent aphasic groups were significantly more accurate than the fluent group. There were no differences between the nonfluent and non-brain-damaged groups.

For the right hemisphere groups, the anterior and posterior groups were significantly more accurate in the normal than the delayed theme condition, regardless of the presence of the contextual picture. There were no differences between the two right hemisphere groups. The non-brain-damaged group was significantly more accurate than both right

Table 11-4. Mean overall accuracy scores for the normal and delayed theme conditions

Theme Condition	Group		
	Right	Left	Normal
Normal theme	27.8[a]	25.4	30.1
Delayed theme	16.7	23.8	30.0

[a]Maximum score equals 32 (number of questions across the picture condition).

Table 11-5. Mean overall accuracy scores for the normal and delayed theme conditions for the left and right hemisphere subgroups

Theme Condition	Group				
	Right Hemisphere			Left Hemisphere	
	Anterior	Posterior	Normal	Fluent	Nonfluent
Normal theme					
Picture	14.3[a]	14.2	15.1	13.8	14.9
No picture	13.6	13.4	15.0	13.9	14.7
Delayed theme					
Picture	8.2	7.5	14.9	13.5	14.6
No picture	8.6	8.2	15.2	13.3	14.6

[a]Maximum score equals 16 (number of questions per condition).

hemisphere groups in all conditions, except when the picture accompanied normal theme organization for the narratives.

The second analysis consisted of determining the number of narratives for which subjects chose the most central theme. Although some of the brain-damaged subjects, particularly those with aphasia, may be able to identify main ideas in a narrative, it was hypothesized that they may not consistently choose the central theme or main gist of the text. As can be seen in Table 11-6, results were similar to the pattern observed for overall accuracy.

Table 11-7 is a display of data on central theme identification for the aphasic and right hemisphere subgroups. For the aphasic analysis, theme organization did not affect the performance of any group. The non-brain-damaged group identified significantly more central themes than the fluent aphasic group. There were no significant differences between the non-brain-damaged and nonfluent group or between the two aphasic groups.

For the right hemisphere groups, the anterior and posterior groups identified significantly more central themes under the expected than

Table 11-6. Mean central theme identification performance for the normal and delayed theme conditions.

Theme Condition	Group		
	Right	Left	Normal
Normal theme	5.4[a]	6.8	7.3
Delayed theme	2.8	6.3	7.5

[a]Maximum score equals 8 (number of narratives across the picture condition).

Table 11-7. Mean central theme identification for the normal and delayed conditions for the left and right hemisphere subgroups

Theme Condition	Group				
	Right Hemisphere		Normal	Left Hemisphere	
	Anterior	Posterior		Fluent	Nonfluent
Normal theme	6.0[a]	4.8	7.3	6.8	6.8
Delayed theme	3.0	2.4	7.5	5.8	6.8

[a]Maximum score equals 8 (number of narratives across the picture condition).

delayed condition. Non-brain-damaged subjects identified significantly more central themes than both right hemisphere groups regardless of theme organization condition. There were no significant differences between the two right hemisphere groups. The presence of the central theme picture had no influence on central theme identification for any of the three overall groups or the subgroups.

The next analysis dealt with the pattern of error choices for both theme conditions. As can be seen in Table 11-8, both the non-brain-damaged and aphasic subjects primarily chose the unrelated plausible and related implausible responses, with extremely small proportions of nonsensical responses. This pattern was observed regardless of theme condition. For the right hemisphere group, the pattern of errors was different for the two theme conditions. For the normal theme condition, the right hemisphere subjects chose a very high proportion of unrelated plausible responses with a small proportion of related implausible responses. However, for the delayed theme condition, they chose a very high proportion of nonsensical responses.

Table 11-8. Mean proportion of error choices in the normal and delayed theme conditions

Theme Condition	Group		
	Right	Left	Normal
Normal theme			
Unrelated plausible	.825	.575	.479
Related implausible	.144	.425	.503
Nonsensical	.031	.010	.018
Delayed theme			
Unrelated plausible	.012	.535	.502
Related implausible	.252	.446	.486
Nonsensical	.736	.019	.012

SUMMARY AND DISCUSSION

The main finding was that the right hemisphere brain-damaged groups had more difficulty comprehending narratives, especially when the central theme was presented at the end of the text. This was observed regardless of lesion location. These results support the findings of Gardner et al. (1983) and others (Brownell et al., 1986; Wapner et al., 1981; Weylman et al., 1989) who have investigated various aspects of right hemisphere adults' understanding of discourse. Our right hemisphere subjects displayed a greater deterioration in performance when narrative information was presented in an unexpected format (e.g., delayed theme). Delis et al. (1983) observed that right hemisphere subjects performed significantly worse than non-brain-damaged controls on a task requiring the arrangement of sentences in paragraphs. As in our investigation, Delis et al. found that the right hemisphere subjects had difficulty comprehending paragraphs when the order of presentation of narrative propositions was unexpected.

Left hemisphere brain-damaged and non-brain-damaged adults were not affected by organization of the central theme in regard to their comprehension of the narratives. The adults with aphasia appeared to be able to integrate semantic information prior to determining meaning of a narrative without regard to the order of this information. However, as a group, the left hemisphere subjects performed significantly poorer than the non-brain-damaged group on narrative comprehension. These findings are in contrast to Brookshire and Nicholas (1984) and Stachowiak et al. (1977) who attributed the good performance of their subjects to redundancy of information in the narratives. In our study, attempts were made to reduce information redundancy of the experimental stimuli through controlling the amount of information conveyed in regard to propositions. This may account for the different results between studies. Fluent individuals may perform more poorly than other aphasic adults because they do have some difficulty with the integration and comprehension of complex information.

Overall, the presence of a picture depicting the narrative central theme did not affect performance of any group. This finding was in accordance with Waller and Darley's (1978) results with aphasic individuals in which no improvement in comprehension was observed when a picture accompanied presentation of a narrative. Pierce and Beekman (1985) found that extralinguistic picture cues aided comprehension of subsequent sentential information for low comprehending aphasic adults. The contrastive findings may be due to the length of the linguistic material. Pierce and Beekman used sentences whereas we and Waller and Darley (1978) employed paragraph-length narratives. In Pierce and Beekman (1985), the pictures cues may have been of benefit to the aphasic adults because the experimental stimuli were not long enough for subjects to apprehend the contextual cohesion observed in paragraphs.

Persons with right hemisphere brain-damage frequently have been observed to experience difficulty in processing visual-spatial material. However, in our study, the theme picture did not influence narrative comprehension. Therefore, problems with integration of complex linguistic units into coherent wholes may be independent of visual-spatial information processing.

VARIABLES INFLUENCING NARRATIVE THEME COMPREHENSION AND CONCLUSIONS

This last section of the chapter examines some variables that may play a role in brain-damaged adults' comprehension of narrative themes.

ORGANIZATIONAL SKILLS

Adults with right hemisphere brain-damage may be impaired in the integration of information in conversation and in narratives, especially when an organizing theme does not occur at the beginning of the discourse. They appear unable to use the macrostructure as an organizer in apprehending a paragraph, particularly when theme presentation does not follow a canonical organization. Consequently, they retain isolated pieces of data rather than integrating this information to deduce the meaning of the narrative. The unexpected narrative organization appears to be the specific variable that interferes with story processing. In fact, recently, it has been observed that right hemisphere adults perform at a level comparable to non-brain-damaged adults in comprehending stories that follow an expected form (Rehak et al., 1992).

Unlike aphasic and non-brain-damaged adults, right hemipshere individuals are poor at imposing macrostructure when it does not initially exist. This impairment appears to contribute to these adults' noted problems in following a conversation, as this type of discourse often has variable theme organization. Rehak et al. (1992) found that right hemisphere brain-damaged adults functioned normally in canonically directed conversation. However, when the organization of the conversation was disrupted through presentation of blocking or tangential statements, performance on interpreting conversations deteriorated.

The ability to organize language at the narrative level may depend on intact right hemisphere processing. Although aphasic subjects may perform more poorly than non-brain-damaged adults on narrative comprehension, this decrement appears to result from the linguistic demands of the narrative task, rather than from narrative-level organizational deficits. Both right and left hemisphere brain-damaged adults appear to rely more on the macrostructure than the microstructure in text comprehension (Huber, 1990). Although left hemisphere brain-damaged adults have compromised linguistic skills, however, they appear to retain an organizing principle for narrative comprehension. We continue to support the idea of a special role for the right hemisphere in text comprehension skills and a separation of narrative-level deficits from those specific to other language levels.

ATTENTION ALLOCATION AND ATTENTIONAL SKILLS

Another variable that may influence the comprehension of narrative themes is the adequacy of attentional skills. Specifically, is theme comprehension dependent on the activation and/or allocation of attentional resources, particularly when thematic information is presented in a variable or unexpected manner? In our study, the aphasic adults' narrative comprehension was unaffected by the order of presentation of the narrative theme. Yet, it has been hypothesized that aphasic adults present with a pervasive deficit in the distribution of attentional resources (McNeil, Odell, & Tseng, 1990; McNeil & Kimelman, 1986), thereby resulting in performance variability on linguistic processing tasks. Why, then, are aphasic adults successful in comprehending delayed theme narratives? Pierce (1991) has suggested that the allocation of attentional resources as a function of the redundancy of narrative information may account for aphasic adults' high level of performance. It is possible that repetition of the key lexical items in the narratives (i.e., nouns) yields enough redundancy to enable aphasic adults to distribute their processing resources adequately so as to meet the demands of the thematic comprehension task. That is, by the time they hear the thematic sentence at the end of the narrative, the key lexical items representing the characters and events are familiar, thus requiring less attention. Furthermore, repetition of the key lexical items leads to expectations about possible narrative outcomes. More resources can then be focused on integrating the delayed theme with other narrative information. Narratives that vary along a redundancy continuum should be utilized with brain-damaged adults to determine whether degree of contextual redundancy influences allocation of attentional resources and subsequently, comprehension performance.

Unlike the aphasic adults, our right hemisphere brain-damaged subjects showed a significant decrement in performance when narrative theme presentation was delayed. In general, damage to the right hemisphere has been associated with deficiencies in directed attention and allocation of attentional resources (Heilman, Valenstein, & Watson, 1984; Mesulam, 1981; Posner, Walker, Friedrich, & Raphal, 1984). Attentional impairments may account for our subjects' difficulty in apprehending narrative thematic cues, particularly when these cues are noncanonical. Perhaps the effort to retain and integrate narrative information without the aid of a central theme consumes the attentional resources that are available to the right hemisphere individual. Consequently, this inefficiency in allocation yields little attention that can be devoted to comprehending narrative information when the theme is presented in noncanonical order at the end of the narrative. Or, it is possible that right hemisphere individuals have difficulty retaining and integrating narrative information when theme presentation is delayed because of insufficient activation of attentional mechanisms, particularly for comprehending complex constructs. Comprehending linguistic information presented in noncanonical or unexpected format is a difficult task requiring effortful and controlled activation of processing resources. Right hemisphere adults may perform poorly because they continue to rely on processing strategies that are only appropriate for more automatic tasks; thus, attentional activation is not sufficient for the task demands.

INFERENCING ABILITIES

Inference is the identification of key features of a situation and the ability to recognize the relationship of these features to one another and to other cues in a particular context or situation (Morrow et al., 1990; Myers, 1990). Inference allows us to interpret the intended meaning of a particular context and has been identified as a major process employed by the executive control system (Burns, 1985). Inferencing skills have been found to be adequate in most adults with aphasia (Chapey, 1986; Foldi, Cicone, & Gardner, 1983). It has been hypothesized that inference failure may represent a central underlying basis for most right hemisphere communication disorders (Myers, 1990). However, not all researchers have observed inference deficits in right hemisphere brain-damaged adults (Joanette, Goulet, & Hannequin, 1990). This controversy may be related to the nature of the task or, at a more basic level, the definition of inference itself.

Can inference failure account for the poor performance of right hemisphere brain-damaged adults in comprehending delayed narrative themes? One way to investigate this is by examining the nature of the task and its reliance on inferencing abilities. As mentioned previously, to comprehend a narrative, a listener must construct a model of the situations described through integration of information from each narrative sentence. This is accomplished by applying world knowledge of the situation to the narrative; integrating what is heard with what is known. When theme presentation is delayed, the individual must still begin the process of narrative interpretation, initially without the aid of a central theme. Consequently, when the theme is introduced at the end of the narrative, the individual must then make an inference regarding the intended meaning of the narrative. That is, they must determine the relationship between (1) the narrative interpretation developed before the theme was presented and (2) the presented central theme. Right hemisphere adults appear to have difficulty recognizing the relationship between these two elements. The result is often retention of isolated pieces of narrative data rather than understanding the intended meaning, in other words, a lack of inference or faulty inference.

Another way to investigate whether inference failure is the basis for reduced performance on delayed narrative theme comprehension may be to examine error patterns on the comprehension task. As mentioned previously, when theme presentation was in the expected format, right hemisphere patients primarily chose plausible foils. However, when theme presentation was delayed, error choices were primarily nonsensical responses. These results suggest that for expected theme organization, the right hemsiphere adults can maintain the "script" of the situation. Although they are sometimes incorrect, they make plausible interpretations of the narrative information. However, when the information is presented in noncanonical form, the right hemisphere adults have difficulty recognizing the relationship between the key elements in the narrative and the relationship between these elements and the situation presented. Consequently, they choose the nonsensical, unrelated response. That is, they make the wrong inference because they never seem to acquire the "script" of the situation. So, inference failure may account for difficulties in comprehending information presented noncanonically for our right hemisphere brain-damaged adults. The consistency and extent of this phenomenon in the right hemisphere population in general, however, appears to be related to the nature of the input, the complexity of the task, and the nature of the inference.

REFERENCES

Arvedson, J., & McNeil, M. (1988, November). *Response interference of auditory processing with left/right hemisphere lesions.* Paper presented at the American Speech-Language-Hearing Association convention, Boston, MA.

Baddeley, A. (1986). *Working memory.* Oxford: Oxford University Press.

Bihrle, A. M., Brownell, H. H., Powelson, J., & Gardner, H. (1986). Comprehension of humourous and nonhumourous materials by left and right-brain-damaged patients. *Brain and Cognition, 5,* 399–411.

Bransford, J. D., & Johnson, M. K. (1972). Contextual prerequisites for understanding: Some investigations of comprehension and recall. *Journal of Verbal Learning and Behavior, 11,* 717–726.

Brookshire, R. (1987). Auditory language comprehension disorders in aphasia. *Topics in Language Disorders, 8,* 11–23.

Brookshire, R., & Nicholas, L. (1984). Comprehension of directly and indirectly stated main ideas and details in discourse by brain-damaged and non-brain-damaged listeners. *Brain and Language, 21,* 21–36.

Brownell, H., Michel, D., Powelson, J., & Gardner, H. (1983). Surprise but not coherence: Sensitivity to verbal humor in right hemisphere patients. *Brain and Language, 18,* 20–27.

Brownell, H., Potter, H., Bihrle, A., & Gardner, H. (1986). Inference deficits in right brain-damaged patients. *Brain and Language, 27,* 310–321.

Burns, M.S. (1985). Language without communication: The pragmatics of right hemisphere damage. In M. S. Burns, A. S. Halper, & S. I. Mogil (Eds.), *Clinical management of right hemisphere dysfunction.* Rockville, MD: Aspen.

Cannito, M., Jarecki, J., & Pierce, R. (1986). Effects of thematic structure on syntactic comprehension in aphasia. *Brain and Language, 27,* 38–49.

Cannito, M., Vogel, D., & Pierce, R. (1991). Contextualized sentence comprehension in nonfluent aphasia: Predictiveness and severity of comprehension impairment. In T. Prescott (Ed.), *Clinical aphasiology* (vol. 20). Austin, TX: Pro-Ed.

Cannito, M., Vogel, D., Pierce, R., & Hough, M. (1991). Time post-onset and contextualized sentence comprehension in nonfluent aphasia. In M. Lemme (Ed.), *Clinical aphasiology* (vol. 21). Austin, TX: Pro-Ed.

Caplan, D., & Evans, K. (1990). The effects of syntactic structure on discourse comprehension in patients with parsing impairments. *Brain and Language, 39,* 206–234.

Caramazza, A., & Miceli, G. (1991). Selective impairment of thematic role assignment in sentence processing. *Brain and Language, 41,* 402–436.

Caramazza, A., & Zurif, E. (1976). Dissociation of algorithmic and heuristic processes in language comprehension: Evidence from aphasia. *Brain and Language, 3,* 572–582.

Chapey, R. (1986). Cognitive intervention: Stimulation of cognition, memory, convergent thinking, divergent thinking and evaluative thinking. In R. Chapey (Ed.), *Language intervention strategies in adult aphasia* (pp. 215–238). Baltimore: Williams & Wilkins.

Clark, A., & Flowers, C. (1987). The effect of semantic redundancy on auditory comprehension in aphasia. In R. Brookshire (Ed.), *Clinical aphasiology conference proceedings* (pp. 174–179). Minneapolis: BRK Publishers.

Dale, E., & Chall, J. (1948). A formula for predicting readability. *Educational Research Bulletin, 27*, 37–54.

Delis, D. C., Wapner, W., Gardner, H., & Moses, J. A. (1983). The contribution of the right hemisphere to the organization of paragraphs. *Cortex, 19*, 43–50.

Deloche, G., & Seron, X. (1981). Sentence understanding and knowledge of the world: Evidence from a sentence-picture matching task performed by aphasic patients. *Brain and Language, 14*, 57–69.

Dooling, D. J., & Lachman, R. (1971). Effects of comprehension on retention of prose. *Journal of Experimental Psychology, 88*, 216–222.

Fletcher, C. R., & Bloom, C. P. (1988). Causal reasoning in the comprehension of simple narrative texts. *Journal of Memory and Language, 27*, 235–244.

Foldi, N. (1987). Appreciation of pragmatic interpretations of indirect commands: Comparison of right and left hemisphere brain-damaged patients. *Brain and Language, 31*, 88–108.

Foldi, N., Cicone, M., & Gardner, H. (1983). Pragmatic aspects of communication in brain-damaged patients. In S. Segalowitz (Ed.), *Language functions and brain organization* (pp. 51–86). New York: Academic Press.

Gardner, H., Brownell, H. H., Wapner, W., & Michelow, D. (1983). Missing the point: The role of the right hemisphere in the processing of complex linguistic materials. In E. Perecman (Ed.), *Cognitive processing in the right hemisphere* (pp. 169–191). New York: Academic Press.

Germani, M. J., & Pierce, R. (1992). Contextual influences in reading comprehension in aphasia. *Brain and Language, 42*, 308–319.

Glanzer, M. (1972). Storage mechanisms in recall. In G. H. Bower & J. T. Spence (Eds.), *The psychology of learning and motivation*. New York: Academic Press.

Glanzer, M., & Cunitz, A. R. (1966). Two storage mechanisms in free recall. *Journal of Verbal Learning and Verbal Behavior, 5*, 351–360.

Grossman, M. (1982). Reversal operations after brain-damage. *Brain and Cognition, 1*, 331–359.

Heilman, K., Scholes, R., & Watson, R. (1976). Defects of immediate memory in Broca's and conduction aphasia. *Brain and Language, 3*, 201–208.

Heilman, K., Valenstein, E., & Watson, R. (1984). Neglect and related disorders. *Seminars in Neurology, 4*, 209–219.

Hirst, W., LeDoux, J., & Stein, S. (1984). Constraints on the processing of indirect speech acts: Evidence from aphasiology. *Brain and Language, 23*, 26–33.

Hough, M. S. (1990). Narrative comprehension in adults with right and left hemisphere brain-damage: Theme organization. *Brain and Language, 38*, 253–277.

Hough, M., Pierce, R., & Cannito, M. (1989). Contextual influences in aphasia: Effects of predictive versus nonpredictive narratives. *Brain and Language, 36*, 325–334.

Huber, W. (1990). Text comprehension and production in aphasia: Analysis in terms of micro- and macrostructure. In Y. Joanette & H. Brownell (Eds.), *Discourse ability and brain-damage: Theoretical and empirical perspectives* (pp. 154–179). New York: Springer-Verlag.

Huber, W., & Gleber, J. (1982). Linguistic and nonlinguistic processing of narratives in aphasia. *Brain and Language, 16*, 1–18.

Joanette, Y., Goulet, P., & Hannequin, D. (1990). *Right hemisphere and verbal communication*. New York: Springer-Verlag.

Joanette, Y., Goulet, P., Ska, B., & Nespoulous, J. (1986). Informative content of narrative discourse in right-brain-damaged right-handers. *Brain and Language, 29*, 81–105.

Kaplan, J. A., Brownell, H. H., Jacobs, J. R., & Gardner, H. (1990). The effects of right hemisphere damage on the pragmatic interpretation of conversational remarks. *Brain and Language, 38*, 315–333.

Katsuki-Nakamura, J., Brookshire, R., & Nicholas, L. (1988). Comprehension of monologues and dialogues by aphasic listeners. *Journal of Speech and Hearing Disorders, 53*, 408–415.

Kintsch, W., & van Dijk, T. (1978). Toward a model of text comprehension. *Psychological Review, 85*, 363–394.

Kudo, T. (1984). The effect of semantic plausibility on sentence comprehension in aphasia. *Brain and Language, 21*, 208–218.

McDonald, S., & Wales, R. (1986). An investigation of the ability to process inferences in language following right hemisphere brain damage. *Brain and Language, 29*, 68–80.

McNeil, M., & Kimelman, M. (1986). Toward an integrative information processing structure of auditory comprehension and processing in adult aphasia. In L. LaPointe (Ed.), *Seminars in speech and language: Aphasia: Nature and assessment* (pp. 123–146). New York: Thieme-Stratton.

McNeil, M., Odell, K., & Tseng, C. (1990). Toward the integration of resource allocation into a general theory of aphasia. In T. Prescott (Ed.), *Clinical aphasiology* (vol. 20, pp. 21–39). Austin, TX: Pro-Ed.

Mesulam, M. M. (1981). A cortical network for directed attention and unilateral neglect. *Annals of Neurology, 10*, 309–325.

Millar, J. M., & Whitaker, H. A. (1983). The right hemisphere's contribution to language: A review of the evidence from brain-damaged subjects. In S. J. Segalowitz (Ed.), *Language functions and brain organization* (pp. 87–113). New York: Academic Press.

Morrow, D., Bower, G., & Greenspan, S. (1989). Updating situation models during narrative comprehension. *Journal of Memory and Language, 28*, 292–312.

Morrow, D., Bower, G., & Greenspan, S. (1990). Situation-based inferences during narrative comprehension. In A. Graesser & G. Bower (Eds.), *Inferences and text comprehension* (pp. 123–135). New York: Academic Press.

Morrow, D. G., Greenspan, S. L., & Bower, G. H. (1987). Accessibility and situation models in narrative comprehension. *Journal of Memory and Language, 26*, 165–187.

Moscovitch, M., & Umilta, C. (1990). Modularity and neuropsychology: Implications for the organization of attention and memory in normal and brain-damaged people. In M. Schwartz (Ed.), *Modular processes in dementia* (pp. 1–59). Cambridge, MA: MIT/Bradford.

Mross, E. (1990). Text analysis: Macro- and microstructural aspects of discourse processing. In Y. Joanette & H. Brownell (Eds.), *Discourse ability and brain-damage: Theoretical and empirical perspectives* (pp. 50–68). New York: Springer-Verlag.

Myers, P. (1984). Right hemisphere impairment. In A. Holland (Ed.), *Language disorders in adults*. San Diego: College-Hill Press.

Myers, P. (1986). Right hemisphere communication impairment. In R. Chapey (Ed.), *Language intervention strategies in adult aphasia*. Baltimore: Williams & Wilkins.

Myers, P. (1990). Inference failure: The underlying impairment in right-hemisphere communication disorders. In T. Prescott (Ed.), *Clinical aphasiology* (vol. 20). Austin, TX: Pro-Ed.

Myers, P., & Linebaugh, C. W. (1981). Comprehension of idiomatic expressions by right-hemisphere-damaged adults. In R. Brookshire (Ed.), *Clinical aphasiology conference proceedings*. Minneapolis: BRK Publishers.

Pierce, R. (1988). Influence of prior and subsequent context on comprehension in aphasia. *Aphasiology, 2,* 577–582.

Pierce, R. (1989). Linguistic context and aphasia treatment. In R. Pierce & M. J. Wilcox (Eds.), *Seminars in speech and language: Pragmatics in aphasia*. New York: Thieme-Stratton.

Pierce, R. (1991). Contextual influences during comprehension in aphasia. *Aphasiology, 5,* 1–3.

Pierce, R., & Beekman, L. (1985). Effects of linguistic and extralinguistic context on semantic and syntactic processing in aphasia. *Journal of Speech and Hearing Research, 28,* 250–254.

Pierce, R., & DeStefano, C. (1987). The interactive nature of auditory comprehension in aphasia. *Journal of Communication Disorders, 2,* 15–24.

Pierce, R., & Wagner, C. (1985). The role of context in facilitation of syntactic decoding in aphasia. *Journal of Communication Disorders, 18,* 203–214.

Posner, M.J., Walker, J.A., Friedrich, F.J., & Raphal, R.D. (1984). Effects of parietal lobe injury on covert orienting of visual attention. *Journal of Neuroscience, 4,* 1863–1864.

Puskaric, N., & Pierce, R. (1991, November). *Reading comprehension in aphasia: Effects of prediction and expectation*. Paper presented at the American Speech-Language-Hearing Association annual convention, Atlanta, GA.

Rehak, A., Kaplan, J., & Gardner, H. (1992). Sensitivity to conversational deviance in right hemisphere-damaged patients. *Brain and Language, 42,* 203–217.

Rehak, A., Kaplan, J., Weylman, S.T., Kelly, B., Brownell, H., & Gardner, H. (1992). Story processing in right hemisphere brain-damaged patients. *Brain and Language, 42,* 320–336.

Rosenthal, V., & Bisiacchi, P. (1992). *Tacit integration and referential structure in the language comprehension of aphasics and normals*. Manuscript submitted for publication.

Schwanenflugel, P., & Shoben, E. (1985). The influence of sentence constraint on the scope of facilitation for upcoming words. *Journal of Memory and Language, 24,* 232–252.

Schwanenflugel, P., & LaCount, K. (1988). Semantic relatedness and the scope of facilitation for upcoming words and sentences. *Journal of Experimental Psychology: Learning, Memory, and Cognition, 14,* 344–354.

Sherman, J., & Schweickert, J. (1989). Syntactic and semantic contributions to sentence comprehension in agrammatism. *Brain and Language, 37,* 419–439.

Simpson, G., Peterson, R., Casteel, M., & Burgess, C. (1989). Lexical and sentence context effects in word recognition. *Journal of Experimental Psychology: Learning, Memory, & Cognition, 15,* 88–97.

Speelman, C. P., & Kirsner, K. (1990). The representation of text-based and situation-based information in discourse comprehension. *Journal of Memory and Language, 29,* 119–132.

Stachowiak, F. J., Huber, W., Poeck, K., & Kerschensteiner, M. (1977). Text comprehension in aphasia. *Brain and Language, 4*, 177–195.

Thorndyke, P. (1977). Cognitive structures in comprehension and memory of narrative discourse. *Cognitive Psychology, 9*, 77–110.

Tompkins, C., & Mateer, C. A. (1984). Factors influencing paragraph comprehension by subjects with left or right hemisphere involvement. In R. Brookshire (Ed.), *Clinical aphasiology conference proceedings* (pp. 202–207). Minneapolis: BRK Publishers.

Ulatowska, H., Allard, L., & Chapman, S. (1990). Narrative and procedural discourse in aphasia. In Y. Joanette & H. Brownell (Eds.), *Discourse ability and brain damage: Theoretical and empirical perspectives* (pp. 180–198). New York: Springer-Verlag.

van Dijk, T., & Kintsch, W. (1983). *Strategies of discourse comprehension.* New York: Academic Press.

Waller, M., & Darley, F. (1978). The influence of context on the auditory comprehension of paragraphs by aphasic subjects. *Journal of Speech and Hearing Research, 21*, 732–745.

Waller, M., & Darley, F. (1979). Effect of pre-stimulation on sentence comprehension by aphasic subjects. *Journal of Communication Disorders, 12*, 461–469.

Wapner, W., Hamby, S., & Gardner, H. (1981). The role of the right hemisphere in the apprehension of complex linguistic materials. *Brain and Language, 14*, 15–33.

Wegner, M. L., Brookshire, R., & Nicholas, L. (1984). Comprehension of main ideas and details in coherent and noncoherent discourse by aphasic and nonaphasic listeners. *Brain and Language, 21*, 37–51.

Weylman, S. T., Brownell, H., Roman, M., & Gardner, H. (1989). Appreciation of indirect requests by left-and right-brain-damaged patients: The effects of verbal context and conventionality of wording. *Brain and Language, 36*, 580–591.

CHAPTER 12

Conceptual Processing of Discourse by a Right Hemisphere Brain-Damaged Patient

CARL H. FREDERIKSEN AND BRIGITTE STEMMER

When individuals suffer a right hemisphere brain lesion, deficits in the comprehension and production of natural language discourse have been reported to occur. It has been hypothesized that right hemisphere brain-damaged (RHD) patients have difficulties that are specific to tasks requiring text-level processing. However, the range of discourse tasks is extensive, and the number and kind of reported dysfunctions is diverse. Therefore, it is extremely difficult, based on the existing research, to specify precisely what specific processes in the comprehension and/or production of discourse are affected or are not affected in RHD patients. Although there are a number of explanations extant in the literature concerning the effects of right hemisphere damage on discourse processing, it is not clear from the published literature just how to evaluate these hypotheses based on the methods that have been employed to assess discourse processing. The problem, essentially, is that the comprehension and production of discourse are complex cognitive processes, and observed deficits in discourse behavior can have multiple explanations.

To better understand the nature of dysfunctions in discourse comprehension and production in RHD patients, we need to monitor processing at multiple levels during comprehension or production so that we can evaluate dysfunctions in specific component processes and their contributions to the organized processing of discourse. The psychological study of the cognitive processing and representation of discourse in comprehension and production tasks has resulted in models of these component processes and representations that can make such monitoring of cognitive processing in RHD patients possible. The present case study represents an attempt to use current cognitive models and methods for assessing discourse processing in order to identify specific dysfunctions in the comprehension and production of discourse in RHD patients.

MODELS OF DISCOURSE PROCESSING

The study of discourse as a psychological phenomenon may be seen historically as a succession of models of discourse and discourse processing in which the language units that are processed in comprehending (or producing) discourse and the types of cognitive representations that are constructed by a language user in processing discourse have been successively expanded. Initially, discourse was viewed as consisting of a sequence of *sentence units*, each of which is processed in terms of its *lexical and syntactic structure*. To account for the observation that individuals do not remember the form of sentences in comprehending discourse, but rather their meaning, this model had to be expanded to include the *propositional meaning units* that are encoded in sentences, and the processes by which sentences are interpreted semantically (i.e., in terms of the propositional content they encode; Frederiksen, 1975; Kintsch & van Dijk, 1978). The set of propositions representing the semantic content of a text was referred to as the *discourse microstructure* by Kintsch and van Dijk (1978).

It also was observed that in comprehending discourse, readers normally create and retain a representation of a text's meaning that includes large numbers of *inferred propositions*. In recall and summarization tasks, subjects were found to produce propositions that relate propositions in a text, or that delete, generalize, elaborate, or are entailed by text propositions. Furthermore, they are often unaware of which of their propositions were explicitly stated in a text and which were the result of inferences. Therefore, a model of discourse comprehension had to include inferential processes that relate the semantic content of a current sentence (i.e., its propositions) to the propositional content of discourse that precedes the sentence. Consequently, the language unit that had to be considered must be longer than an individual sentence—a *coherent text unit* consisting of a sentence together with its prior discourse context. Furthermore, the propositional representations associated with a text also had to be expanded to include these inferred propositions.

Kintsch and van Dijk (1978) referred to this expanded propositional representation as the *discourse macrostructure*.

Subsequent research established that this purely text-based view of comprehension is incomplete. It was found that when texts are understood, propositional information is acquired and inferences are made selectively. Inferences reflect not only the propositional content of a text, but also the structure of the conceptual knowledge being communicated through the text as well as the reader's prior conceptual knowledge. Thus, discourse comprehension reflects not only the propositional content of a text, but also the *conceptual knowledge structure* that is represented both explicitly and implicitly by the text, or that readers already possess when they understand a text (Frederiksen, 1986). Although this conceptual knowledge may be thought of as existing independently of a text, it may be reflected in a text in several ways—through the explicit propositional content of the text, through the sequential and topical organization of that content in the text, and through the inferences that must be made by readers to construct a representation of the conceptual knowledge from the propositional meanings that are expressed explicitly in the text.

During reading, a conceptual representation (i.e., a "mental model") is constructed by a reader using both text propositions and prior knowledge. This *knowledge construction process* is guided by the organization and sequencing of the conceptual information in the discourse, and by the structure of the reader's prior knowledge. In addition, it has been shown that during comprehension, readers also may derive conceptual knowledge from the context, that is, the *situation* of which the discourse is a part, and that this context can be important in establishing a reader's purposes and uses of text information. A reader's purpose is important in establishing plans or meta-comprehension strategies that he or she may use to direct and control the processing of discourse.

Thus, in addition to requiring text-based processing, discourse comprehension also requires conceptual knowledge-based processing. The units of information that are processed include language structures within the discourse itself, the propositions interpreted on the bases of these language structures, propositions that are derived from these propositions by means of inferences, the semantic and conceptual knowledge structures expressed by the text propositions, and the context or situation of which the text is a part.

In current theories of discourse comprehension, conceptual processing has been explained in two ways. In one theory, readers use so-called *schema or frame-based processes*, applying their prior conceptual knowledge structures (e.g., schemata, frames, scripts, etc.) during comprehension and modifying them as necessary to incorporate available text information. In the alternative theory, readers use *constructive processes*, applying structure-generating rules, reasoning, and inferences to generate conceptual structures and integrate them into a coherent conceptual representation (e.g., situation model, mental model, conceptual frame, etc.). In so doing they use the available text propositions, their prior knowledge, and contextual information available to them in the situation.

Discourse, then, is currently viewed as a sequence of natural language expressions that is produced by a speaker or writer to represent coherent conceptual knowledge and communicate it to a listener or reader in a context. As a complex language structure, discourse consists of lexical and syntactic units, a sequential structure, a referential structure of cohesive relations that link lexical and syntactic elements across sentences (Halliday & Hasan, 1976; Tutin, 1992), and a topical or thematic structure (Grimes, 1975). These linguistic structures express semantic content and represent conceptual structures at multiple levels including propositional meaning units, semantic relations that link propositions into connected networks, and both local and global conceptual frame structures. Discourse processing is viewed as a complex, multi-layered cognitive process that involves constructing and operating simultaneously on linguistic, propositional, semantic, and conceptual frame representations.

The development and use of explicit models of discourse structures, and of the propositional and conceptual information represented by discourse, have made possible the study of the multiple representations and levels of processing that are involved in discourse comprehension and production. These models can be used to analyze individual differences in discourse processing and, as we will show in this article, differences in the processing of particular narratives by RHD individuals (see Mross, 1990, and Frederiksen, Bracewell, Breuleux, & Renaud, 1990, for surveys of these models and methods).

THE RIGHT HEMISPHERE IN DISCOURSE BEHAVIOR

In recent years, evidence from studies with RHD individuals has accumulated which suggests that the right hemisphere (RH) is not only involved in visuospatial, attentional, and emotional disorders (de Renzi, 1982; Heilman, Bowers, Valenstein, & Watson, 1986) but also plays a role in discourse comprehension and production (for a survey see Joanette, Goulet, & Hannequin, 1990; Millar & Whitaker, 1983). Researchers have explored the interpretation and organization of narratives, conversations, or specific texts such as "non-literal" language by RHD patients (for a survey see Joanette, Goulet, & Hannequin, 1990). However, despite the numerous studies to this end, no clear picture as to the role of the RH in discourse comprehension and production has emerged, and the descriptive or explanatory account of the discursive behavior of RHD individuals is in many cases diverse.

DEVIANT DISCOURSE BEHAVIOR IN RHD PATIENTS RELATIVE TO NORMAL CONTROLS

One of the few observations that seems to be uniform is the description of the RHD patients' *conversational or narrative style* in free conversation or narrative production as embellishing, rambling, tangential, non-informative, irrelevant, repetitive, confabulatory and/or intrusive (Hough, 1990; Moya, Benowitz, Levine, & Finkelstein, 1986; Roman, Brownell, Potter, Seibold, & Gardner 1987; Sheratt & Penn, 1990; Wapner, Hamby, & Gardner, 1981).

The exploration of *microstructural aspects* of narrative discourse has brought about controversial results. In a story retelling task, RHD patients produced fewer text words, fewer T-units and fewer complete but more incomplete cohesive markers (Uryase, 1988). However, Joanette, Goulet, Ska, and Nespoulous (1986) did not find differences of the number of words or T-units produced in the narrative production of RHD patients. In a scrambled story test, RHD patients performed similarly on high and low cohesion versions of stories relative to normal controls (Huber & Gleber, 1982). Brownell, Carroll, Rehak, and Wingfield (1992), on the other hand, found that RHD patients made greater than normal use of the presence or absence of anaphoric pronominal cohesive ties in a multiple-choice judgment task.

Studies investigating the *macrostructural level* of discourse seem even more diverse with regard to the tasks chosen, the phenomena investigated and the findings reported. RHD individuals have been shown to behave differently relative to normal controls in the re-arrangement of sentences to form a coherent paragraph despite the presence of temporal, spatial, or thematic cues (Delis, Wapner, Gardner, & Moses, 1983; Huber & Gleber, 1982; Schneiderman, Murasugi, & Saddy, 1992; Wapner, Hamby, & Gardner, 1981). RHD patients have further been described as having difficulties with reporting or judging the main idea of a narrative when the central theme was shifted to the end of the narrative but not when the theme occurred at the beginning of the narrative; or with selecting an appropriate title or summary for a story (Hough, 1990; Moya, Benowitz, Levine, & Finkelstein, 1986; Rehak, Kaplan, Weylman, et al., 1992). On the other hand, in sentence judgment tasks on the content of stories, RHD patients performed in a manner similar to normal controls and were shown to remember main ideas better than details (Brookshire & Nicholas, 1984). Rehak, Kaplan, Weylman, et al. (1992) found that the performance of RHD patients was similar to that of normal controls in their judgments about a statement referring to the main clue of a story.

Some authors reported a poorer performance of RHD patients in the production or judgments of discourse components (Joanette, Goulet, Ska, & Nespoulous, 1986; Sherratt & Penn, 1990; Uryase, 1988; Uryase, Liles, & Duffy, 1989). RHD individuals demonstrated some difficulty in interpreting redundant conversations and considerable difficulties with tangential conversation in interpreting and/or responding to advancers and blockers in conversational discourse (Rehak, Kaplan, & Gardner, 1992).

It has further been observed that RHD individuals seem to have problems with *re-evaluating information*. RHD patients did not alter their initial interpretation of a sentence although the following context rendered the interpretation as implausible (Brownell, Potter, Bihrle, & Gardner, 1986). In story recall and story arrangement tasks, RHD patients had difficulties in assessing the appropriateness of various facts, situations, and characterizations (Wapner, Hamby, & Gardner, 1981). RHD patients were able to judge a story's affective appeal appropriately, but they had difficulties in making plausible predictions as to the continuation of the story if no clue or trigger was present (Rehak, Kaplan, Weylman, et al., 1992).

RHD individuals have further been described as having difficulties comprehending or producing specific texts involving *"non-literal" language* such as that found in indirect speech acts, idioms, proverbs, metaphors or humor (Bihrle, Brownell, Powelson, & Gardner, 1986; Brownell, Michel, Powelson, & Gardner, 1983; Foldi, 1987; Heeschen & Reischies, 1979; Hirst, LeDoux, & Stein, 1984; Kaplan, Brownell, Jacobs, & Gardner, 1990; Stemmer, Giroux, & Joanette, in press; Weylman, Brownell, Roman, & Gardner, 1989). However, just as for studies investigating the narrative behavior of RHD individuals, the findings reported and the conclusions drawn in these studies are not always uniform and need to be evaluated with care (cf. Joanette, Goulet, & Hannequin, 1990; Stemmer, in press).

EXPLANATIONS

Various attempts have been made to account for the observed verbal behavior of RHD individuals in terms of processes that are assumed to be affected. Some authors have hypothesized that the underlying problem is due to an *impairment at the level of inferential processing*. However, studies to this end are not conclusive. Whereas Read (1981) and Caramazza, Gordon, Zurif, and DeLuca (1979) have observed problems with logical inferencing or syllogistic reasoning, Joanette and Goulet (1987) did not find such problems. Moya, Benowitz, Levine, and Finkelstein (1986) observed that RHD patients had difficulties with drawing inferences from narrative passages. Other researchers have reported problems with evaluating incorrect inferences, or rejecting false statements but no problems with judging correct inferences (Brownell, Potter, Bihrle, & Gardner, 1986;

Joanette & Goulet, 1987; McDonald & Wales, 1986). A preserved ability to make plausible predictions for the continuation of suspense stories (Rehak, Kaplan, Weylman, et al., 1992) would seem to support the view that situation-specific inferencing mechanisms are intact. Against these stands the observation that RHD individuals had difficulties with making plausible predictions when confronted with surprise stories.

One reason that no conclusive statements concerning inferencing processes have emerged may be that the various studies explored inferencing at different levels. As has been discussed in the previous sections, inferencing is a process that relates the semantic content (propositions) within a sentence and across sentences to the context and the situational circumstances in which the text is embedded and as such entails the activation and integration of various types of conceptual knowledge. Thus, the use of prior conceptual knowledge structures such as scripts, schemata, or frames, or the use and construction of conceptual models (which have been referred to as situation models, mental models, or conceptual frames), have been shown to be fundamental to comprehending, producing and processing discourse. Therefore, it is not surprising that several researchers have suggested that the impairment is at a higher conceptual level.

Problems of RHD patients in appropriately organizing the episodes in a story, or using components of a story structure (as defined by a "story grammar" analysis) have been interpreted as pointing to an *impairment at the level of a narrative schema or frame* (Uryase, 1988; Uryase, Liles, & Duffy, 1989; Wapner, Hamby, & Gardner, 1981). However, Roman, Brownell, Potter, Seibold, and Gardner (1987) demonstrated that in a script-completion task and judgment task of scripts elements, the RHD patients exhibited a generally preserved knowledge of highly routinized information such as that contained in scripts.

Wapner, Hamby, and Gardner (1981) characterized RHD subjects' difficulties in appreciating the relations among the key points of a story or joke, or their inability to assess plausibility, as problems in acquiring a sense of the overall gestalt or form of linguistic entities, that is, *integrating information or conceptualizing the unit as a whole*. Delis, Wapner, Gardner, and Moses (1983) arrived at a similar conclusion; however, they viewed the observed deficit in integrating complex units into coherent wholes as being manifested not only across language but also across visual-spatial modalities. Schneiderman, Murasugi, and Saddy (1992) argued against such a view and ascribed the problems to a general impairment in formulating macro-structures in the sense of van Dijk & Kintsch (1983).

A *breakdown at the level of processes that construct new conceptual models*, such as mental models, has been proposed by Rehak, Kaplan, and Gardner (1992). These authors reported that RHD subjects had difficulties interpreting and/or responding to blockers in conversation and interpreted this as a breakdown of those components of the mental model that deal with judging intention and appropriateness in conversation. Similarly, Stemmer, Giroux, and Joanette (in press) have speculated that the difficulties of RHD patients in appropriately applying and evaluating non-conventionally indirect requests may reflect a breakdown at the level of planning, monitoring, or integrating two or more mental models (in the sense of Johnson-Laird, 1983).

Despite these rather diverse and sometimes contradictory findings, the picture that emerges seems to suggest that a right hemisphere lesion may—in some patients—affect processing mechanisms at a higher conceptual level. Our inability to provide a more coherent and precise account of these mechanisms may lie in several shortcomings encountered in many of the studies such as: (1) a lack or inaccuracy in defining the units of analysis, (2) a disregard for the need to investigate multiple levels of discursive behavior in the same RHD individual, and (3) a lack of formulating hypotheses and interpreting empirical findings within the framework of a precise model of the discourse and its processing. What is thus needed is a more comprehensive assessment of multiple aspects of discourse comprehension and discourse processing in RHD patients. In the following section we will introduce discourse and conceptual processing models that will allow us to monitor and evaluate these aspects of discourse.

USING DISCOURSE MODELS TO MONITOR DISCOURSE PROCESSING

MULTIPLE LEVELS OF REPRESENTATION AND PROCESSING OF DISCOURSE

In the present study, we will use a stratified model of discourse representation and processing in which it is assumed that during discourse comprehension, a reader or listener constructs a cognitive representation which encompasses knowledge structures at multiple levels, including propositional, semantic, and conceptual information (cf., Frederiksen, 1975, 1986; Frederiksen, Bracewell, Breuleux, & Renaud, 1990; Frederiksen & Donin, 1991; Frederiksen, Donin, Décary, Emond, & Hoover, 1992).[1] As a strategy for studying this knowledge construction process, texts presented to subjects are analyzed by applying formally specified models to generate what we will call a *text model*. A text model includes representations of the multiple structures that may be constructed by subjects in comprehending the texts. These representations include propositional, semantic network, and conceptual frame structures. The representations specified in a text model

---

[1] The reader is referred to these references for a more complete description of the model.

are taken as *hypotheses* about the cognitive representations that must be constructed by a reader to comprehend a text. If, in comprehending a discourse, a subject is found to infer or selectively acquire propositional, semantic, or conceptual frame information specified by the hypothetical text model for the discourse, then this is interpreted as evidence for processing activity at the level or of the type needed to generate cognitive representations similar to those specified in the text model. Thus, representations of information that are specified in a text model serve two functions. They are used to: (1) make predictions that reflect processing operations at various levels, and (2) analyze and interpret verbal protocols produced by subjects who are attempting to understand and use text information.

In the following sections we will illustrate how a text model is constructed by analyzing one of the stories that we developed for this study, the airplane text, in terms of its propositional and conceptual frame structures. This text model of the airplane story will serve as a reference structure against which the verbal recall protocols of the subjects will be matched. These matches are used to infer the processing activity of the subjects during the comprehension and production of a recall of the airplane story.

THE DEVELOPMENT OF A TEXT MODEL: THE AIRPLANE TEXT

Propositional Analysis

The three stories[2] that were used in the present study were designed to require semantic or conceptual processing at several levels (for an example of one of the stories see Appendix A). At the most basic level, the stories had to be represented at a propositional level, and a propositional analysis was carried out for each story to model its propositional structure. At the level of microproposition inferences, the propositional content of many sentences was incomplete. Therefore, the propositional analysis included identification of empty 'slots' that could be filled by information provided by the subjects. Since many different contextual inferences could be made on the basis of these propositions, contextual inferences were evaluated for each subject by analyzing the propositions the subject generated and their relations to text-specified propositions.

---

[2] The three stories were the Airplane Text, the Lottery Text, and the Moon Colony Text. The first story was designed in such a way that two problem structures, a "real" thematic content and an "imaginary" thematic content, had to be linked in order to resolve a discontinuity or discrepancy in the story. The second story also required a reconceptualization of events that had taken place in the first part of the story to reconcile later events in the story. In the Moon Colony Text, on the other hand, no discrepancy had to be resolved. This story thus was regarded as a control story and will not be discussed further in the present paper.

The propositional analysis of the texts was carried out sentence-by-sentence with the help of a computer program that assists the user in applying rules to generate a propositional representation for a text (Décary & Frederiksen, in preparation). Propositions are defined by a set of grammar rules that may be applied to a sentence to "parse" it semantically. Table 12-1 presents the first sentence of the Airplane Text, the propositions generated to represent its semantic content, and the parse tree for each proposition. For example, the first proposition (1.1) in the sentence consists of case and other semantic relations that define the components of a processive proposition (i.e., a "System"): a *Process* (feel), the *Patient* of the process ("Laura"), the *Theme* of the process (an embedded proposition representing "what she felt"), a *Tense* associated with the process (PAST), and a *Truth Value* (POSITIVE). The second proposition (1.2) represents an Event consisting of an *Action* ("rise"), an *Affected Object* ("airplane") which is a determined object that is definite (DEF) and singular (SING), an *Aspect* (CONTINUOUS: "rising"), and a *Truth Value* (POSITIVE). For each proposition, the parse tree lists the choices made in applying rules to create the proposition (see Frederiksen et al., 1990).

A simplified and summarized version of the propositional structure of the entire Airplane Text is given in Table 12-2. Here, individual propositions are represented by their identification numbers (the first number is the segment number in the text, the second the number of the proposition for the particular segment). Each number is accompanied by a word or words that help identify its content. When propositions are linked to other propositions, this is indicated by a labeled link that describes the nature of the link. When a proposition is embedded in a slot in another proposition, it is enclosed in parentheses. For example, the propositions 1.1 ("Laura felt") and 1.2 ("airplane rising") given in Table 12-1, are shown in Table 12–2 as being linked by a *Theme* (THM) relation. Furthermore, proposition 1.2 is embedded in proposition 1.1 as indicated by parentheses. If more than one proposition is embedded in another proposition, then a branch is used in the diagram to represent the link between the two embedded propositions and the proposition in which they are embedded. For example, both propositions 2.3 ("sunny skies") and 2.4 ("wind") are *Agents* (AGT) embedded in the Event Proposition 2.2 ("clear away fog"). By following the diagram of Table 12–2 while reading the corresponding text segments (in Appendix A), the reader can get a sense of the propositional structure that is fully specified in the list of propositions for the text.

Conceptual Frame Structure

Narrative Frame Structure. The Airplane Text reflects more than one kind of conceptual frame structure. At one level, the states, processes,

Table 12–1. Propositions for sentence 1 from the Airplane Text[a]

(1) *Laura felt the airplane rising swiftly.*

Proposition (1.1) (representing the process: *Laura felt*):
(System <1.1>: (Process <felt>), (Patient.Rel (Object <Laura>)), (Theme.Relation.Process <1.2>), (R.Tense <PAST>), (Truth.Value <POS>))

Parse Tree:
Proposition (System
  (Prop.Number <1.1>)
  (Process.Slot (Process (Process.Identifier <felt>)))
  (Processive.Frame (Patient.Rel (Patient* (Object (Proper.Noun.Identifier <Laura>)))))
  (Process.Identifying.Relation* (Theme.Relation.Process (Theme*
    (Proposition.Label* (Prop.Number <1.2>)))))
  (R.Tense (Tense <PAST>))
  (Truth.Value* <POS>))

Proposition (1.2) (representing the event: *the airplane rising*):
(Event <1.2>: (Act <rising>), (Object.Rel (Object <airplane>) (Determiner <DEF>) (Number <SING>)), (R.ASPECT <CONT>), (Truth.Value <POS>))

Parse Tree:
Proposition (Event
  (Prop.Number <1.2>)
  (Act.Slot (Act (Act.Identifier <rising>)))
  (Resultive.Frame (Object.Rel (Affected.Obj* (Object (Determined.Object
    (Object.Identifier <airplane>) (Determiner (Non.Generic (Ng.Determiner <DEF>)
    (Ng.Quantifier (Number <SING>)))))))))
  (Act.Identifying.Relation* (Attribute.Relation.Act (Attribute.Act
    (Attribute.Identifier <swiftly>))))
  (R.Aspect (Continuous <-ing>))
  (Truth.Value* <POS>))

[a] An asterisk denotes a rule that may be applied repeatedly.

and events described in the text are organized as a *narrative frame structure* in which events and processes within the text are linked by *temporal order relations* that represent the sequence in which they occur in time within the story. In addition, narrative conceptual structures represent *causal* (CAU) and conditional (COND) relationships between events, *elapsed time* between events (DIFF:TEM), and *descriptions* of the situations in which the events occur. The principal components of the airplane narrative are indicated in Table 12–2 by headings. The narrative begins with a situation description (Situation 1: "Laura is flying to New York," etc.). This is followed by the Event Sequence 1 involving the plane (an explosion, a storm, rapid descent of the plane, etc.). Then there is a second event sequence (Event Sequence 2) describing Laura's actions and what

Table 12-2. Summary of propositional structure of the Airplane Text

SITUATION 1

1.1 Laura felt—THM->(1.2 airplane rising)
2.1 beautiful day
(2.3 sunny skies)
(2.4 wind)———————|—AGT->2.2 clear away fog

2.6—ORD:LOC— { GR (2.5 fog hung) / L over city

3.1 announced—THM—>(3.4 —AND— (3.3 scrape —OBJ— { (3.5 SE tip)) / (3.6 of UK))) (3.2 heading northwest))

4.1 DIFF:TEM = 2hrs — { there / (4.2 land—RSLT->(4.3 LOC in NY)) (3.7 flying towards Greenland))

EVENT SEQUENCE 1

5.3 sounded— { R.ACT->(5.1—RSLT->(5.2 awful noise)) / THM—>(5.4 —PROX— { (5.1) / explosion

6.1 Laura puzzled
6.2 Laura looked out window
7.1 Laura heard—R.PROC->(7.2 rain)
7.3 saw—R.ACT->(7.4 trees bend—AGT->(7.5—CAU— { ANT (7.6 wind)) / CONSQ force))

8.2—CAU— { CONSQ (8.1 her horror) / ANT (8.3 seemed—THM->(8.4 something caught fire))
9.1 L.felt—R.PROC->(9.2 plane tumbling, 9.3 plane descending)
10.1 passengers started screaming
10.2 others tossed around in aisle *continued*

Key to symbols: **AGT**: agent of an action; **AND**: and relation; **ANT**: antecedent of a causal or conditional relation; **CAU**: causal relation; **COND**: conditional relation; **CONSQ**: consequent of a causal or conditional relation; **DIFF:TEM**: difference in time relation; **EQUIV**: equivalence relation; **GOAL**: goal of an action or process; **GR**: greatest; **L**: least; **LOC**: location; **OBJ**: object affected by an action; **ORD:LOC**: ordered locations; **ORD:TEM**: temporal order; **PAT**: patient of a process; **PROX**: proximity relation; **R.ACT**: action related to a process; **R.OBJ**: object related to a process; **R.PROC**: related process; **R.THM**: theme resulting from an action; **RSLT**: result of an action; **TEM**: time; **THM**: theme of a process or object.

Table 12-2. *(continued)*

EVENT SEQUENCE 2

11.1 fear striken
11.2 not know—THM->(11.3 what she was doing)
11.4 she tried—GOAL->(to get up)

12.1 too late
13.1 collapsed—OBJ->(13.2 parts of ceiling)
13.3 she felt suffocating
14.1 surrounded by water—PAT->(14.2 her body)
14.3 water ice cold
15.1 voice yelling at her
15.2 someone tried—GOAL->(15.3 pull her—RSLT->(15.4 out))
16.1 she struggled—GOAL->(16.2 regain—RSLT->(consciousness))

17.1 knew-THM->(17.2—COND- | ANT(17.4 understand-THM->(17.5 event))
                          | CONSQ (17.3 she want to live)

SITUATION 2

                                | AGT->husband)
18.1 she heard—R.PROC->(18.2 yell— | LOC->outside)
                                | R.THM->(18.3, 18.4, 19.1))

18.3 wake up (2X)
18.4 you have been dreaming
18.5 her husband

19.1—COND— | CONSQ (19.2 we won't survive the night)
                 | ANT (19.3 storm keeps on)

18.6—PROX— | outside
                 | tent

EVENT SEQUENCE 3

20.3—EQUIV— | TEM (20.1 he pulled—R.OBJ->(20.4 her arm))
                 | TEM (20.2 he screamed—R.THM->(21.1-2, 22.1-2))

21.1 tent already collapsed
21.2 water pouring in
22.1 we must hurry

22.2—COND— | ANT (empty)
                 | CONSQ (22.3 we'll be blown—RSLT->(22.4 off cliff))

happened to her (she tried to get up, etc.). Then there is a shift to a new situation description (Situation 2: her husband yelling from outside the tent, etc.), and this is followed by a final event sequence (Event Sequence 3: he pulled her arm, etc.). Evidence of processing the text as a narrative structure would be the production of inferred propositions that elaborate and link events to one another to construct and elaborate a narrative frame structure for the text.

Problem Frame Structure. As is true for most stories, many of the events of the airplane story can be interpreted in terms of the underlying motives of the protagonists as they attempt to solve problems posed by situations in the story. Events initiated by characters in the story often correspond to the characters' plans and the actions they take to achieve goals. A *problem frame* is a sequence of events that reflect the enactment of characters' plans. Events are linked to particular procedures within a plan and these are specified in terms of types of activities carried out in applying the procedure to solve the problem (e.g., adopting a goal, interpreting a situation, making a decision, planning or carrying out an action, testing conditions for an action, or evaluating a result; see Frederiksen & Donin, 1991).

The airplane text consists of two problem frames. The main goal of the first is to save oneself in the situation of an airplane accident, while the main goal of the second is to escape from the storm. The airplane accident frame involves sub-procedures of "regaining consciousness" (propositions 16.1–2, 17.1), "getting up" (11.1–4, 12.1–13.3), "getting out of the plane" (15.1–4), and "getting out of the water" (14.1–3). The 'storm' problem frame consists of three sub-procedures: "getting out the tent" (18.1–6, 19.1–3, 20.1–4, 21.1–22.1), "moving away from the cliff" (22.1–4), and "getting out of the storm" (not mentioned). Evidence of processing the text in terms of the problem frame would be selective recall of information pertinent to the problem, production of propositions that specify subgoals that elaborate the frame (at various levels in the frame hierarchy), and description of various types of activities associated with these subgoals.

The Dream Frame. A salient characteristic of the conceptual structure of the airplane text is the difficulty in relating the two problem structures that we have just described. The resolution of this problem for the reader is to apply what might be called the Dream Frame to *re-conceptualize* the content of the first situation and event sequences (i.e., the airplane accident) as the imaginary thematic content of a dream. In other words, the first problem frame (the airplane accident) can be embedded in the real situation and event structure of the second problem frame (the dream). In addition, there can be parallels between the real situation and the imaginary situation, and these can be inferred analogically.

Evidence for the construction of such a high-level conceptual frame would be the production of propositions that explicitly embed the first narrative within the Dream Frame, and that specify similarities or causal links between real events and imaginary events. It should be noted that the Dream Frame could be used to re-conceptualize the text information, whether or not events were interpreted in terms of characters' plans.

EVALUATION OF COGNITIVE PROCESSING USING EXPLICIT TEXT MODELS

Coding Recall of Propositions and Inferential Operations on Propositions

First, subjects' recall protocols were segmented into clausal or sentence units. Then, each segment was coded against a listing of the propositions for the text. The parse tree representations of propositions were used in coding since these included rules that were not applied. These were represented as empty slots that could be filled by means of inferences by the subject. Segments that matched entire propositions (*whole proposition matches*), or parts of propositions (*fragment matches*) were coded, and all inferred information that filled or modified the contents of slots within propositions was coded. If the segment included new propositions that were inferentially related to that proposition, the proposition was coded as *inferred*. From the coded data it is thus possible to determine which propositions were literally paraphrased from the text, which propositions were modified using microproposition inferences, and which propositions were linked to inferred propositions generated by the subjects.

Analysis of Inferred Propositions

Inferred propositions were analyzed in terms of their relationships to the text propositions. By studying the structure of these inferred propositions, their links to text propositions, and to each other, it was possible to construct a model of the connected semantic structure that the subject produced for the text. The extent and patterns of links provide means for studying subjects' contextual inferences in processing the text.

Analysis of Conceptual Structure

The construction of a narrative structure, of problem frames, or of the Dream Frame as conceptual representations of the text is indexed by the types of inferred propositions that the subjects produced in their protocols.

Evidence of narrative frame processing would be production of temporal or causal links between events, and events that "bridge" events in the text narrative. Evidence of construction of a problem frame representation would be production of propositions that refer to new (unmentioned) subgoals or procedures, or to planning and other types of activities associated with characters' generation and use of procedures to solve their problems. Finally, evidence of use of the Dream Frame would be generation of inferred propositions that explicitly state the embedding relationship referred to previously, and that describe analogical links between the imaginary and the real situations.

OBJECTIVES

The main objective of the present study was to explore whether using a particular cognitive approach and explicit models of discourse structure and discourse processing would help us identify more accurately the particular processes that may be impaired and those that function normally in the comprehension and production of narrative texts by one RHD patient. On the basis of the reported findings concerning the comprehension and production of discourse by RHD individuals, we predicted that the RHD patient would behave similarly to the normal control subject with respect to local linguistic and proposition-level semantic processing of sentences within a discourse. However, we expected that the RHD patient would exhibit problems at a more global conceptual level of discourse processing. Our approach to testing this hypothesis was to use the techniques outlined above to analyze the discourse processing of a RHD patient in comparison to that of a normal patient. In this way, we could localize processing dysfunctions in terms of particular levels of processing or types of processing operations that are affected. To pursue our objective, it was thus necessary to: (a) design texts that require particular levels of representation and processing for their comprehension, (b) develop models of text representations at local propositional, semantic, and conceptual levels, and (c) use the text models to monitor processing at different levels and evaluate the conceptual representations constructed by the subject in comprehending the text.

Specific objectives of the study may be summarized as follows: (1) to apply models of discourse to evaluate the representation and processing of two examples of narrative discourse by a RHD patient and a normal control subject; (2) to identify evidence of processing at different levels by analyzing the verbal protocols of these subjects; (3) to identify sources of deviant discourse processing in the RHD patient by making an inter-subject comparison of the results obtained for the two subjects for each narrative discourse; (4) to identify aspects of normal or deviant discourse processing that are generalizable (i.e., replicable) across the two texts by making an intra-subject comparison of the results obtained for the two narrative texts for each subject; and (5) on the basis of these results, to test the above hypotheses concerning the specific cognitive processes that are affected in the RHD patient.

METHODS

SUBJECTS

Selection of the Patient

The RHD patient (A.W.) was a right-handed (a score of 100 on the Edinburgh Handedness Scale), 79-year-old female native speaker of English (with some knowledge of French) who had left school after grade 5 and later enrolled in a 2-year evening program for secretarial work. The patient had suffered a CT documented unifocal hemorrhagic infarct in the right middle cerebral artery region 4 months prior to data collection (Figure 12–1). An EEG performed 3 months after the infarct showed a slowing of the alpha rhythm over the right temporal region and no signs of epilepsy. At the time of data collection the patient clinically presented with a slight dysarthria, left hemiplegia, left hemianopia, and left hemisensory loss.

Selection of the Control Subject

The control subject was a hospitalized non-brain-damaged 76-year-old right-handed female with a high-school diploma. Her native language was English and she had some knowledge of French. Neither the RHD nor the control subject had any previous brain lesions, no psychiatric, drug or alcohol history, nor did they take any medication known to influence mental ability.

Neuropsychological Assessment of the Patient

The patient (A.W.) obtained a score of 29/30 on the Mini Mental State (Folstein, Folstein, & McHugh, 1975) which was performed about 1 month after the stroke. More detailed neuropsychological evaluation was performed 3 and 4 months after the infarct. The patient's visuo-constructional abilities were assessed using the following tasks: copying a house, drawing a clock, constructing a two-dimensional star and a dice with matches

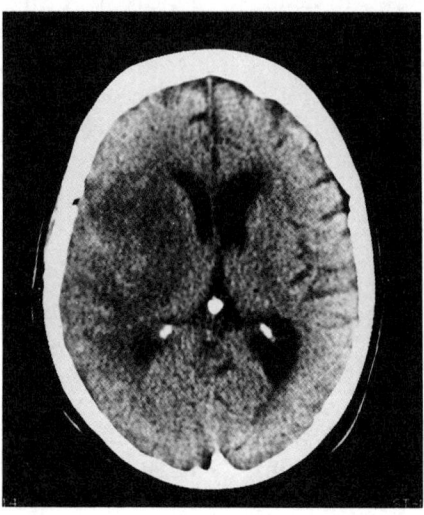

Figure 12–1. Axial CT scan showing a region of hypodensity in the right frontal, temporal and parietal lobes due to hemorrhagic infarction in the middle cerebral artery territory, and mass effect with compression of the right lateral ventricle.

according to a model, and copying the REY Figure (the patient obtained a score of 8 which may be compared to a norm of 32.9). Results on these tasks were indicative of a severe visuo-constructional apraxia. The patient exhibited a left visual hemineglect as shown in her performance on the Bells test (Gauthier, Dehaut, & Joanette, 1989) (the patient obtained a score of 16/35, and all bells in the columns left of the midline were omitted) and in a complex geometrical form discrimination test (Agniel, Joanette, Doyon, Duchein, in press). The Bells test and the drawing of the house were repeated a month later and the results were indicative of an improvement (the Bells score increased to 25/35, and all bells in the third outer column and 2 out of 5 bells in the second outer column were omitted). In addition, the patient performed poorly on the WAIS-R picture completion task (7/20) and was unable to do the picture arrangement task, the object assembly task, the block design and the Benton Line Orientation Task. The patient did not show any impairment in visual object identification or in orientation, naming, reasoning, simple calculation, and memory abilities.

MATERIALS

Two narrative texts (the Airplane Text and the Lottery Text) were designed so as to require particular levels of conceptual representation and processing for their comprehension. The Airplane Text tells the story of a woman experiencing an airplane crash (Appendix A). The final paragraph of the text introduces a turning-point from which it could be deduced that the woman was dreaming. There are two versions of the Airplane Text which differ in the wording used to present the turning point of the story in the final paragraph. In Version 1 the wording was less explicit than in Version 2 concerning the theme of this paragraph. The second story, the Lottery Text, presents a man who thinks he may lose his job. He meets the director of a bank to discuss certain matters. In the final paragraph of the story we learn that he has won a million-dollar prize.

PROCEDURE

The patient (A.W.) was seen over a total of 13 sessions, each session lasting between 60 to 90 minutes. Four sessions were reserved for collecting the data on the Airplane and the Lottery Texts, that is, two separate sessions for each text. These sessions always started with a 15-minute warm-up during which nonverbal neuropsychological testing was performed. In the first session, the procedure for both texts was the same: Each text was first read paragraph by paragraph to the patient in an even, unemotional voice. After each paragraph, the patient was instructed to retell in her own words what she had understood was going on in the story. The story was then read a second time to the patient without interruption, and the patient was asked to give a summary of the story.

In the first "airplane" session, which corresponded to the second meeting with the patient, Version 1 of the Airplane Text was presented. Version 2 was introduced 5 days later. The first session for the Lottery Text corresponded to the third meeting with the patient. In the second session, which took place 5 days later, the Lottery Text was presented a second time in order to ask specific questions about the story. This time the entire story was read to the patient right away and no recall was asked for. The four sessions in which the Airplane and the Lottery Texts were presented were audiotaped. The other 9 sessions were used for further neuropsychological assessment.

RESULTS: THE AIRPLANE TEXT

The analyses of both texts, that is, the Airplane Text and the Lottery Text, showed similar results as to the processing activities which were inferred from comparing the analyzes of the RHD patient's protocol with the one of the control subject. As we have previously described the analysis of the Airplane Text in detail, we will present the results obtained with this text, and, more specifically, the results that pertain to the RHD patient's and the control subject's processing of the text at the levels specified previously, namely: (1) interpretation of the propositional content of sentences, (2) inferences that modify propositions ("micro-proposition inferences"), (3) inferences that generate new propositions based on the explicit propositional content of the text ("macro-proposition inferences"), (4) inferences that reflect the generation of a narrative frame structure for the text, (5) inferences that reflect the production of a problem frame structure, and (6) inferences that reflect the use of the Dream Frame.

PROPOSITIONS RECALLED

In comparing segments from the subjects' protocols to text propositions, a proposition could be coded as: (a) *whole recall* (if at least two slots and a defining relation for the proposition were recalled), (b) *fragment recall* (if a fragment of the proposition was recalled), or (c) *linked to inferred propositions* (if the proposition was not recalled but the protocol contained a proposition inferentially related to the proposition). The frequencies of these three categories of response for each section of the text are given in Table 12–3.

The measure indexing the extent of processing of text propositions is the frequency of whole proposition recall. As may be seen in Table 12-3, this measure was higher for the patient than for the control subject for all sections of the text except for Situation 2 (which introduced the crucial shift in situation and the narrative discontinuity into the passage). Overall, 28.75% of the RHD patient's total coded propositions consisted

Table 12–3. Propositions matched by segments in subjects' paragraph recall protocols for the Airplane Text, version 2

Text Section	Number in Text	Matched to RHD Patient				Matched to Control			
		Whole	Frag.[a]	Infer.[b]	Total	Whole	Frag.[a]	Infer.[b]	Total
Situation 1	18	4	4	2	10	0	1	1	2
Event Sequence 1	21	8	2	5	15	2	3	2	7
Event Sequence 2	22	3	1	1	5	0	2	2	4
Situation 2	9	2	1	1	4	2	3	0	5
Event Sequence 3	10	6	0	0	6	0	1	1	2
Total	80	23	8	9	40	4	10	6	20
Percent	100	28.75	10.0	11.25	50.0	5.0	12.5	7.5	25.0

[a]fragment
[b]inferred

of whole recalls, whereas only 5% of the control subject's coded propositions were whole recalls. Thus, the control subject recalled *less* of the propositional content of the text than did the RHD patient.

MICROPROPOSITION INFERENCES

The extent of modification of propositions—by filling empty slots or modifying the contents of slots in propositions—is reflected in the proportion of the propositions recalled (*whole recall*) for which there was modification of the contents of the propositions by means of "slot inferences" of various kinds. As an example of micro-proposition (slot) inference, the first proposition for sentence 3 of the Airplane Text (*The pilot announced that they were heading northwest* . . .) is:

Event 3.1
  (Act (announced)),
  (Agent.Rel (Object <pilot> (Determiner <DEF>) (Number <SING>))),
  {Instrument.Rel < >},
  {Recipient.Rel < >},
  (Res.Theme.Rel <3.4>),
  {Goal.Rel < >},
  {Act.Identifying.Relation < >},
  (R.Tense <PAST>),
  {R.Aspect < >},
  {Modality < >},
  (Truth.Value <POS>)).

This proposition includes the following unfilled slots (marked by enclosing the slots relation name in curly brackets: {. . .}): *{Instrument.Rel}* (e.g., with the microphone, with the PA system . . .), *{Recipient.Rel}* (e.g., to the passengers), *{Goal.Rel}* (e.g., to inform them, to reassure them . . .), *{Act.Identifying.Relation}* (e.g., calmly, firmly . . .), *{R.Aspect}* (e.g., was announcing (continuous), had announced (completive) . . .), and *{Modality}* (e.g., could have announced . . .). These slots could be filled in numerous ways other than by the examples given. The patient's protocol for the Airplane Text, Version 2, included the following segment:

The pilot had told <u>them where they were going</u> (segment 40, underline added).

In this segment the following micro-proposition (i.e., slot) inferences were made: *Recipient: them, R.Aspect: had* (completive), and the proposition contained in the *Res.Theme.Rel* slot (*they were heading northwest*) was replaced with a proposition (*where they were going*) that is related inferentially to it. Such microproposition inference is a common feature of normal subjects' protocols.

To measure the extent to which these two subjects processed propositions by means of microproposition inferences, a further subcategorization of the propositions that had been previously coded as whole proposition recall was made to identify those propositions that were modified by means of slot inferences, and those that were not. The results revealed that of the 23 whole propositions that were recalled by the RHD patient, 16 (69.6%) were modified by means of slot inferences and 7 were not modified. For the control subject, 3 out of 4 propositions classified as whole recall (75%) were modified by slot inferences. Both the patient and the control, therefore, were unlikely to simply paraphrase the literal semantic content of propositions. Rather, they modified propositions by operating on their "arguments" (i.e., slots), making inferences that filled empty slots or modified the contents of existing filled slots. Thus there was evidence of use of microproposition inferences by both subjects.

MACROPROPOSITION INFERENCES

The extent to which a subject generated inferred propositions that linked, summarized, elaborated, or in other ways augmented or connected the explicit propositional structure of the text is indexed by the percent of propositions for which there were related inferred propositions present in the subjects' protocols. The presence of fragments of propositions in subjects' protocols always occured in the presence of an inferred proposition that used the fragment. Thus the sum of Fragments and Inferred Propositions is a measure of the extent to which text propositions were used in macroproposition inferences. This sum can be expressed as a percent of Total Propositions matched in coding a subject's protocol. The percent figure for the RHD patient was 42.5% (17/40 propositions), whereas for the control subject is was 80% (16/20). While the total number of propositions that were recalled by the control subject (20) was half that recalled by the patient (40), this was accompanied by a rate of production of inferred propositions that was nearly twice that of the patient. The control subject, therefore, produced a larger percent of inferred propositions that were related to the text propositions, whereas the RHD patient produced larger total numbers of propositions that were explicitly given by the text (albeit, modified by means of inferences on their arguments).

To study the structure of these inferred propositions, that is their pattern of links to text propositions and to each other, a *qualitative model* of the semantic macrostructure that each subject produced was constructed on the basis of the propositional coding and a propositional analysis of their inferred propositions. The results of this analysis is given in Figure 12–2 (a, b) for the RHD patient, and in Figure 12–3 for the control subject. In these figures, text propositions are represented as proposition numbers accompanied by short verbal descriptors (as in Table 12–2), inferred propositions (produced by the subjects) are represented by short descriptors surrounded by ellipses, and links between propositions are represented by labeled directional relations. If a link is represented by a dotted line, it was not explicitly stated by the subject but was reflected in a previous "match" done in the propositional coding.

Labels on relational links in Figure 12–3 correspond to types of relations in the propositional representation. Examples ot types of links found in the subjects protocols are:

COND (conditional link; Patient, segment 02: *they must have been in England because there was there had been a heavy fog the night before . . .*; Control, segment 31: *. . . if they didnt hurry up and get out that they would be trapped in the rain . . .*);

GOAL (link from a proposition to another proposition which fills a goal slot within the proposition; Patient, segment 01: *Laura and her husband they want to go to New York*);

RSLT (points to a proposition which is the result of an event proposition; Patient, segment 04: *they were gonna fly to New York*; segment 32: *she must have been rescued . . . to this tent*);

SOURCE [points from an event to a proposition specifying the state or situation prior to the event taking place; Patient, segment 02: *Laura and her husband want to go to New York (01) and they must have been in England (02)*);

AGT (points from a proposition which specifies the immediate cause or agent of an event to the event; Patient, segments 10–11: *it (fire) got to the gas tank*);

CAU [points from a proposition which represents a cause of another proposition; Patient, segment 08: *she knew was gonna be in the Southern part of England (07) cause the pilot had explained that (08)*];

AND [conjoining relation; Control, segments 09–12: *there had to be some kind of a similarity there (09) the water (10) and the plane going down (11) and the trees (12)*];

LOC (location relation; Patient, segment 02: *they must have been in England . . .*);

THM (theme of a cognitive event or process; Patient, segment 07: *she knew was gonna be in the southern part of England*);

R.PROC [a process that is related to another process, Patient, segments 12–13: *she could feel the plane descending (12) falling actually (13)*];

ATT (attribute relation; Patient, segment 11: *it (fire) wouldnt have been too bad . . .*);

ORD:TEM [temporal order relation; Patient, segments 07–09: *she knew was gonna be in the southern part of England (07) cause the pilot had explained that (08) and then she heard an explosion (09)*];

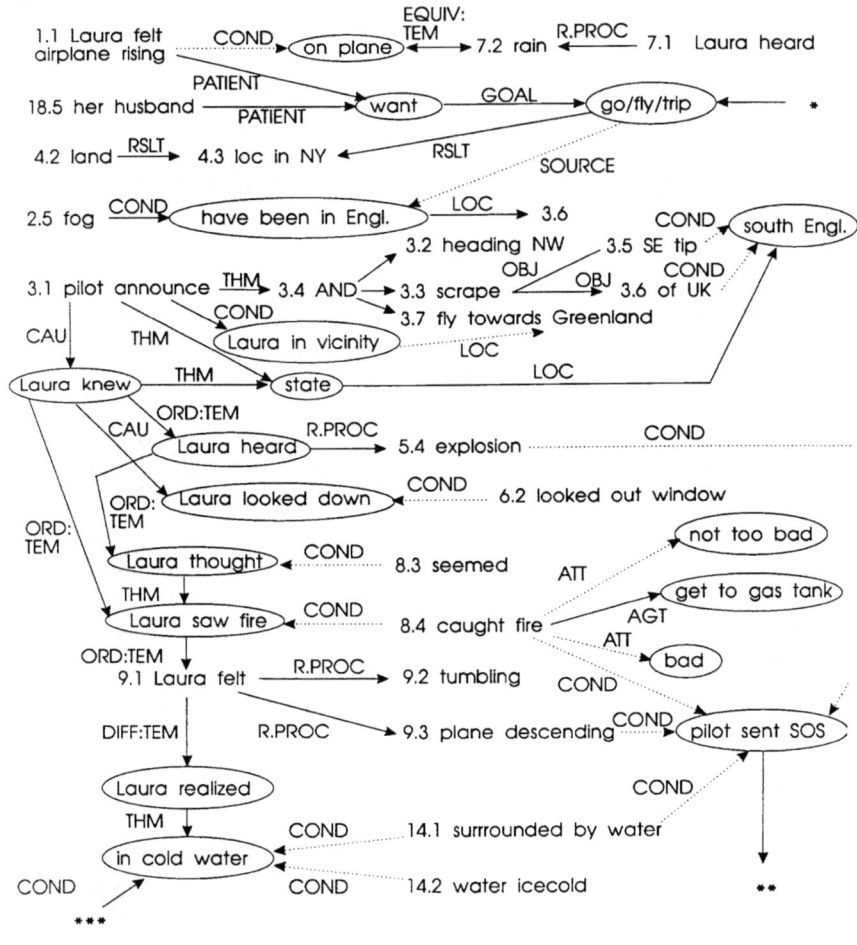

Figure 12–2a. Propositional structure inferred by the RHD patient for the Airpla Text, Version 2.

EQUIV:TEM [equivalence in time; Patient, segments 37–38: *she was the tent on the edge of a cliff* (36) <u>and</u> *her husband was pulling her arm* (37) *c saying he was afraid that they were going to get blown right off* (38); segme 19–20: *they must have gone to see if they could rescue the people* (19) <u>and t was when</u> *she could hear people shouting* (20)];

PART (part of an object, action, or process; Patient, segment 36: *was in the tent on <u>the edge of a cliff</u>*);

IDENT [identity relation; Patient, segments 33–34: *she started to dre after that experience* (33) *she had a <u>nightmare</u> actually* (34)];

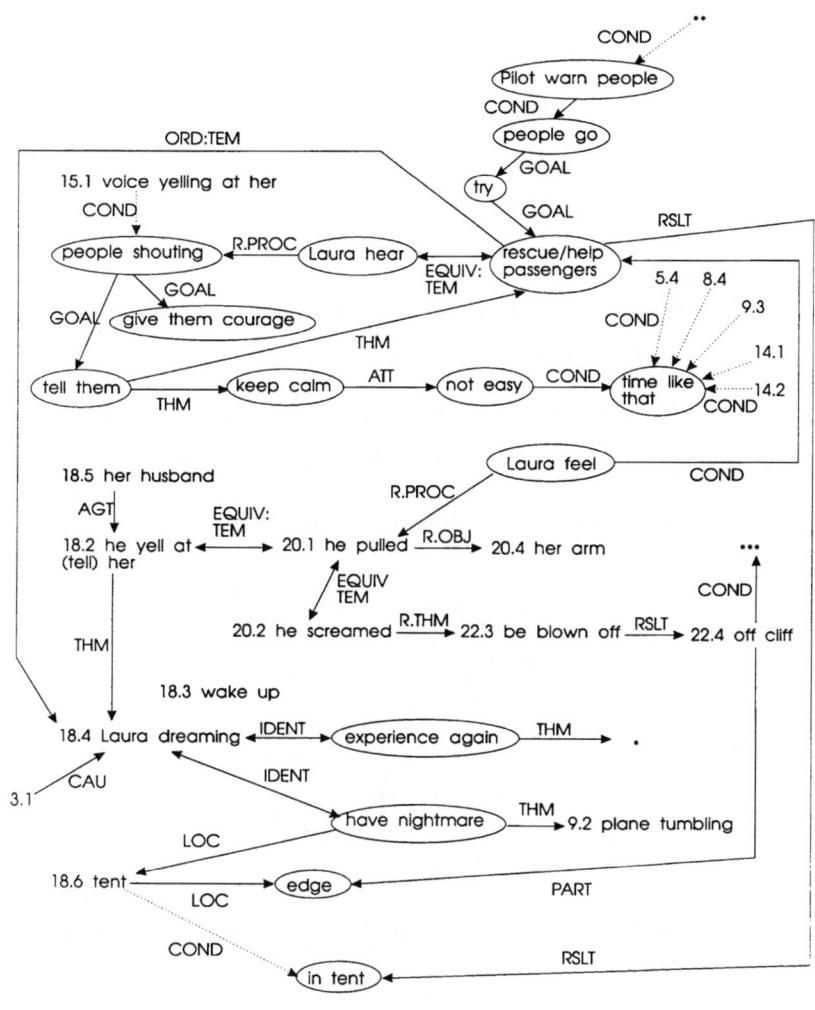

Figure 12–2b.

PROX [proximity relation linking propositions that are similar with respect to a multidimensional attribute (e.g., location) or multiple attributes (e.g., similarity): Control, segment 09: *she knew that it was a storm (07) and the trees were bending (08)* <u>*so there had to be some kind of a similarity there*</u> *(09) the water (10)* . . .; segment 23: it *(explosion)* <u>*could have been*</u> thunder or lightening and rain].

These qualitative models of the macrostructures produced by each subject reveal the extent and types of relational structures generated by

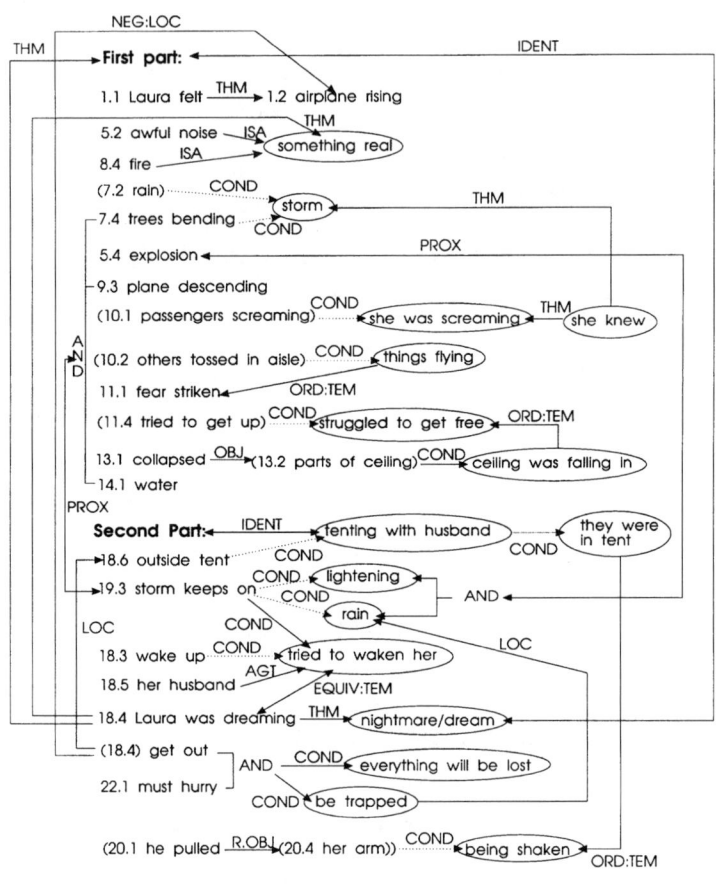

Figure 12–3. Propositional structure inferred by the control subject for the Airplane Text, Version 2.

each subject for the text. The extent of macro-structure generation is reflected in the *number* of connections (links) made between propositions in the structure. Examination of the particular *types* of inferred structures generated by the subjects reveals the types of conceptual representations they were constructing for the text. With respect to the extent of connections, it is apparent from Figures 12–2 and 12–3 that both subjects constructed a highly connected propositional macro-structure for the text. However, for the first part of the text, the control subject (Figure 12–3) generated propositions *summarizing* the text propositions, providing few details about the events and situation. The RHD patient, in contrast, stayed "close to the text," providing elaborative and bridging inferences that either elaborated the situations and events, or connected events from the first situation to those associated with the second situation. Thus, both subjects generated a connected propositional macro-structure for the text, but they did so in very different ways.

NARRATIVE FRAME STRUCTURE

Evidence for the construction of a narrative frame structure for the text would be the production of inferred propositions that (a) provide *temporal, causal*, or *conditional* links between events in the story; and (b) consist of additional events that have been inferred to *"bridge"* gaps between events in the story. Inspection of the propositional macro-structures depicted by the graphs in Figures 12–2 and 12–3 ought to reveal the extent to which each subject was constructing these types of propositional structures. As may be seen in Table 12–4, the RHD patient produced 10 temporal links, 6 conditional links between events or processes, 5 causal or result links, and 17 inferred propositions that "bridged" events and processes in the story by contributing to chains of causally, conditionally, or temporally related propositions. In contrast, the control subject produced 4 temporal links, 4 conditional links, no causal links, and only four "bridging" propositions. Thus, there is evidence from selective inferencing that the RHD patient was processing the text propositions in terms of a *narrative frame structure*, and that in contrast, for the control subject, the narrative frame structure was less important in controlling the subject's inferences.

PROBLEM FRAME STRUCTURE

The problem frames for this text were relatively simple. Nevertheless, an indicator of the use of a problem frame (i.e., a goal structure) to explain events initiated by the characters in the story is the explicit production of inferred goal relations and goal propositions to link events and processes

Table 12–4. Indicators of inferences narrative reflecting structure for Airplane Text, version 2

Type of Relation/Link	RHD Patient	Control Subject
Temporal Relations	10	4
Conditional Relations	6	4
Causal or Result Relations	5	0
Bridging Propositions*	17	4

* connect events or processes through Causal/Conditional/Temporal Chains

in the story. The RHD patient produced five explicit goal relations in her protocol, providing evidence that the narrative structure she was constructing also was organized in terms of an underlying conceptual representation of the goals the characters used to motivate their actions. In contrast, the control subject did not produce any explicit goal links. Thus, there is no evidence that the control subject was actively constructing problem frames to represent story events.

THE DREAM FRAME STRUCTURE

Evidence of use of the Dream Frame in constructing a conceptual representation of this text would be (a) the generation of inferred propositions that explicitly state the embedding relationship in which Situation 1 and Event Sequences 1 and 2 are *embedded as themes* of the event *dreaming* (proposition 18.4) in Situation 2; and (b) the generation of *analogical relations* that explicitly relate events, processes, and states in the dream to those in the "storm" situation (Situation 2 and Event Sequence 3). A summary of links the subject constructed that reflect use of the Dream Frame to "reconcile" the discontinuity in the story (that is to relate Situation 1 and its events, to Situation 2 and its events) is given in Table 12–5.

The control subject produced three explicit thematic links that indicated that the information in Situation 1 was the thematic content of the dream event (e.g., *she was dreaming and that she went through the first part of it in the dream*). Furthermore, this subject explicitly marked analogical relations between the imaginary events of Situation 1 and the real events of Situation 2 as follows. This subject produced: (a) two statements of similarity (PROX) relations comparing events across the two situations (e.g., *so there had to be some kind of a similarity there . . .*); (b) one explicit contradiction (*everything would be lost not from an airplane but from a tent . . .*); (c) one identity (*she went through the first part of it in a dream*) and two sub-categorization (ISA) relations (*the noise and the fire could have been something very real that she was dreaming*); and (d) three "bridging" propositions that linked the imaginary to the real events (e.g., *something real, it was a real nightmare*).

In contrast, the RHD patient acknowledged the thematic relationship of Situation 1 events to the dream in Situation 2 only at the end of her protocol and in response to a probe question from the experimenter (*she was just experiencing the same thing all over again*), and she generated one bridging proposition (*experiencing the same thing over again*). In fact, from the complete transcript (only the relevant excerpt is given in Appendix 4) it is obvious that the experimenter had mistakenly assumed that, after the keyword "dream" had been elicited, the RHD patient had discovered the thematic relationship of Situation 1 and 2. The experimenter

Table 12–5. Indicators of use of the dream frame by the RHD patient and the control subject for the Airplane Text, version 2

Type of Relation/Link	RHD Patient	Control Subject
Theme Relation	2	3
Similarity (Proximity) Relation	0	2
Contradiction (NEG)/Contrast	0	1
Identity/ISA Relations	0	3
Bridging Propositions	1	3

thus kept referring to the 'dream' and probing the subject (at times by explicitly repeating the relevant text segments) to try and find parallels between events in the 'dream' and events in the 'storm' situation. However, despite this, the subject did not identify any contradictions or contrasts, proximity (similarity) relations, or identity (or category) relations to link the two situations analogically. Instead, she assumed that all of the events were real and she constructed the narrative bridge referred to previously. Therefore, the patient did not use the Dream Frame to reconceptualize the events in the story, but instead responded to the discontinuity introduced in Situation 2 by constructing a set of plausible events that could have bridged the two situations.

DISCUSSION

In the present study we have made an attempt to account for the complex multi-layered nature of the cognitive processes involved in understanding or producing discourse as they function in individuals with right hemisphere brain damage. We applied a particular method of discourse analysis and model of discourse processing to analyze specific narratives and the verbal productions generated by one RHD and one control subject in recalling these narratives. In doing so, we were able to monitor the subjects' processing of discourse at multiple levels. Specifically, we investigated the subjects' interpretation of the propositional content of sentences, and their performance at a micropropositional level, at a macropropositional level, and at a conceptual processing level during discourse comprehension and during subsequent production of recall protocols. Our methods led us to identify discursive behavior of the RHD subject that differed from that of the non-brain-damaged control subject in such a way as to indicate problems at the level of cognitive processes that construct new conceptual representations of the text.

PROPOSITIONAL INTERPRETATION AND MICROPROPOSITION INFERENCES

Our results indicated that, relative to the control subject, the RHD patient recalled more of the literal *propositional content* of the text, that is propositions which were literally paraphrased from the text. There also was compelling evidence that both subjects modified propositions by using microproposition inferences to fill or modify slots within propositions. Thus there was *no* evidence of impairment of semantic processing at a "micropropositional" level, and in fact evidence of a *greater* amount of processing at this level in the RHD patient.

Our findings do not corroborate studies reporting fewer use of text words, T-units, or complete cohesive markers in RHD subjects' recalls, insofar as these units are assumed to reflect *semantic* processing. Inconsistent findings of such studies may reflect the failure of these studies to employ semantic units (text propositions) in evaluating subjects' story retelling protocols. Furthermore, since an important component of micro-proposition inference is to resolve anaphoric elements within propositions, our results appear to be consistent with research which reports that the number of anaphoric referential ties in a story can influence the RHD patient's ability to interpret utterances at the sentence level. These findings make sense if one considers that the RHD patient is not impaired at this microstructural level of processing and consequently may rely more on a 'literal' processing of text propositions. The RHD patient may be using *nonimpaired* processes of semantic interpretation and microproposition inference in discourse comprehension or production to compensate for difficulties in processing the text at higher levels of conceptual structure.

MACROPROPOSITION INFERENCES

At the macrostructural level, *both* subjects constructed highly connected propositional macrostructures for the text. They differed, however, in the ways in which they built their macrostructures for the text. Whereas the control subject produced inferred propositions that *summarized* the text, giving few details, the RHD patient stayed "close to the text," inferring propositions that *elaborated* and *bridged* propositions that were explicitly represented in the text. There was virtually no evidence of impairment of processing at a macropropositional level. The qualitative differences observed appeared to reflect the combined consequences of a greater emphasis on processing at a micropropositional level in the RHD patient, and differences between the two subjects in their processing of the text at a conceptual frame level.

Explanatory attempts ascribing observed difficulties in the verbal behavior of RHD patients to an impairment of inferencing processes at a macrostructural level would not appear to be corroborated by our findings. "Contradictory" evidence cited in support of such a claim, in our opinion, needs to be re-evaluated in terms of the tasks and measures used to support the claim. Unfortunately these tasks and measures often are more ambiguous than they may appear to be at first glance. For example, sentence rearrangement tasks may reflect processing of the text at a number of levels including both macro-structural and conceptual frame levels, and judgments of the main idea of a text also are complex and may reflect multiple aspects of the linguistic structure of the text (e.g., its thematic structure) as well as the propositional macrostructure and the structure of the conceptual knowledge expressed by a text.

CONCEPTUAL FRAME STRUCTURES

An analysis of the propositions which were selectively inferred by the subjects to construct a *narrative frame* structure showed that the RHD subject relied more on this narrative frame structure than did the control subject in order to control or guide the conceptual processing of the text propositions. This use of a narrative frame by the RHD patient may at least partially explain what has been described in the literature as an "embellishing," "tangential," "confabulatory," and so on, *narrative style* of RHD patients. Similarly, whereas the RHD patient explicitly constructed problem frames to represent story events, the control subject obviously was less dependent on the underlying conceptual representation of the goals the characters used to motivate their actions in order to construct a narrative frame structure. Thus, there was no evidence of an impairment in the conceptual processing of the story events in terms of narrative and problem frame structures by the RHD patient.

Differences in the way the subjects constructed a conceptual representation of the story were most obvious in the use of the *Dream Frame*. Instead of using the Dream Frame to *reconceptualize* the events in the story, as was explicitly done by the control subject, the RHD patient did not produce thematic nor analogical links between the imaginary and the real events. Instead she used bridging inferences to generate plausible links between the two discontinuous sets of events, thus incorporating them into a single narrative structure.

Thus, we did not find any evidence as to our RHD patient's inability to integrate information or conceptualize the unit as a whole, or use schema or frame structures. However, we did find evidence suggesting that the breakdown occurs at the level of processes that construct *new* conceptual models. In other words, the patient *is* able to build a mental model, but it is *how* this model is built and integrated with other mental models that seems to be affected.

Given that the RHD patient did not exhibit any impairment in understanding the story events and situations in terms of a narrative conceptual structure, why did she show such a dramatic difference in terms of use of the Dream Frame? The explanation of this finding that we favor is that the construction of a Dream Frame representation of the text required a greater degree of independence from the text in interpreting its conceptual structure. Thus, what we may be seeing is a reflection of *impairment of autonomous conceptual functions*. Emphasis on micropropositional and narrative processing would, under this hypothesis, reflect reliance by the RHD patient on levels of text processing that are more "text-driven" and less dependent on autonomous conceptual processing and frame-based inferences. That the findings of this study were not restricted to particular subject-matter knowledge is supported by the fact that we found similar results when this same patient and control subject performed similar tasks with the Lottery text, which also required a "forced" reconceptualization of text information when information was presented that was inconsistent with the "obvious" interpretation of events in the story. In this case as well, the RHD patient was unable to reinterpret events in terms of a new conceptual representation.

Given this complex picture of ways and means of operating at a conceptual level in comprehending text, the at times confusing findings reported in the literature are thus not surprising. One reason for this may be that in these studies no task analyses were performed to describe in detail the underlying structures of the narratives, the manner in which the narrative structures were represented in the text, or the cues or stimuli used in the task. For example, in the judgment or production tasks involving "thematic cues" or discourse "components," we do not know in what way the themes or discourse components were related to the narrative, and therefore, what processes may have been required to perform the tasks.

The limits of the present study as to its generalizability are clear. More stimulus material needs to be developed, validated, and tested on a larger number of patients before valid statements as to the processes affected by a RH lesion can be advanced. However, we have demonstrated the feasibility, usefulness, and indeed the necessity, of applying multi-layered and explicit models of discourse processing to pinpoint more accurately the particular processes that may be affected by a RH lesion.

ACKNOWLEDGMENT

We wish to thank Dr. Joel Walters, Bar Ilan University, Israel, for his support and practical help in getting this project started during his sabbatical year at McGill University.

REFERENCES

Agniel, A., Joanette, Y., Doyon, B., Duchein, C. (in press). *Protocole d'évaluation des gnosies visuelle Montréal-Toulouse—PEGV*. Isbergues, France: Ortho-Edition.

Bihrle, A. M., Brownell, H. H., Powelson, J. A., & Gardner, H. (1986). Comprehension of humorous and non-homorous materials by left and right brain-damaged patients. *Brain and Cognition, 5*, 399–411.

Brownell, H. H., Carroll, J. J., Rehak, A., & Wingfield, A. (1992). The use of pronoun anaphora and speaker mood in the interpretation of conversational utterances by right hemisphere brain-damaged patients. *Brain and Language, 43*, 121–147.

Brownell, H. H., Michel, D., Powelson, J., & Gardner, H. (1983). Surprise but not coherence: Sensitivity to humor in right hemisphere patients. *Brain and Language, 18*, 20–27.

Brownell, H. H., Potter, H. H., Bihrle, A. M., & Gardner, H. (1986). Inference deficits in right brain-damaged patients. *Brain and Language, 27*, 310–321.

Caramazza, A., Gordon, J., Zurif, E. B., & DeLuca, D. (1976). Right-hemispheric damage and verbal problem solving behavior. *Brain and Language, 3*, 41–46.

Décary, M., & Frederiksen, C. H. (in preparation). *Representation of structured texts for computer-based learning environments: Beyond the notion of hypertext*. Montréal, Canada: McGill University, Laboratory of Applied Cognitive Science.

Delis, D. C., Wapner, W., Gardner, H., & Moses, J. A. (1983). The contribution of the right hemisphere to the organization of paragraphs. *Cortex, 19*, 43–50.

De Renzi, E. (1982). *Disorders of space exploration and cognition*. New York: Wiley.

Foldi, N. S. (1987). Appreciation of pragmatic interpretations of indirect commands: Comparison of right and left hemisphere brain-damaged patients. *Brain and Language, 31*, 88–108.

Folstein, M.F., Folstein, S.E., & McHugh, P.R. (1975). "Mini-Mental State": A practical method for grading the cognitive state of outpatients for the clinician. *The Journal of Psychiatric Research, 12*, 189–198.

Frederiksen, C. H. (1986). Cognitive models and discourse analysis. In C. R. Cooper & S. Greenbaum (Eds.), *Written communication annual, vol. I: Sudying writing: Linguistic approaches* (pp. 227–267). Beverly Hills, CA: Sage.

Frederiksen, C. H. (1975). Representing logical and semantic structure of knowledge acquired from discourse. *Cognitive Psychology, 7*, 371–458.

Frederiksen, C. H., Bracewell, R. J., Breuleux, A., & Renaud, A. (1990). The cognitive representation and processing of discourse: Function and dysfunction. In Y. Joanette & H. Brownell (Eds.), *Discourse ability and brain damage: Theoretical and empirical perspectives* (pp. 19–44). New York: Springer Verlag.

Frederiksen, C. H., & Donin, J. (1991). Constructing multiple semantic representations in comprehending and producing discourse. In G. Denhière & J.-P. Rossi (Eds.), *Texts and text processing* (pp. 19–44). Amsterdam: North-Holland.

Frederiksen, C. H., Donin, J., Décary, M., Emond, B., & Hoover, M. (1992). Semantic discourse processing and tutoring systems for second language learning. In M. L. Swartz & M. Yazdani (Eds.), *The bridge to international communication: Intelligent tutoring systems for foreign language learning* (pp. 103–121). New York: Springer Verlag.

Gauthier, L., Dehaut, F., & Joanette, Y. (1989). The Bells Test: a quantitative and qualitative test for visual neglect. *International Journal of Clinical Neuropsychology, 11*, 49–54.

Grimes, J. (1975). *The thread of discourse*. The Hague: Mouton.

Halliday, M. A. K., & Hasan, R. (1976). *Cohesion in English.* London: Longman.
Heeschen, C., & Reischies, F. (1979). *On the ability of brain damaged patients to understand indirect speech acts.* Unpublished manuscript, Freie Universität, Berlin, Institut für Physiologie.
Heilman, K. M., Bowers, D., Valenstein, E., & Watson, R. T. (1986). The right hemisphere: Neuropsychological functions. *Journal of Neurosurgery, 64,* 693–704.
Hirst, W., Le Doux, J., & Stein, S. (1984). Constraints on the processing of indirect speech acts: Evidence from aphasiology. *Brain and Language, 23,* 26–33.
Hough, M. S. (1990). Narrative comprehension in adults with right and left hemisphere brain-damage: Theme organization. *Brain and Language, 38,* 253–277.
Huber, W., & Gleber, J. (1982). Linguistic and nonlinguistic processing of narratives in aphasia. *Brain and Language, 16,* 1–18.
Joanette, Y., & Goulet, P. (1987). *Inferencing deficits in right brain-damaged: Absence of evidence.* Paper presented at the 10th European Conference of the International Neuropsychological Society, Barcelona, Spain.
Joanette, Y., Goulet, P., & Hannequin, D. (1990). *Right hemisphere and verbal communication.* New York: Springer Verlag.
Joanette, Y., Goulet, P., Ska, B., & Nespoulous, J.-L. (1986). Informative content of narrative discourse in right-brain-damaged right-handers. *Brain and Language, 29,* 81–105.
Joanette, Y., & Goulet, P. (1990). Narrative discourse in right-brain-damaged right-handers. In Y. Joanette & H. H. Brownell (Eds.), *Discourse ability and brain damage* (pp. 131–153). New York: Springer Verlag.
Johnson-Laird, P. N. (1983). *Mental models: towards a cognitive science of language, inference, and consciousness.* Cambridge, England: Cambridge University Press.
Kaplan, J. A., Brownell, H. H., Jacobs, J. R., & Gardner, H. (1990). The effects of right hemisphere damage on the pragmatic interpretation of conversational remarks. *Brain and Language, 38,* 315–333.
Kintsch, W., & van Dijk, T. A. (1978). Towards a model of text comprehension and production. *Psychological Review, 85,* 363–395.
McDonald, S., & Wales, R. (1986). An investigation of the ability to process inferences in language following right hemisphere brain damage. *Brain and Language, 29,* 68-80.
Millar, J. M., & Whitaker, H. A. (1983). The right hemisphere's contribution to language: A review of the evidence from brain-damaged subjects. In S. J. Segalowitz (Ed.), *Language functions and brain organization* (pp. 87–113). New York: Academic Press.
Moya, K. L., Benowitz, L. I., Levine, D. N., & Finkelstein, S. (1986). Covariant deficits in visuospatial ablities and recall of verbal narrative after right hemisphere stroke. *Cortex, 22,* 381–397.
Mross, E. F. (1990). Text analysis: Macro- and microstructural aspects of discourse processing. In Y. Joanette & H. H. Brownell (Eds.), *Discourse ability and brain damage: Theoretical and empirical perspectives* (pp. 50–68). New York: Springer Verlag.
Nespoulous, J.-L., Lecours, A. R., Lafond, D., Lemay, A., Puel, M., Joanette, Y., Cot, F., & Rascol, A. (1992). *Protocole Montréal-Toulouse d'examen linguistique de l'aphasie.* (Module standard initial: M1β, Version 1992). Isbergues, France: L'Ortho-Edition.
Read, D. E. (1981). Solving deductive reasoning problems after unilateral temporal lobectomy. *Brain and Language, 12,* 92–100.
Rehak, A., Kaplan, J. A., & Gardner, H. (1992). Sensitivity to conversational deviance in right hemisphere-damaged patients. *Brain and Language, 42,* 203–217.

Rehak, A., Kaplan, J. A., Weylman, S. T., Kelly, B., Brownell, H. H., & Gardner, H. (1992). Story processing in right hemisphere brain-damaged patients. *Brain and Language*, *42*, 320–336.

Roman, M., Brownell, H. H., Potter, H. H., Seibold, M. S., & Gardner, H. (1987). Script knowledge in right hemisphere-damaged and in normal elderly adults. *Brain and Language*, *31*, 151–170.

Schneiderman, E. I., Murasugi, K. G., & Saddy, D. J. (1992). Story arrangement ability in right brain-damaged patients. *Brain and Language*, *43*, 107–120.

Sherratt, S. M., & Penn, C. (1990). Discourse in a right hemisphere brain-damaged subject. *Aphasiology*, *6*, 539–560.

Stemmer, B. (in press). A pragmatic approach to neurolinguistics: speech acts (re-)considered. *Brain and Language*.

Stemmer, B., Giroux, F., & Joanette, Y. (in press). Production and evaluation of requests by right brain-damaged individuals. *Brain and Language*.

Tutin, A. (1992). *Etude des anaphores grammaticales et lexicales pour la génération automatique de textes de procédures*. Unpublished doctoral dissertation, Université de Montréal, Montréal, Canada.

Uryase, D. (1988). *Analysis and description of narrative discourse in right hemisphere-damaged adults: A comparison to neurologically normal and left-hemisphere-damaged aphasic adults*. Unpublished manuscript, Storrs, Connecticut, University of Connecticut.

Uryase, S. D., Liles, B. Z., & Duffy, R. J. (1989, November). *Story grammar analysis of retellings by right hemisphere-damaged adults*. Paper presented at the Annual Convention of the Americal Speech-Language-Hearing Association, St. Louis, MO.

van Dijk, T. A., & Kintsch, W. (1983). *Strategies of discourse comprehension*. New York: Academic Press.

Wapner, W. A., Hamby, S., & Gardner, H. (1981). The role of the right hemisphere in the apprehension of complex linguistic materials. *Brain and Language*, *14*, 15–33.

Weylman, S. T., Brownell, H. H., Roman, M., & Gardner, H. (1989). Appreciation of indirect requests by left- and right-brain-damaged patients: The effects of verbal context and conventionality of wording. *Brain and Language*, *36*, 580–591.

APPENDIX A

The Airplane Text, Version 2

(1) Laura felt the airplane rising swiftly. (2) It was a beautiful day. Sunny skies and a slight wind had cleared away the fog which had hung over the city earlier in the morning. (3) The pilot announced that they were heading Northwest and would scrape the Southeastern tip of England flying towards Greenland. (4) From there it would only be a couple of hours until the plane would finally land in New York.

(5) Then there was an awful noise which sounded like an explosion. (6) Puzzled, Laura looked through the window. (7) She could hear the rain battering against the window and see the trees bending by the force of the strong wind. (8) To her great horror something seemed to have caught fire. (9) She felt the airplane tumbling and descending with an incredible speed. (10) Some of the passengers had started screaming and others were tossed around in the aisle.

(11) Fear stricken and not knowing what she was doing, she desperately tried to get up. (12) But is was too late. (13) Parts of the ceiling had collapsed and she felt like suffocating. (14) Then suddenly her body was surrounded by ice cold water. (15) A voice was yelling at her and someone tried to pull her out. (16) She struggled to regain consciousness. (17) She knew if she wanted to live she had to understand what was going on.

(18) "Wake up! Wake up!", she heard her husband yell, "you have been dreaming!" Her husband was yelling from outside the tent. (19) "We won't survive the night if this storm keeps on." (20) As he pulled her arm, he screamed hysterically: (21) "The tent has already collapsed and water is pouring in! (22) We better hurry or we'll be blown right off the cliff."

APPENDIX B

Recall Protocol of Patient

S: 1) well Laura and her husband they want to go to New York 2) and they must have been must have been in England because there was there had been a heavy fog the night before ^ 3) and I figured they were in England 4) and they were gonna fly to New York ^^^
E: uhum very good ^ and then?
S: 5) and ^ while they were on the plane Laura heard ^ could see that it was raining 6) and it was a strong wind cause she could see the trees bending over
E: why did she? can you normally see the trees when you're looking out of [a
S: oh] when you're looking down ^ yes probably
E: okay
S: 7) ^^ and she might have looked down because she knew was gonna be in the Southern part ^of eh England ^ 8) cause the pilot had explained that ^^ 9) and then she heard an explosion (?) 10) and she thought she ^ saw fire 11) ^ I don't know if she saw ^ but it wouldn't have been too bad only until unless it got to the gas tank ^^ 12) and then she could feel the plane descending ^ 13) falling actually ^^ 14) and and in no time she she she realized she was in icy cold water ^ 15) and it seemed that he was saying they were going North ^ to Greenland ^ 16) then she must have been somewhere in the vicinity ^ 17) and ^ the people the pilot probably sent an SOS 18) and and the people ^ were warned ^ 19) and they must have gone to see if they could ^ rescue the people ^ 20) and that and that was when she could that's when she could hear people shouting
E: what were the people shouting?

S: 21) I don't know exactly what 22) but they were trying to give them courage ^ 23) to tell them that they were gonna help them ^ 24) that's what they were shouting ^^ 25) to keep calm (?) 26) but that's easier said then done ^ in a time like that ^ 27) and they did get rescued cause she could feel something pulling her 28) pulling her arm
E: yeah ^ who do you remember who was pulling her arm?
S: 29) her husband was pulling her arm
E: yeah and what did [he
S: 30) but] that was when and he tell her she ^ she was dreaming 31) but ^ I ^ that she wasn't dreaming she might have 32) she must have been rescued according to this tent 33) and that's when she started to dream after that experience ^ 34) she had a nightmare actually
E: yeah ^ what was the nightmare all about?
S: 35) about the plane falling
E: right ^ and where was she? when she had the nightmare
S: 36) she was in the tent on the edge of a cliff 37) and ^ her her husband was pulling her arm 38) and saying he was afraid that they were going to get blown right off 39) and they'd be back in the water I guess ^^
E: okay good ^ and now that you say you said she was having a nightmare she was dreaming about this airplane crash
S: right
E: now do you remember details(!) ^ in you know what she was dreaming which could refer to her being in this tent in a storm ^ why she was dreaming certain things now
S: 40) well she was dreaming because the pilot had told them where they were going to start with ^^ 41) and she she must have forgotten all about her trip to New York ^ 42) and she was just ^ experiencing the the the same thing all over again

E = experimenter
S = subject
^ = pause
? = rising intonation of preceding word or phrase
(?) = incomprehensible production or best guess of preceding word or phrase
[ ] = turn overlap
(!) = emphasis of preceding word or phrase

APPENDIX C

Recall Protocol of Control Subject

S: 1) things flying 2) and then ehm ^^^ she starts to feel a fear 3) but before she could even struggle to get free 4) the the something was falling in (!) on her like the ceiling ^ 5) and she knew she was screaming 6) and there was a storm 7) she knew that it was a storm 8) and the trees were bending ^ 9) so there had to be some kind of a ^ a a similarity there 10) the water 11) and the plane going down 12) and the trees 13) and then then all of a sudden she was being shook ^ 14) and ehm ^^ my version of it that it she was dreaming 15) and that she went through the first part of it in the dream 16) and the second part that they were probably ehm ^ eh ^ tenting 17) or out on a ^ eh ^ with her husband 18) and he was trying to waken her 19) because of the storm ^ 20) that they that they if they didn't hurry up and get out everything would be lost ^ 21) not from an airplane (laughs) but from a tent ^ 22) so that it was partially a dream

E: uhum right ^ would you see now parallels between her experience like being in the tent doing camping ^ what happened there actually and what she was dreaming ^ do you see any connections between what she was dreaming about and what was happening in the tent while she was sleeping ^^^ like let me give you an example ^ in the story it said there was an explosion what could that have been? ^^ in reality? ^ while she was in the tent

S: 23) it could have been thunder or lightening and rain ^ 24) and there seem to be the the overall thing that they were comfortably (?) in this tent 25) and then all of a sudden he is shaking her 26) and that she is dreaming all this is happening 27) and ^ the noise

(?) the fire could have been really something very real ^ 28) that she was dreaming 29) it was a real nightmare ^ 30) when he was awakening her ^ 31) and that if they didn't hurry up and get out that they would be trapped in the ^ rain and whatever

CHAPTER 13

Narrative Expressive Deficits Associated with Right-Hemisphere Damage

PENELOPE S. MYERS

Acquired right hemisphere damage (RHD) leaves linguistic functions essentially intact but may disrupt communication, including narrative expression. For this reason, narratives produced by RHD patients present a unique opportunity to observe breakdowns in some of the cognitive operations requisite to informative and efficient discourse production. Not all RHD adults have communication deficits, but for those who do, narrative output is generally characterized by reduced informative content, lack of specificity, tangential comments, and difficulty in getting to the point (Bloom, Borod, Obler, & Gerstman, 1992; Cimino, Verfaellie, Bowers, & Heilman, 1991; Diggs & Basili, 1987; Joanette, Goulet, Ska, & Nespoulous, 1986; Myers, 1979; Myers & Brookshire, in press; Sherratt & Penn, 1990; Urayse, Duffy, & Liles, 1991; Wapner, Hamby, & Gardner, 1981).

Typically, investigators are interested in the quality of narrative output which is measured by counting the amount and type of content produced. Content is often defined by the number of concepts, "message-units," or propositions mentioned. The amount and type of content mentioned by RHD subjects is then compared to that mentioned by non-brain-damaged (NBD) controls.

A few studies have elicited narratives by asking subjects to retell events from their personal lives or by engaging them in conversation (Cimino et al., 1991; Sherratt & Penn, 1990). In general, however, it is easier to measure narrative output across subjects using constrained stimulus input. For this reason, most investigators elicit narratives by asking subjects to tell a story about pictured scenes or to retell verbally presented stories (Bloom et al., 1992; Myers, 1979; Myers, 1992; Myers & Brookshire, in press; Hough, 1990; Joanette et al., 1986; Rivers & Love, 1980; Sherratt & Penn, 1990; Wapner et al., 1981). Occassionally subjects have been asked to report the events contained in a short film (Urayse et al., 1991; Wapner et al., 1981). Pictured stimuli are used more often than verbally presented stories because they elicit more spontaneous narratives and place fewer demands on short-term memory. Regardless of whether the stimuli are verbal or visual, narrative expression in most studies may be as much a reflection of subjects' comprehension of the stimuli as it is their ability to convey narrative level information.

The next section reviews RHD narrative expressive deficits as described in the literature. The last section explores their possible source. As the discussion unfolds, it should be kept in mind that narrative expression represents one's perception and comprehension of external events as well as one's ability to organize and relate internally generated information.

DEFICIT DESCRIPTION

The following narratives are taken from a study by Myers and Brookshire (in press) in which subjects were asked to tell what was happening in a series of Norman Rockwell illustrations. The examples represent descriptions of a scene depicting three people waiting in a hosptial or doctor's office sometime in the early 1950s. Two men and a boy are seated apart from one another on a bench on the right side of the picture. All three are staring ahead. One of the men has his head bandaged. A "Silence Please" sign is printed on the wall beside him. The other man is leaning forward with his chin in his hands. Next to him is a table containing a full ashtray, magazines, and a newspaper. The boy in the middle sits upright with his hands clasped.

WAITING ROOM SCENE: SAMPLE RESPONSES

Representative NBD Response

"It's people waiting in a waiting room for a doctor to look after them. One man has a bandage. The little boy is quite tense. He's sitting with his legs very close together and his hands held. And the third person is tense, too. He is leaning over, and they're all waiting to be called."

Sample RHD Responses

Example 1. "There are two brothers and a man. They appear to be looking at television. The man apparently is smoking because the ashtray is full of cigarette butts."

Example 2. "This looks like a bench. They're sitting down on a bench, but I don't know if it's a doctor's office or a house, or what. But I know one of them may be day-dreaming."

Example 3. "Well, it could be a baseball game. They all seem so interested."

Example 4. "These two boys are—perhaps their father or their uncle has a bandage around his head—possibly returned from a war. They could be sitting in a church pew. . . . The boys have very serious thoughts on their mind. . . . I suppose wondering what their fate might be."

Example 5. "They're at the movies and they're watching a moving picture. Probably an action picture."

Example 6. "There are three people waiting, sitting on a bench. An older man. It looks like he has a bandage on his head. And the boy in the middle has his hands clenched in his lap. He's wearing blue shorts, white shoes with striped socks. And the man on the end of the bench is wearing leather shoes. And the boy on this end of the bench, I guess he's between the two of them in age. And he has a cigarette tray right by him. And he looks a little anxious. He's got his elbows on his knees. He's got his chin in his hand. He's wearing a khaki suit. The boy's wearing a short sleeved shirt, blue shorts. The man's wearing a dark suit with a tie and the man has a bandage on his head."

Example 7. "In a doctor's office. Father and son and maybe an uncle with his head bandaged up, waiting to have something done about it."

What do these examples tell us? The narratives seem linguistically adequate, in terms of vocabulary, structure, semantics, and linguistic fluency. RHD subjects appear to be aware of the objects and people depicted. Yet, most of them fail to communicate the intended meaning of the scene. The examples typify the three major narrative expressive deficits reported in the literature, namely: (1) reduced level of informative content; (2) reduced efficiency; and (3) impaired development of a macrostructure. These deficits will be addressed in the sections that follow. Throughout the chapter reference will be made to the examples from the "Waiting Room" scene.

REDUCED INFORMATIVE CONTENT

The concept of a "waiting room" is a central concept in explaining the scene described above. Of the concepts mentioned, it probably conveys the most information about the scene. Its omission in the narratives of

RHD subjects is a good example of the nature of reduced informative content found in the literature. As Example 7 demonstrates, not all RHD subjects have difficulty recognizing and expressing main concepts. Conversely, not every NBD control accurately interprets verbal or visual narratives. However, Myers and Brookshire (in press) found that over 80% of the 30 NBD subjects in their study stated that the scene took place in a waiting room, whereas less than 29% of the 24 RHD adults did so.

This result reflects the finding that RHD subjects' narratives may not contain core or central information. Joanette et al. (1986) and Myers and Brookshire (in press) compared the core information produced in the narratives of NBD and RHD subjects. Joanette et al. asked subjects to tell a story based on a picture sequence. They compiled a list of "core" propostions or concepts mentioned by at least 20% of both RHD and NBD subjects. Not surprisingly, they found that RHD subjects mentioned fewer of these "core" concepts than NBD subjects. Myers and Brookshire (in press) asked subjects to explain the events depicted in eight Norman Rockwell scenes, including the "Waiting Room" scene mentioned above. They compiled a list of "major" concepts which were defined as those mentioned by at least 30% of the NBD subjects. Again, RHD subjects mentioned significantly fewer of these "major" or core concepts than did NBD subjects. Other studies have found a general reduction in the number of "message units" (Diggs & Basili, 1987) or "content elements" (Bloom et al., 1992) produced by RHD subjects when describing or telling stories about pictured scenes.

Several studies have analyzed narratives in terms of their completeness, that is, number of episodes included. RHD subjects' narratives contained fewer episodes and important details than those of NBD subjects in studies by Rivers and Love (1980) and Urayse et al. (1991). In the latter study, the episodes included by RHD subjects were themselves judged less complete than those of NBD controls. Episodic completeness was measured along several dimensions including the initiating event, the setting, the internal response, the internal plan, and the direct consequence and reaction. Failure to include some of these important dimensions suggests that although they remembered certain episodes, they did not fully interpret them.

Superficial reporting of narrative events (versus their interpretation) has been noted by several other investigators. Wapner et al. (1981) reported that in retelling narratives, RHD subjects frequently reported pieces of the story verbatim, rather than paraphrasing or interpreting the action. Joanette et al. (1987) found among the "core" concepts frequently omitted by RHD subjects was one that was considered the "gist" or the "substance" of the story.

Some studies have asked RHD subjects to recall episodes from their personal lives. Their narratives have been rated by independent judges as significantly less specific (Cimino et al., 1991) and as containing more empty phrases and non-informative elements (Sherratt & Penn, 1990) than those of NBD adults.

In general, RHD subjects in these studies produce the same number or more words as NBD controls (Bloom et al., 1992; Joanette et al., 1986; Myers & Brookshire, in press). Thus, they may say as much, but convey less. Reporting fewer concepts or fewer episodes from a story accounts for a reduction in informative content. But as the next section suggests, RHD subjects may also include intrusive, tangential, and irrelevant information in their narratives. This tendency results in expression that is less efficient as well as less informative than that of NBD subjects.

REDUCED EFFICIENCY

A fairly consistent characterization of RHD narrative expression is that it contains trivial, tangential, and seemingly unrelated information. Example 6 is a good example of focus on irrelevant detail. The subject describes clothes at the expense of action and never interprets the gist of the scene. Inefficiency in RHD narratives is characterized by two types of extraneous information: (1) tangential and even confabulatory comments; and (2) insignificant but related detail.

Many investigators have commented on the intrusive additions in the narrative expression of some RHD patients. For example, Wapner et al. (1981) noted that RHD subjects embellished stories three times as often as NBD controls. In some cases they confabulated endings or explanations for characters' actions that were not consistent with the narrative. Some of the stories presented by Wapner et al. were designed to be "noncannonical," that is, the story endings were surprising, and did not follow from the expectations set up in the body of the story. For example, a farmer, angry at the laziness of a hired hand, ends up giving him a raise. While NBD subjects shook their heads in confusion as they retold this story, RHD subjects tended to justify the farmer's action by making additions to the story (i.e., invoking possible but improbable motives for his action).

In a paragraph interpretation study, Hough (1990) also reported that RHD subjects produced significantly more confabulations and embellishments than NBD controls. Again, some of the stimuli were designed to be unusual in that the theme in half of the stimuli was delayed until the end of the paragraph. Interestingly, RHD subjects produced significantly more embellishments and confabulations in retelling delayed-theme than non-delayed theme paragraphs.

These findings suggest that RHD patients resort to confabulation when perplexed by narrative content or the intention of questions. Clinical observation of RHD patients supports this possibility. Asked to describe the events depicted in a pictured scene as part of a standard language evaluation, one RHD patient described the picture's plastic coating, the type of ink used, and the weight of the paper on which the drawing was printed. He did not describe the scene itself until the clinician was able to more fully explain the nature of her request. Patients tend to respond in a straightforward manner to inquiries about things they are certain of, but may give elaborate and often inaccurate responses when confronted by uncertainty. Thus, they may be able to relate distant events appropriately, but anxious to cover confusion about their present circumstances, they may respond to questions about their future plans in exquisite, but unfounded detail (i.e., an elaborate explanation of what they will be doing on their return to work tomorrow— when a return to work at all is out of the question).

Not all RHD patients' narratives are inefficient, as Examples 3, 5, and 7 demonstrate. Not all inefficient narratives are characterized by confabulation or comments tangential to the task. The second type of inefficiency, noted in Example 6, results from focus on insignificant detail. Mackisack, Myers, and Duffy (1987), for example, eliminated tangential comments from the analysis of subjects' explanations of pictured scenes and still found that RHD subjects produced twice as many words and labeled twice as many objects compared to NBD controls. That is, subjects tended to list but not interpret what they saw, as if they were taking "object inventories" rather than explaining the depicted events.

As this discussion suggests, uninformative content may be characterized not only by lack of information, but by excessive information in the form of intrusive comments and attention to information not considered relevant to the overall theme of the narrative. Asked what had brought him into the hospital, one RHD patient who had had a stroke on a Sunday morning reported in chronological order all the events, large and small, that had occurred in his life from the previous Saturday morning on—including what he had had for breakfast. He ended his report by quoting his wife who said, "Marvin's had a stroke." He got his message across and answered the question, but was hardly efficient in doing so. Resorting to such a level of unnecessary detail and to a chronological order of events in which to cast his story, suggests that this patient's inefficiency may have been related to a deficit in establishing a macrostructure for his narrative. Impairments in generating a macrostructure for narrative expression are discussed in the following section.

MACROSTRUCTURE IMPAIRMENTS

A macrostructure reduces narrative content to its essential message (Schneiderman, Murasugi, & Saddy, 1992). Without a macrostructure, narrative expression may become unfocused and rambling. The expression of unnecessary detail and the laborious path taken by some RHD patients to make a point suggests problems in generating a macrostructure. According to Brownell (1988) and Hough (1990), developing a macrostructure for narrative discourse involves the extraction of meaning from individual sentences and their integration into the context supplied by the other sentences. Similarly, to understand the macrostructure for pictured stories, individually depicted items must be extracted and integrated. It is assumed that adequate discourse production depends on this same process of selection and integration of units of information internal to the subject.

Right-hemisphere damage may create problems in these operations. For example, Delis, Wapner, Gardner, and Moses (1983) found RHD subjects impaired relative to NBD controls in arranging printed sentences into coherent paragraph-length stories even though the stories were preceded by a sentence containing the central theme. RHD subjects appeared to ignore this macrostructure cue in ordering the sentences that followed into a story. In a similar story arrangement task, Schneiderman et al. (1992) included a theme sentence in only some of the stimuli. They found that theme sentences had a beneficial effect on LHD and NBD, but not on RHD subjects' performance.

Hough (1990) found that, unlike the performance of NBD and LHD subjects, RHD subjects' paragraph interpretation deteriorated when a central theme sentence was delayed until the end of the paragraph. According to Hough, RHD subjects "appeared unable to utilize the macrostructure as an organizer in apprehending a paragraph" (p. 271). She goes on to explain:

> These individuals retained isolated pieces of paragraph data rather than integrating this information to deduce the meaning of the narrative . . . this often resulted in the "listing" of information rather than generating an overall theme. (p. 271)

"Listing" behavior echoes Mackisack et al.'s finding that RHD subjects appear to take object inventories rather than integrating objects and actions into an overall theme when explaining pictured stories. Wapner et al. (1981) also cited excessive focus on isolated events as a factor in RHD impairments in inferring the morals of stories. Finally, relating deficits on an inference task to narrative impairments, Brownell, Potter, Bihrle, and Gardner (1986) concluded,

> Where normal listeners are concerned to weave a coherent interpretation of an entire discourse so that each component jibes with the broader reality, RHD patients are often stuck with, or are satisfied with, a limited and piecemeal understanding. (p. 319)

Thus, there is considerable speculation that RHD subjects' narrative discourse suffers from impaired generation of macrostructures. Examples 1, 3, 4, and 5 demonstrate generation of inacurrate macrostructures. Example 6 demonstrates the verbal floundering that may occur in the absence of a macrostructure. As Wapner et al. (1981) state, lack of an "organizing principle" may result in difficulty judging "which details matter."

A macrostructure is essentially an inference about the "gist" of a narrative. An inference may be considered a "hypothesis about sensory data such that input is not only sensed, but interpreted" (Myers, 1992). Based on inference, sensory input is transformed from one level of meaning to another. In the "Waiting Room" scene the macrostructure or gist of the picture is contained in the phrase "In a doctor's office" (Example 7). Generation of this inference depends on lesser inferences that serve as building blocks for the macrostructure. For example, one infers from the bandage that one man is injured. Further inferences are made by integrating individual elements with one another. In isolation, the sign "Silence Please" might suggest a library, but in combination with other contextual features, such as the wounded man, it suggests a medical facility. As Brownell (1988) and Joanette et al. (1986) explain, the links between sentences in a story or between actions and objects in pictured scenes are not necessarily explicitly stated or depicted, so one must infer the connections between them.

Difficulty in generating inferences both about a macrostructure and about individual elements that lead to a macrostructure has been investigated in several studies which measured inference generation in response to pictured scenes (Mackisack et al., 1987; Myers, 1979, 1992; Myers & Brookshire, in press). In these studies, narratives were elicited by asking subjects to explain what was happening in the scenes, and the numbers of inferential and non-inferential concepts were counted and compared to those of NBD controls. Non-inferential concepts were defined as ones whose meaning was independent of contextual information. The meaning of inferential concepts, however, relied on context. Thus, in the waiting room scene the term "man" would be considered non-inferential, whereas "patient" would be considered "inferential." Inferential concepts depended on the recognition and integration of other contextual cues.

Myers (1979) and Myers and Linebaugh (1980) elicited narratives from explanations of the "cookie theft" picture from the Boston Diagnostic Aphasia Examination (Goodglass & Kaplan, 1976). A list of concepts generated by a sample of NBD subjects was obtained from a study by Yorkston and Beukelman (1980) and divided by judges into those that were inferential and those that were not. Thus, "woman" was judged to be non-inferential, whereas "mother" was judged as inferential because it depended on the integration of contextual features (i.e., kitchen appliances, children, the activity of wiping dishes etc.). Based on this list of concepts, both studies found that RHD subjects produced significantly fewer inferred concepts than NBD subjects.

Using definitions for "inferred" and "pictured" noun phrases similar to those in Table 13–1, Mackisack et al. (1987) found that RHD subjects produced significantly fewer inferred noun phrases than NBD subjects in

Table 13–1. Noun phrase categories

Pictured Accurate:	A noun phrase that accurately refers to a person or object depicted in the picture
Pictured Wrong:	A noun phrase that inaccurately or imprecisely refers to a person or object in the picture
Inferred Accurate:	A noun phrase that refers to a person, object, or abstract concept whose function or meaning is accurately inferred from the context of the picture
Inferred Wrong:	A noun phrase that refers to a person, object, or abstract concept whose function or meaning is inaccurately inferred from the context of the picture

Source: Adapted from Myer, P. S. (1992). The effect of visual and inferential complexity on the verbal expressions of non-brain-damaged and right-hemisphere-damaged adults. (Doctoral dissertation, University of Minnesota.) *Dissertation Abstracts International*, 53, 03B.

explaining the events in Norman Rockwell illustrations. In addition, as mentioned earlier, RHD subjects produced twice as many "pictured" noun phrases as did NBD controls, suggesting the tendency, noted in Example 6, to identify objects rather than integrating them into the rest of the context.

Interested in whether RHD subject's problems in developing inferences from pictured scenes were caused by the visual or by the inferential complexity of the stimuli, Myers (1992) manipulated levels of both in a study of narrative expression. Visual complexity was defined as the number of objects and people depicted in a scene, while inferential complexity was defined as the number of inferences necessary to understand the scene. A series of validation studies yielded eight pictures on which 10 independent judges agreed on levels of inferential and visual complexity. There were two pictures in each of the following four categories: (1) visually simple-inferentially simple; (2) visually simple-inferentially complex; (3) visually complex-inferentially simple; and (4) visually complex-inferentially complex. Noun phrases were analyzed according to the operational definitions in Table 13–1. Comparing responses within groups across levels of inferential and visual complexity, it was found that the number and accuracy of both "inferential" and "pictured" noun phrases were not affected by visual complexity. Inferential complexity, on the other hand, had a significant effect on narratives of both RHD and NBD subjects in that they made significantly fewer and significantly less accurate inferences in response to inferentially complex than in response to inferentially simple pictures. Comparisons across groups revealed that RHD subjects produced fewer accurate inferences than NBD subjects. However, both groups were highly accurate and did not differ from each other in their production of "pictured" noun phrases.

These results suggest several things. First, RHD subjects are able to identify objects and people depicted in complex scenes as readily as

NBD subjects. Second, visual complexity does not affect inference generation. Third, increased levels of inferential complexity has a deleterious effect on the narrative expression of RHD subjects.

These results held as well for the number of concepts produced by subjects (Myers, 1992; Myers & Brookshire, in press). Increased levels of inferential, but not visual complexity, resulted in a reduced number of the "major" concepts mentioned by NBD subjects. Thus, the level of inference required in narrative discourse appears to have a significant effect on narrative output.

Taken together, these studies and those reviewed earlier in this section suggest that impaired inference generation may affect the development of a macrostructure and the degree to which narrative expression is informative and efficient. As we have seen, inferences at any level are based on the process of attending to and selecting relevant bits of information, and on integrating them with one another and with one's store of personal and world knowledge. Deficits in any one of these operations may result in a general inference deficit that impairs narrative expression and comprehension. The explanation for narrative expressive deficits, then, appears to be related to a pervasive inference impairment. Support for this hypothesis comes from areas outside the narrative realm in which deficits in the operations necessary for inference generation have been found. These non-narrative level inference impairments are discussed in the following section.

DEFICIT EXPLANATION

INTEGRATION OF INDIVIDUAL ELEMENTS

As noted earlier, integration of bits of information with one another is an important step in generating inferences. There is evidence of problems in integrating information subsequent to RHD at both the perceptual and cogntive levels of processing.

Perceptual integration deficits have been noted in drawing or copying objects and geometric forms. Drawings by RHD patients tend to be spatially disorganized and fragmented. Object parts may not be oriented properly within the framework of the object (i.e., a chimney drawn at right angles to a house, or the hands and numbers drawn outside the face of a clock). These impairments are considered deficits in spatial organization and integration as opposed to a motor execution or programming deficit.

Impaired *spatial* integration of features may be related to impairments in *cognitive* integration. For example, Moya, Benowitz, Levine, and Finklestein (1986) and Benowitz, Moya, and Levine (1990) found RHD subjects were impaired at inferring the overall theme, the relationships between characters and events, and the motivation of characters in short narratives. These deficits were significantly correlated in both studies with impairments in the number of details included and in the spatial organization of RHD subjects' drawings of geometric forms and simple objects. As Benowitz et al. (1990) state, these findings

> suggest the possibility that the appreciation of spatial configurations and the comprehension of interrrelationships among elements in narrative material may to some extent require a common mechanism. (p. 240)

Problems in integrating information in the verbal realm abound. For example, RHD subjects may have difficulty in interpreting sarcasm, "white lies," and idiomatic expressions because of a problem in integrating these forms of speech with preceding context (Kaplan, Brownell, Jacobs, & Gardner, 1990; Myers & Linebaugh, 1981; Van Lancker & Kempler, 1987). For example, Myers and Linebaugh (1981) found RHD subjects were significantly impaired relative to NBD controls in interpreting two sentence stories in which the outcome turns on a figure of speech. Understanding the story depended on integrating the idiomatic expression with the context supplied by the first sentence.

Similarly, Brownell et al. (1986) found RHD subjects impaired relative to NBD controls in generating inferences from sentence pairs, particularly when misleading information was presented in the first, as opposed to the second, sentence. Taken in isolation, the first sentence in the misleading condition lead to an erroneous inference. For example, "Barbara became too bored to finish the history book. She had already spent five years writing it." RHD subjects had trouble integrating the sentences into a unit and, as a result, had problems revising the expectations generated by the first sentence.

Other deficits in integrating contextual features include impairments in interpreting "indirect requests" (Foldi, 1987; Hirst, LeDoux, & Stein, 1984; Weylman, Brownell, Roman, & Gardner, 1989). Interpreting the question, "Could you open the window?" as a request versus an inquiry into one's physical capacity depends on the context in which the question is asked. That is, the ability to transcend the referential meaning of the question is partly dependent on integrating it with other contextual information such as the temperature of the room, the facial expression of the speaker, and so on. An equally important factor is the ability to relate the request and the context in which it is made to one's previous experience of such requests. Incorporating personal knowledge plays a significant role in interpreting and producing narrative expression.

INTEGRATION OF ELEMENTS WITH PERSONAL KNOWLEDGE

Impairments in the ability to retrieve or utilize personal experience have been found in studies in which contextual processing was not a factor.

For example, some RHD adults are impaired in appreciating the connotative (versus denotative) meaning of single words (Brownell, Potter, Michelow, & Gardner, 1984; Brownell, Simpson, Bihrle, Potter, & Gardner, 1990; Gardner & Denes, 1973; Winner & Gardner, 1977). Denotative meanings are similar to dictionary definitions. To take the example of Myers (in press) the denotative meaning of "lion" might be "animal that lives in Africa." Its connotative meanings might include "ferocious," "King of the jungle," and even "MGM." Connotative meanings can be considered alternates to the dictionary definitions of words that everyone would agree on. As the above example illustrates, one must bring personal knowledge to bear in the process of arriving at the connotation of a word.

Another source of evidence for problems in retrieving and integrating personal knowledge into an ongoing situation comes from studies of "verbal fluency" that ask subjects to generate as many members as they can for a given category. RHD subjects have been found particularly impaired at generating members of uncommon categories such as "uses for a brick" (Diggs & Basili, 1987) or "things to take on a camping trip" (Hough, May, & DeMarco, in press). Presumably, these categories rely on less automatic retrieval than do categories typically used in verbal fluency takes (i.e., "animals"). Diggs and Basili (1987) found RHD subjects produced significantly fewer uses for common objects compared to NBD controls. Hough et al. (1992) found RHD subjects did not differ from NBD controls in generating members of common categories, but were significantly impaired in the uncommon category condition. As the authors point out, subjects had to appeal to their store of previous and personal experience in the uncommon category condition. These studies suggest that the effort required for inference generation plays a significant role in RHD discourse production.

EFFORTFUL VERSUS AUTOMATIC INFERENCE

Just as they may be able to manage simple scripts, stories, and procedural discourse (Ostrove, Simpson & Gardner, 1990; Rehak, Kaplan, Weylman, Kelley, & Brownell, 1992; Roman, Brownell, Potter, & Seibold, 1987), RHD patients may be able to manage simple inferences. Thus, subjects in the study by Myers (1992) were generally able to infer the meaning of a scene depicting Thanksgiving dinner, but had more difficulty in inferring the macrostructure for the "waiting room" scene. McDonald and Wales (1986) found that RHD subjects could manage simple inferences from two verbal premises. For example, they were not impaired in inferring "a bird is under the table" based on the premises that the bird is in the cage and the cage is under the table. However, as noted, verbal inferences that are more complex, more contextually dependent, and more effortful may present problems (Brownell et al., 1986).

Evidence of deficits in effortful versus automatic inference generation also comes from investigations of visuoperceptual deficits. Studies of object recognition have shown that RHD patients are able to recognize and identify familiar objects and pictures of objects presented in prototypic view (Damasio, 1985; DeRenzi & Spinnler, 1966; Kertesz, 1983; Layman & Green, 1988; Warrington & James, 1967), but deficits may emerge if stimuli have been degraded in some way, making recognition more difficult. These deficits include problems in identifying figures that are overlapping, incomplete, fragmented, or that are depicted in unusual orientations or size (DeRenzi, Scotti, & Spinnler, 1969; DeRenzi & Spinnler, 1966; Hier & Kaplan, 1980; Humphries & Riddoch, 1984; Layman & Green, 1988; Myers, 1979; Myers, Linebaugh, & Mackisack, 1985; Warrington & James, 1967; Warrington & Taylor, 1973, 1978).

A common feature of the tasks used to elicit object recognition deficits is the forced reliance on a limited set of depth cues (Myers, 1991). Use of this limited set of cues imposes three-dimensions or depth to the drawings, which enables one to disambiguate them. For example, identifying overlapping figures forces subjects to use the single cue of occlusion or interposition to infer that one figure is in front of another. Identifying incomplete figures also requires use of the cue of occlusion—in this case, one must infer an imaginary occluder that hides parts of the figure. The cues of shading, luminance, and texture changes enable one to match a prototypically depicted object to one depicted in an unusual rotation (i.e., rotated in the plane).

As Myers (1991) suggests, assigning depth to the two-dimensional images that impinge on the retina is a form of inference. Images are transformed from two to three dimensions in an automatic process that involves combinations of the multiple and redundant depth cues available in the real world. However, when depth cues are limited, the inference of three dimensionality is more effortful. The visual puzzles described above are not automatically resolved. Subjects must make use of limited information to transform what appears to be a jumble of lines or blotches on a page into recognizable objects or figures. Reduction of cues stresses the system, and it appears that when the system is stressed by limited information, the process of inference breaks down even at the perceptual level. This possibility suggests that impairments in inference generation may be a general consequence of RHD affecting multiple levels of processing. The source of these deficits may lie in one of the major symptoms of RHD—attentional impairments.

ATTENTION DEFICITS

The most salient attention deficit associated with RHD is the syndrome of unilateral neglect in which patients fail to report, respond, or orient to stimuli in contralesional and occassionally in ipsilesional space despite the motor and sensory capacity to do so (Gainotti, D'Erme, Monteleone, & Silveri, 1986; Heilman, Watson, Valenstein, & Damasio, 1983). RHD in general, and neglect in particular, are associated with various types of attention deficits that include impairments in the following: (1) *arousal and vigilance* (Coslett, Bowers, & Heilman, 1987; Dee & Van Allen, 1973; Heilman, Schwartz, & Watson, 1978; Howes & Boller, 1975; Morrow, Vrtunsk, Kim, & Boller, 1981); (2) *sustained attention* (Bub, Audet, & LeCours, 1990); (3) *disengaging and shifting covert attention* (Farah, Wong, Monheit, & Morrow, 1989; Posner, Snyder, & Davidson, 1980; Posner, Walker, Friedrich, & Raphal, 1984; Robin & Rizzo, 1989); and (4) *selective attention* (Mesulam, 1981; Rapcsak, Verfaellie, Fleet, & Heilman, 1989).

Deficits in arousal and vigilance may make RHD patients less responsive to information that signals the context within which discourse takes place and may increase the effort needed to organize internal information. Impairments in sustained attention may affect the ability to maintain attention to extralinguistic information such as facial expression, gesture, and prosodic contour during complex interactions. Deficits in disengaging and shifting attention may have an impact on mental flexibility such that the ability to generate alternate meanings or change initial interpretations is impaired. Impaired selective attention may make it difficult to filter distracting stimuli and to focus on significant and relevant information both internal to the patient and in the external environment. Thus, attentional impairments may have profound impact on many of the cognitive operations involved in discourse production.

Evidence of the impact of attention disorders on narrative discourse can be found by investigating relationship between neglect on narrative production. The studies by Myers (1992) and Myers and Brookshire (in press) mentioned earlier, found that neglect was strongly related to the generation of both major concepts and inference and that the relationship was independent of visual processing per se. RHD subjects were divided according to their scores on a battery of neglect tests. Subjects with high levels of neglect produced significantly fewer accurate inferred noun phrases than subjects with low levels of neglect. In addition, subjects with high levels of neglect, unlike those with low neglect, produced fewer accurate concepts in all conditions of visual and inferential complexity compared to NBD subjects. Yet, there was no difference between the NBD and the high neglect group on accuracy of "pictured" noun phrases, suggesting that neglect was not related to recognizing visual information. In addition, performance of neglect patients was not affected by levels of visual complexity in the scenes, but was affected by their level of inferential complexity. Finally, both RHD and NBD groups mentioned the same number of concepts from either side of the midline of the scenes. These results suggest that neglect affects the attentional and cognitive processes involved in generating concepts and inferences in narrative expression.

CONCLUSION

Narrative production deficits may occur as a consequence of RHD and may be described as an impairment in the comprehension as well as in the expression of narrative level discourse. These deficits are characterized by reduced levels of informative content, reduced efficiency, and reduced ability to form a macrostructure, all of which appear to be related to one another. They also appear to be related to an impaired ability to select and integrate relevant bits of information with one another and with personal knowledge, operations considered crucial in generating inferences. RHD discourse impairments may be associated with a general impairment in inference generation, reflected in tasks as diverse as narrative discourse and visuoperceptual processing. The exact nature of this impairment is not yet understood, but it appears to have a relationship to task difficulty and to deficits in attention. The influence of attention on RHD communication deficits needs further investigation as does the hypothesis that RHD results in a pervasive inference deficit affecting multiple levels of processing, including narrative expression. What is certain is that some RHD patients have problems in generating efficient and informative discourse, and that these problems are related to cognitive rather than to linguistic deficits.

REFERENCES

Benowitz, L. I., Moya, K. L., & Levine, D. N. (1990). Impaired verbal reasoning and constructional apraxia in subjects with right hemisphere damage. *Neuropsychologia, 28*, 231–141.

Bloom, R. L., Borod, J. C., Obler, L. K., & Gerstman, L. J. (1992). Impact of emotional content on discourse production in patients with unilateral brain damage. *Brain and Language, 42*, 153–164.

Brownell, H. H. (1988). The neuropsychology of narrative comprehension. *Aphasiology, 2*, 247–250.

Brownell, H. H., Potter, H. H., Bihrle, A. M., & Gardner, H. (1986). Inference deficits in right brain-damaged patients. *Brain and Language, 27*, 310–321.

Brownell, H. H., Potter, H. H., Michelow, D., & Gardner, H. (1984). Sensitivity to lexical denotation and connotation in brain damaged patients: A double dissociation? *Brain and Language, 22*, 253–265.

Brownell, H. H., Simpson, T. L., Bihrle, A. M., Potter, H. H., & Gardner, H. (1990). Appreciation of metaphoric alternative word meanings by left and right brain-damaged patients. *Neuropsychologia, 28*, 375–383.

Bub, D., Audet, T., & Lecours, A. R. (1990). Re-evaluating the effect of unilateral brain damage on simple reaction time to auditory stimulation. *Cortex, 26*, 227–237.

Cimino, C. R., Verfaellie, M., Bowers, D., & Heilman, K. M. (1991). Autobiographical memory: Influence of right hemisphere damage on emotionality and specificity. *Brain and Cognition, 15*, 106–118.

Coslett, H. B., Bowers, D., & Heilman, K. M. (1987). Reduction in cerebral activation after right hemisphere stroke. *Neurology, 37*, 957–962.

Damasio, A. R. (1985). Disorders of complex visual processing: Agnosias, achromatopsia, Balint's syndrome, and related difficulties of orientation and construction. In M. Mesulam (Ed.) *Principles of behavioral neuroglogy* (pp. 259–288). Philadelphia: F. A. Davis.

Dee, H. L., & Van Allen, M. W. (1973). Speed of decision-making processes in patients with unilateral cerebral disease. *Archives of Neurology, 28*, 163–166.

Delis, D., Wapner, W., Gardner, H., & Moses, J. (1983).The contribution of the right hemisphere to the organization of paragraphs. *Cortex, 19*, 43–50.

DeRenzi, E., Scotti, G., & Spinnler, H. (1969). Perceptual and associative disorders of visual recognition. *Neurology, 19*, 634–642.

DeRenzi, E., & Spinnler, H. (1966). Visual recognition in patients with unilateral cerebral disease. *Journal of Nervous and Mental Disease, 142*, 515–525.

Diggs, C., & Basili, A. G. (1987). Verbal expression of right cerebrovascular accident patients: Convergent and divergent language. *Brain and Language, 30*, 130–146.

Farah, M. J., Wong, A. B., Monheit, M. A., & Morrow, L. A. (1989). Parietal lobe mechanisms of spatial attention: Modality-specific or supramodal? *Neuropsychologia, 27*, 461–470.

Foldi, N. S. (1987). Appreciation of pragmatic interpretation of indirect commands: Comparison of right and left hemisphere brain-damaged patients. *Brain and Language, 31*, 88–108.

Gainotti, G., D'Erme, P., Monetleone, D., & Silveri, M. C. (1986). Mechanisms of unilateral spatial neglect in relation to laterality of cerebral lesions. *Brain, 109*, 599–612.

Gardner, H., & Denes, G. (1973). Connotative judgements by aphasic patients on a pictorial adaptation of the semantic differential. *Cortex, 9*, 183–196.

Goodglass, H., & Kaplan, E. (1976). *The Boston diagnostic aphasia examination*. Philadelphia: Lea and Febiger.

Heilman, K. M., Schwartz, H. D., & Watson, R. T. (1978). Hypo-arousal in patients with the neglect syndrome and emotional indifference. *Neurology, 28*, 229–232.

Heilman, K. M., Watson, R. T., Valenstein, E., & Damasio, A. (1983). Localization in neglect. In A. Kertez (Ed.), *Localization in neuropsychology* (pp. 471–492). New York: Academic.

Hier, H., & Kaplan, J., (1980). Verbal comprehension deficits after right hemisphere damage. *Applied Psycholinguistics, 1*, 279–294.

Hirst, W., LeDoux, J., & Stein, S. (1984). Constraints on the processing of indirect speech acts: Evidence from aphasiology. *Brain and Language, 23*, 26–33.

Hough, M. S. (1990). Narrative comprehension in adults with right and left hemisphere brain-damage: Theme organization. *Brain and Language, 38*, 253–277.

Hough, M. S., May, M. J., & DeMarco, S. (in press). Categorization skills in right hemisphere brain-damage for common and goal-derived categories. In M. Lemme (Ed.), *Clinical aphasiology* (vol. 22). Austin, TX: Pro-Ed.

Howes, D., & Boller, F. (1975). Simple reaction time: Evidence for focal impairment from lesions in the right hemisphere. *Brain, 98*, 317–332.

Humphries, G. W., & Riddoch, M. J. (1984). Routes to object constancy: Implications from neurological impairments of object constancy. *The Quarterly Journal of Experimental Psychology, 36A*, 385–415.

Joanette, Y., Goulet P., Ska, B., & Nespoulous, J-L. (1986). Informative content of narrative discourse in right-brain-damaged right-handers. *Brain and Language, 29*, 81–105.

Kaplan, J., Brownell, H., Jacobs, J. R., & Gardner (1990). The effects of right hemisphere damage on the pragmatic interpretation of conversational remarks. *Brain and Language, 38*, 315–333.

Kertesz, A. (1983). Right-hemisphere lesions in constructional apraxia and visuospatial deficit. In A. Kertesz (Ed.), *Localization in neuropsychology* (pp. 445–470). New York: Academic.

Layman, S., & Green, E. (1988). The effect of stroke on object recognition. *Brain and Cognition, 7*, 87–114.

Mackisack, E. L., Myers, P. S., & Duffy, J. R. (1987). Verbosity and labeling behavior: The performance of right hemisphere and non-brain-damaged adults on an inferential picture description task. In R. H. Brookshire (Ed.), *Clinical aphasiology* (vol. 17, pp. 143–150). Minneapolis: BRK Publishers.

McDonald, S., & Wales, R. (1986). An investigation of the ability to process inferences in language following right hemisphre brain damage. *Brain and Language, 29*, 68–80.

Mesulam, M. (1981). A cortical network for directed attention and unilateral neglect. *Annals of Neurology, 10*, 307–325.

Morrow, L., Vrtunsk, P. B., Kim, Y., & Boller, E. (1981). Arousal responses to emotional stimuli and laterality of lesion. *Neuropsychologia, 19*, 65–71.

Moya, K. L., Benowitz, L. I., Levine, D. N., & Finklestein, S. (1986). Covariant deficits in visuospatial abilities and recall of verbal narrative after right hemisphere stroke. *Cortex, 22*, 381–397.

Myers, P. S. (1979). Profiles of communication deficits in patients with right cerebral hemisphere damage. In R.H. Brookshire (Ed.), *Clinical aphasiology: Conference proceedings* (pp. 38–46). Minneapolis: BRK Publishers.

Myers, P. S. (1991). Inference failure: The underlying impairment in right-hemisphere communication disorders. In T. Prescott (Ed.), *Clinical aphasiology*, (vol. 20, pp. 167–180). Austin, Texas: Pro-Ed.

Myers, P. S. (1992). The effect of visual and inferential complexity on the verbal expression of non-brain-damaged and right-hemisphere-damaged adults (Doctoral dissertation, University of Minnesota, 1992). *Dissertation Abstracts International, 53*, 03B.

Myers, P. S. (in press). Communication disorders associated with right hemisphere brain damage. In R. Chapey (Ed.), *Language intervention strategies in adult aphasia* (3rd ed.). Baltimore: Williams & Wilkins.

Myers, P. S., & Brookshire, R. H. (in press). The effects of visual and inferential complexity on the picture descriptions of non-brain-damaged and right-hemisphre-damaged adults. In M. Lemme (Ed.), *Clinical Aphasiology* (vol. 22). Austin, TX: Pro-Ed.

Myers, P. S., & Linebaugh, C. W. (1980, November). *The perception of contextually conveyed relationships by right brain-damaged patients.* Paper presented at the American Speech-Language-Hearing Association Convention, Detroit, MI.

Myers, P. S., & Linebaugh, C. W. (1981). Comprehension of idiomatic expressions by right-hemisphere-damaged adults. In R. H. Brookshire (Ed.), *Clinical aphasiology: Conference proceedings* (pp. 254–261). Minneapolis: BRK Publishers.

Myers, P. S., Linebaugh, C. W., & Mackisack, E. L. (1985). Extracting implicit meaning: Right versus left hemisphere damage. In R. H. Brookshire (Ed.), *Clinical aphasiology* (vol. 15, pp. 72–82). Minneapolis: BRK publishers.

Ostrove, J. M., Simpson, T., & Gardner, H. (1990). Beyond scripts: A note on the capacity of right hemisphere-damaged patients to process social and emotional content. *Brain and Cognition, 12,* 144–154.

Posner, M. I., Snyder, C. R., & Davidson, B. J. (1980). Attention and the detection of signals. *Journal of Experimental Psychology: General, 109,* 160–174.

Posner, M. I., Walker, J. A., Friedrich, F. J., & Raphal, R. D. (1984). Effects of parietal lobe injury on convert orienting of visual attention. *Journal of Neuroscience, 4,* 1863–1864.

Rapcsak, S. Z., Verfaellie, M., Fleet, W. S., & Heilman, K. M. (1989). Selective attention in hemispatial neglect. *Archives of Neurology, 46,* 178–182.

Rehak, A., Kaplan, J. A., Weylman, S. T., Kelly, B., & Brownell, H. H. (1992). Story processing in right-hemisphere-brain damaged patients. *Brain and Language, 42,* 320–336.

Rivers, D. L., & Love, R. J. (1980). Language performance on visual processing tasks in right hemisphere lesion cases. *Brain and Language, 10,* 348-366.

Robin, D. A. & Rizzo, M. (1989). The effect of focal cerebral lesions on intramodal and cross modal orienting of attention. In T. Prescott (Ed.), *Clinical aphasiology* (vol. 18, pp. 61–74). Austin, TX: Pro-Ed.

Roman, M., Brownell, H. H., Potter, H. H., & Seibold, M. S. (1987). Script knowledge in right hemisphere-damaged and normal elderly adults. *Brain and Language, 31,* 151–170.

Schneiderman, E. I., Murasugi, K. G., & Saddy, J. D. (1992). Story arrangement ability in right brain-damaged patients. *Brain and Language, 43,* 107–120.

Sherratt, S. M., & Penn, C. (1990). Discourse in a right-hemisphere brain-damaged subject. *Aphasiology, 4,* 539-560.

Urayse, D., Duffy, R. J., & Liles, B. Z. (1991). Analysis and description of narrative discourse in right-hemisphere-damaged adults: A comparison with neurologically normal and left-hemisphere-damaged aphasic adults. In T. Prescott (Ed.), *Clinical aphasiology* (vol. 19, pp. 125-138). Austin, TX: Pro-Ed.

Van Lancker, D. R., & Kempler, D. (1987). Comprehension of familiar phrases by left- but not by right hemisphere damaged patients. *Brain and Language, 32,* 265–277.

Wapner, W., Hamby, S., & Gardner, H. (1981). The role of the right hemisphere in the appreciation of complex linguistic materials. *Brain and Language, 14,* 15–33.

Warrington, E. K., & James, M. (1967). Disorders of visual perception in patients with localized cerebral lesions. *Neuropsychologia, 8,* 457–487.

Warrington, E. K., & Taylor, A. M. (1973). The contribution of the right parietal lobe to object recognition. *Cortex, 9,* 152–164.

Warrington, E. K., & Taylor, A. M. (1978). Two categorical stages of object recognition. *Perception, 7,* 695–705.

Weylman, S. T., Brownell, H. H., Roman, M., & Gardner, H.(1989). Appreciation of indirect requests by left- and right-brain-damaged patients: The effects of verbal context and conventionality of wording. *Brain and Language, 36,* 580–591.

Winner, E., & Gardner, H., (1977). The comprehension of metaphor in brain damaged patients. *Brain, 100,* 719–727.

Yorkston, K. M., & Beukelman, D. R. (1980). An analysis of connected speech samples of aphasic and normal speakers. *Journal of Speech and Hearing Disorders, 45,* 27–36.

PART IV

Narrative Capacities of Patients with Dementia

CHAPTER 14

Narrative Schema in Dementia of the Alzheimer's Type

BERNADETTE SKA AND DOMINIQUE GUÉNARD

Since the 1960s, interest in discourse analysis has grown, and theoretical approaches have become more sophisticated. The general objective in that domain is a better knowledge of the complex cognitive functioning underlying human communication behavior. Models were first developed in normal cognitive psychology (Bobrow & Collins, 1975; Kintsch, 1974). Since then, studies with aged and brain-damaged subjects have begun to contribute to the refinement of the questions on discourse abilities and processing (Joanette & Brownell, 1990).

The theoretical background of discourse studies comes from semantic memory models. In fact, impairment of the semantic system is considered to be among the most prominent problems among diffuse brain-damaged subjects such as those with dementia of the Alzheimer's type (Cardebat, Démonet, Nespoulous, Puel, & Rascol, 1991). From a neuropsychological point of view, the study of discourse production in dementia of the Alzheimer's type is thus relevant to the investigation of semantic alterations due to such disease. On the other hand, from a cognitive point of view, the study of discourse production allows one to test theoretical models. In this context, the goal of this chapter is to propose an analysis and discussion of one particular component of discourse production among dementia of the Alzheimer's type subjects, namely the narrative schema that underlies storytelling, considered from a semantic point of view.

SEMANTIC MEMORY AND DEMENTIA OF THE ALZHEIMER'S TYPE

Discourse production may be studied from two different perspectives: the surface structure or the base structure (Kintsch, 1974). The surface structure of discourse production corresponds to the output of words that have been organized into sentences. The base structure is formed by the abstract entities which express concepts and their relationships, which emerge from semantic memory, and which are translated into the words and sentences of the surface structure. Psycholinguistic theory assumes that the base structure is composed of a number of components that are hierarchically organized as well as dissociable. Kintsch (1985) distinguished the following components of the base structure: the microstructure, the macrostructure, and the superstructure. The **microstructure** of a text is an hierarchically organized list of micropropositions, which are the smallest units of information of a text. The **macrostructure** is derived from the microstructure and expresses the core contents of a text by means of a list of macropropositions. The macropropositions represent the core conceptual units of a text. The **superstructure** corresponds to the way in which a text is organized. All texts, such as scientific reports or narrative stories, have a defined superstructure. In contrast to microstructure or macrostructure, which are content specific, superstructure is a form of abstract knowledge independent of content. In this regard, superstructure shares the same invariant properties of the abstract representations that comprise general human knowledge (Barsalou & Sewell, 1985).

The fact that patients with dementia of the Alzheimer's type have impairments of semantic memory is now well established (Chertkow & Bub, 1990; Huff, Corkin, & Growdon, 1986; Martin & Fedio, 1983). However, the evaluation of these semantic memory deficits is invariably reliant on performance on lexical-semantic tasks such as word fluency, category fluency, picture naming, or naming to description. The most prominent theoretical model underlying these studies is the lexical network model (Chang, 1986) which defines relations between features, items, and categories. Only a few studies with Alzheimer's patients have taken into account the semantic representations underlying the production of discourse more elaborate than the production of single words or sentences. The knowledge representations described as script or narrative schema are other forms of semantic structures that might be impaired in dementia of the Alzheimer's type.

SCRIPT AND DEMENTIA OF THE ALZHEIMER'S TYPE

A **script** is defined as a description of an activity of daily life that is comprised of a number of events occurring in a typical sequence (Mandler, 1984). An often cited example is that of a meal eaten at a restaurant. Associated with a meal at a restaurant is a sequence of events that are generally followed, such as waiting to be seated, reading the menu, ordering the meal, and so on.

Scripts have been employed with adult patients to assess the knowledge representation related to semantic superstructures. Weingartner, Grafman, Boutelle, and Martin (1983) compared patients with Korsakoff's disease, those with dementia of the Alzheimer's type, and normal controls on two tasks related to script knowledge. The first was a script-event discrimination task. Subjects were asked to determine whether two events came from the same script. If the two events were of the same script, the subjects then had to determine whether the events had been presented in the correct sequence. The second task required that subjects generate a script. The subjects had to recall all the events that occurred after they had gotten up in the morning and before they left the house. The results indicated that dementia of the Alzheimer's type patients made more sequence ordering type errors than did the Korsakoff's disease or control subjects on the script discrimination task. Moreover, the errors were more frequent between events that were set close together in time. On the script generation task, dementia of the Alzheimer's type patients produced fewer events than the Korsakoff's disease or control subjects.

Roman, Brownell, Potter, Seibold, and Gardner (1987) compared older adults and right hemisphere brain-damaged patients on tasks of script production, continuation, and judgment. In the script production task, subjects were asked to produce a list of the events, in the appropriate order, related to changing a flat tire and to eating dinner in a restaurant. In the script continuation task, the subjects were required to describe the next step in a script after hearing the title of the story and two correctly sequenced events. In the script judgment task, the subjects were required to judge script event membership, temporal order, and relative importance. The right hemisphere brain-damaged patients and elderly controls demonstrated preserved knowledge of script information in all the tasks. Thus, script knowledge does not seem to be affected by damage to the right hemisphere or by the processes of normal aging.

In a third study, Grafman et al. (1991) examined script retrieval in patients with probable dementia of the Alzheimer's type and compared their performance to both depressed patients and normal controls. The tasks were the same as in the Weingartner et al. (1983) study. The results indicated that the dementia of the Alzheimer's type patients generated scripts that frequently contained implausible events; also, the scripts rarely contained information with a low value of centrality. Values of centrality were provided by normative data and indicated how critical an event was in relation to the definition of the script. As in the Weingartner et al. (1983) study, dementia of the Alzheimer's type subjects produced more sequence errors in the discrimination task than did the depressed subjects or the normal controls.

The results of these studies lend support to the notion that the representation of knowledge as assessed by script generation or script evaluation tasks is impaired in subjects with dementia of the Alzheimer's type (Grafman et al., 1991; Weingarten et al., 1983) and remains intact in normal aged subjects (Roman et al., 1987).

NARRATIVE SCHEMA AND DEMENTIA OF THE ALZHEIMER'S TYPE

The **narrative schema** is the semantic structure corresponding to the sequential arrangement of events in a story (Brewer, 1985). It forms the basis of the production of a story in the same way a script underlies the description of an activity of daily life.

The components of a story schema have been defined by Stein and Glenn (1979) as the conceptual framework which specifies the logical order of occurrence of seven categories of information. The first category of information, *setting*, defines the context of an *initiating event*, the second category of information. This results in the generation of an *internal response* (the third category of information) which expresses a conflict that motivates the creation of an *internal plan*, the fourth category of information. This plan is created to effect a change as a result of the protagonist's subsequent *actions (attempts)*, which can have number of *consequences* (the fifth and sixth categories of information, respectively). These consequences precipitate emotional or cognitive *reactions*, the seventh category of information. Each category of information may be represented by one or more macropropositions, which express the precise content of that schema component.

A number of studies have employed the notion of schema components, as developed by Stein and Glenn (1979), in tasks of narration comprehension and recall in children. Results show that children as young as 6 years of age use schema components in their understanding and recall of narrative stories. The results also demonstrate that they exhibit evidence of such a framework of understanding and recall as early as the age of 4 (Denhière, 1978–79; Fayol, 1985; Stein & Glenn, 1982). However, to date, few studies have attempted to analyze the narrative schema in normal elderly subjects or in persons with dementia of the Alzheimer's type.

Given that the narrative schema is a semantic structure with the same properties as a script, it can be hypothesized that in a narration production task, dementia of the Alzheimer's type subjects would produce fewer schema components yet make more intrusions and sequential-order errors than would normal aged controls.

METHODS

SUBJECTS

Dementia of the Alzheimer's Type Subjects

Six women (M = 64.8 years; s = 7.2) with a diagnosis of possible or probable Alzheimer's disease according to the criteria of the NINCDS-ADRDA Work Group (McKhann et al., 1984) were included in this study. All were outpatients in the early stages of the disease. The first symptoms reported by the subject or her family appeared less than 5 years prior to testing. A comprehensive medical, neurological, and neuropsychological examination was administered to each patient. All subjects were found to be between levels 3 and 4 on the Global Deterioration Scale (Reisberg, Ferris, De Leon, & Crook, 1982).

Control Subjects

Six women (M = 67.5 years; s = 4.8) with no history of neurological, psychiatric, or psychological problems were involved in the study.

TASK

Each subject was required to produce three stories. The first story to be generated was the fairly tale *Little Red Riding Hood* with no visual (pictorial) support. Subjects were required to tell the story relying entirely on personal memory of the tale. The second story was prompted by seven ordered pictures representing the events leading up to and causing a car accident. The third story to be produced relied on a single pictured scene illustrating a bank holdup.

SCORING

The story schema proposed by Stein and Glenn (1979) was used to analyze the story productions. This schema includes seven components: setting, initiating event, internal response(s), internal plan(s), attempt(s), consequence(s), and reaction(s). That there can exist more than one macroproposition per schema component is dependent on the number of individuals in the story.

Evaluation of the Presence of the Schema Components

Prior to testing, the set of necessary macropropositions for each schema component was determined. For each of the theoretical schema components, at least one macroproposition must be present; otherwise, the schema would be considered incomplete. The "method of judges" was used to determine the list of macropropositions. The list of macropropositions corresponding to the schema components of each of the three stories was generated by tabulating the propositions generated by 11 university students. Propositions produced by at least 7 of the 11 students were retained (see Appendix for the list of macropropositions).

To score the subject-generated stories, two aspects of their productions related to the schema components were analyzed. The first was to determine the presence or absence of various schema components for each of the productions. The second aspect of the subject generated stories to be examined was related to the content of the macropropositions. On the basis of the list of macropropositions generated by 7 of 11 university student judges, three classes of information were defined: explicit information, implicit information, and no information. **Explicit information** was information that corresponded directly and unambiguously to the particular schema component. **Implicit information** was information not explicitly related to a schema component, yet which permitted a listener to infer details in order to understand the following episode of the story. **No information** indicated that no macropropositions related to the schema component in question were produced. Subjects' productions (three stories per subject) were analyzed by 2 university student judges who classified the macropropositions as belonging to one of the three categories listed above. Discrepancies were resolved through discussion between the 2 judges.

DEFINITION OF RELEVANT AND IRRELEVANT INFORMATION

The second task was to determine a criterion for distinguishing relevant versus irrelevant information in relation to the content of the stories. This determination was important to establish the presence of intrusive errors in the dementia of the Alzheimer's type subjects' productions. Two types of relevant information were considered, essential and secondary information. An **essential** proposition provided information of fundamental importance with respect to the logical sequence of the story and which corresponded to a macroproposition as determined by the university student judges. **Secondary** information expressed supplementary details which, although not fundamental to the overall understanding of the story, remained relevant and pertinent. All other information was considered to be **irrelevant.** The propositions were classified as essential or secondary based on the judgments made by 7 of 11 university student judges. The subjects' productions (three stories per subject) were analyzed by 2 judges who used the reference list of essential and secondary propositions. Discrepancies were resolved through discussion between the 2 judges.

SEQUENTIAL-ORDER ERRORS

The third parameter to be considered was the sequential order in the narrations. Two types of errors were defined: anticipation and regression. An **anticipation** error occurred when a macroproposition was generated too early in the sequence, whereas a proposition occurring too late in the sequence was deemed a **regression** error.

RESULTS

PRESENCE OF THE SCHEMA COMPONENTS

Table 14–1 provides a summary of the types of information generated by the dementia of the Alzheimer's type and control subjects in their recollection of the *Little Red Riding Hood* story. Each value corresponds to the number of subjects who provided a certain type of information relating to one of the seven schema components and to whether the information provided was explicitly evident or implicitly determined from the story. The results indicate that the dementia of the Alzheimer's type subjects produced fewer explicit details than the normal controls and that among the dementia of the Alzheimer's type subjects two schema components, internal plan and consequences, were never generated. The dementia of the Alzheimer's type subjects produced as many explicit as implicit details, whereas the normal elderly controls produced many more explicit details across all schema components. When explicit and implicit details are considered together, each schema component of the *Little Red Riding Hood* story was produced by at least three of the six control subjects.

Table 14–2 shows the results from subjects' narrative productions to the series of images depicting the Car Accident. In this instance, as in the previous one, control subjects generated more details concerning the events than did the dementia of the Alzheimer's type subjects. The number of explicit details in the control subjects' stories was greater than the number of implicit details. The dementia of the Alzheimer's type subjects, however, showed the opposite pattern of results, that is, the number of implicit details was greater than the number of explicit details. However, when the total number of explicit and implicit details are taken together, more schema components were produced to this story than to the *Little Red Riding Hood* story. Also, for both dementia of the Alzheimer's type subjects and normal controls, two schema components, internal response and internal plan, were generated less often for this story than for the previous one.

Table 14–3 shows the results for the subjects' narrative productions to the single illustration of the Bank Holdup. In this condition, neither control or dementia of the Alzheimer's type subjects generated consequence

Table 14–1. The number of subjects who gave explicit information (EI), implicit information (II), both explicit and implicit information (EI + II), and no information (NI) corresponding to the seven schema components: setting (S), initiating event (IE), internal response (IR), internal plan (IP), attempt(s) (A, A'), consequence(s) (C, C'), and reaction (R) to the story of *Little Red Riding Hood*

	Control Subjects				DAT* Subjects			
	EI	II	EI + II	NI	EI	II	EI + II	NI
S	6	0	6	0	3	1	4	2
IE	5	0	5	1	3	3	6	0
IR	3	0	3	3	1	1	2	4
IP	2	3	5	1	0	0	0	6
A	5	1	6	0	0	1	1	5
A'	6	0	6	0	1	1	2	4
C	2	1	3	3	0	0	0	6
C'	4	1	5	1	1	0	1	5
R	3	0	3	3	0	1	1	5
Total	36	5	41	12	9	8	17	37

* DAT: dementia of the Alzheimer's type

Table 14–2. The number of subjects who gave explicit information (EI), implicit information (II), both explicit and implicit information (EI + II), and no information (NI) corresponding to the seven schema components: setting (S), initiating event (IE), internal response (IR), internal plan (IP), attempt(s) (A), consequence(s) (C), and reaction (R) to the Car Accident story

	Control Subjects				DAT* Subjects			
	EI	II	EI + II	NI	EI	II	EI + II	NI
S	6	0	6	0	4	2	6	0
IE	6	0	6	0	1	4	5	1
IR	0	3	3	3	0	1	1	5
IP	2	0	2	4	0	1	1	5
A	5	1	6	0	2	3	5	1
C	6	0	6	0	1	4	5	1
R	5	0	5	1	0	4	4	2
Total	30	4	34	8	8	19	27	15

* DAT: dementia of the Alzheimer's type

Table 14–3. The number of subjects who gave explicit information (EI), implicit information (II), both explicit and implicit information (EI + II), and no information (NI) corresponding to the seven schema components: setting (S), initiating event (IE), internal response (IR), internal plan (IP, IP', IP"), attempt(s) (A, A', A"), consequence(s) (C), and reaction (R) to the Bank Holdup story

	Control Subjects				DAT* Subjects			
	EI	II	EI + II	NI	EI	II	EI + II	NI
S	4	1	5	1	4	0	4	2
IE	5	1	6	0	4	0	4	2
IR	4	2	6	0	1	3	4	2
IP	2	3	5	1	1	3	4	2
IP'	0	2	2	4	0	0	0	6
IP"	3	3	3	0	0	3	3	3
A	1	0	1	5	0	0	0	6
A'	6	0	6	0	1	5	5	0
A"	5	0	5	1	0	2	2	4
C	0	0	0	6	0	0	0	6
R	0	0	0	6	0	0	0	6
Total	30	12	42	24	11	16	27	39

* DAT: dementia of the Alzheimer's type

and reaction schema components. Moreover, dementia of the Alzheimer's type subjects did not produce internal plan and attempt components. Only one control subject produced an internal plan whereas only two control subjects produced an attempt component. Generally, when schema components are generated the control subjects produced more than the dementia of the Alzheimer's type subjects. In the dementia of the Alzheimer's type subjects' productions, the number of implicit details was again greater than the number of explicit details while the opposite pattern of results was observed in the control subjects' productions.

TYPES OF INFORMATION

Overall, the control subjects' stories imparted more essential information ($n = 170$, see Table 14–4) than do the dementia of the Alzheimer's type subjects' narratives ($n = 65$). Also, the secondary details provided by the control subjects outnumbered those provided by the dementia of the Alzheimer's type subjects ($n = 94$ to $n = 76$, respectively). The production of irrelevant information was much more frequent among the dementia of the Alzheimer's type subjects ($n = 40$) than among the controls ($n = 3$).

In each of the narratives, the control subjects invariably provided more essential information than secondary information (see Table 14–4). This

Table 14–4. The number of times essential information (ES), secondary information (SE), and irrelevant information (IR) were provided by the dementia of the Alzheimer's type and normal elderly control subjects for each of the stories

	Control Subjects			DAT* Subjects		
	ES	SE	IR	ES	SE	IR
Little Red Riding Hood	61	31	3	13	12	11
The Car Accident	61	40	0	26	52	13
The Bank Holdup	48	23	0	26	12	16
Total	170	94	3	65	76	40

* DAT: dementia of the Alzheimer's type

was not the case in the productions of the dementia of the Alzheimer's type subjects. In the story of Little Red Riding Hood, the dementia of the Alzheimer's type subjects produced virtually the same number of essential propositions ($n = 13$) and secondary propositions ($n = 12$). However, in the Car Accident story, the dementia of the Alzheimer's type subjects produced twice as many secondary details ($n = 52$) as essential details ($n = 26$). Whereas in the narrative productions of the Bank Holdup story the results were exactly the opposite, with the dementia of the Alzheimer's type subjects providing 26 essential propositions to 12 secondary propositions.

SEQUENTIAL-ORDER ERRORS

Table 14–5 shows the number of anticipation and regression errors found in both the control subjects' and dementia of the Alzheimer's type subjects' productions. Few errors of either kind were made in the Little Red Riding Hood narratives. In the Car Accident story, the dementia of the Alzheimer's type subjects made five anticipation and two regression errors whereas the controls subjects made only two regression errors. In the Bank Holdup story, the pattern of results was similar for both groups. Generally, regression errors were more frequent than the anticipation errors.

DISCUSSION

STORY SCHEMA COMPONENTS

Overall, the dementia of the Alzheimer's type subjects generated fewer story components than the age-matched controls. This result is consistent with the results obtained in previous studies involving dementia of

Table 14–5. Sequential-order errors: Anticipation errors (A), correspond to information that is provided too early in the sequence of events, and Regression errors (R), which correspond to information that is provided too late in the sequence of events

	Control Subjects		DAT* Subjects	
	A	R	A	R
Little Red Riding Hood	0	1	1	1
The Car Accident	0	2	5	2
The Bank Holdup	1	4	0	4
Total	1	7	6	6

* DAT: dementia of the Alzheimer's type

the Alzheimer's type subjects and script productions (Weingartner et al., 1983). However, the results in the present study suggest that the subjects' performance is determined largely by the nature of the stimuli.

In the story of *Little Red Riding Hood*, internal response, attempts, consequence, and reaction schema components were rarely present in the dementia of the Alzheimer's type subjects' narrative productions (although, internal response, consequence, and reaction components were also less frequent in control subjects' productions). Subjects were asked to generate this story without the assistance of any visual stimuli; thus, the subjects were required to rely only on their long-term memory of the fairy tale. That some of the story elements may have been forgotten could conceivably hamper a subject's ability to respect the schema.

In the Car Accident story, the dementia of the Alzheimer's type subjects' performance was similar to that of the normal control subjects. The chronologically ordered sequence of images provides the essential elements of the story, which constrains the narrative productions. The schema is imposed and thus the story does not need to be reconstructed by the subject. However, two schema components, internal response and internal plan, were produced less frequently. These schema components are representative of affective and cognitive attributes which are not explicitly evident from the depicted scenario. That these two components have to be inferred from the pictures seems to have had an influence on the subjects' productions.

In the Bank Holdup story, two schema components, internal plan and attempts, were rarely produced by members of either group, whereas two components, consequences and reactions, are never produced. These four components were not explicitly depicted; rather, they had to be inferred from the illustration. That the consequences and reaction schema components were never produced suggests that the subjects did not invent an ending to the story. It is conceivable that had more detailed instructions been provided to the subjects, they may have been led to complete the story.

SEQUENTIAL-ORDER ERRORS

The dementia of the Alzheimer's type subjects made more sequential-order errors than the control subjects. In the *Little Red Riding Hood* and the Bank Holdup narratives, dementia of the Alzheimer's type subjects produced as many errors as the controls, although the dementia of the Alzheimer's type subjects' story schemas were more incomplete in these productions. In the Car Accident story, the dementia of the Alzheimer's type subjects produced five anticipation and two regression errors. In this case, the schema productions should have been constrained due to the ordered presentation of the images which provide explicit information with respect to both content and sequence. However, the dementia of the Alzheimer's type subjects were apparently unable to make simultaneous use of both types of information as evidenced by the fact that they produced more sequence errors than content errors. This pattern of performance has also been seen in dementia of the Alzheimer's type subjects' script productions (Grafman et al., 1991; Weingartner et al., 1983).

IRRELEVANT INFORMATION

The dementia of the Alzheimer's type subjects generated more irrelevant information than the control subjects. In contrast to the greater number of sequential-order errors made by the dementia of the Alzheimer's type subjects in the more constrained presentations, the number of intrusion errors was greater in the less constrained scenarios, the *Little Red Riding Hood* and the Bank Holdup stories. Again, this pattern of performance has been seen in dementia of the Alzheimer's type subjects' script productions (Grafman et al., 1991; Weingartner et al., 1983). The production of intrusion errors by dementia of the Alzheimer's type subjects has also been observed in tasks of text recall (Butters, Grandholm, Salmon, & Grant, 1987) and word list learning (Kramer et al., 1988). Butters et al. (1987) have suggested that dementia of the Alzheimer's type patients have an increased sensitivity to interference between different types of information from similar categories. Their conclusions were drawn from observations of dementia of the Alzheimer's type subjects' performance on episodic memory tasks. In semantic memory tasks, such as a story narration, dementia of the Alzheimer's type subjects seem to have difficulties in selecting the most appropriate details to complete the narrative. It was noted that among the dementia of the Alzheimer's type subjects' productions of the *Little Red Riding Hood* story, there was a tendency to include elements from other well-known fairy tales. In the Bank Holdup story, the intrusion errors appear to result from the patients' misinterpretation of the scene. The role and nature of interference in semantic memory tasks remains to be fully understood.

CONCLUSION

The present study assessed the use of story schema in the evaluation of dementia of the Alzheimer's type subjects. The results indicate that the behavior of the dementia of the Alzheimer's type subjects in story production is comparable to their performance in script production. They provide fewer schema components than controls, they make sequential-order errors, and they produce more irrelevant propositions. However, for both dementia of the Alzheimer's type and control subjects, the story productions and the presence or absence of various schema components are greatly influenced by the nature of the narrative to be generated. In the Car Accident story, each schema component was present in at least one of the dementia of the Alzheimer's type subjects' productions and in at least two of the control subjects' productions. In the Bank Holdup story, the composition of the narrative productions of the two subject groups were very similar, including the fact that, in both cases, a number of the schema components were never produced. In the production of the *Little Red Riding Hood* story, in which no visual cues are available, the differences between the two groups were most prominent. Each schema component of this story was produced by at least three of the six control subjects, whereas all the dementia of the Alzheimer's type subjects failed to produce two schema components, internal plan and consequences. In the second situation, the Bank Holdup, the unitary image is the factor that determines a subject's preference for providing a description of events rather than a narration of a story. This is demonstrated by the absence in the subjects' productions of a conclusion to the story which is not illustrated in the picture. Finally, the sequence of pictures for the Car Accident scenario constrains the structure of the story, which resulted in more schema components being generated by all subjects. Paradoxically, the dementia of the Alzheimer's type subjects do not necessarily respect the sequential ordering of the schema components. The dementia of the Alzheimer's type subjects appear to have had difficulty performing the two tasks simultaneously, producing the appropriate components and sequencing them correctly.

Another finding of the present study is that the dementia of the Alzheimer's type subjects generate more details of an implicit nature than do the normal controls. Bayles, Kasniak, and Tomoeda (1987) have proposed that individuals with dementia of the Alzheimer's type have problems with some pragmatic aspects of verbal communication as evidenced by the fact that they do not ensure that they have been understood. Garcia (1991) has shown that dementia of the Alzheimer's type subjects have problems respecting established conversational rules. The relative role of pragmatic and semantic components in narratives remains to be fully understood.

Most of the studies regarding narrative schema have used recall in the evaluation of memory and comprehension. Few studies have used production of narratives to assess memory and comprehension, and even fewer studies have focused on the elderly. This study assessed the utility of using the story schema as developed by Stein and Glenn (1979) in the evaluation of the narrative productions of both healthy elderly subjects and subjects with probable dementia of the Alzheimer's type. Our results suggest that the use of this story schema by normal aged subjects may not be generalizable across various forms of narratives. A greater understanding of the nature of schema components and narrative productions will be necessary to more effectively discriminate between the productions of normal elderly individuals and those of patients with dementia of the Alzheimer's type.

Discourse studies in neuropsychology are meant to provide some insights into the nature of the organization of the cognitive processes underlying human communication. Despite the limits of this study, some conclusions may be drawn about the effects of dementia of the Alzheimer's type on communication. The first one concerns the use of a schema to memorize and recall a text. Bartlett (1932) hypothesized the existence of a "schema" to account for the transformations that occur to stories stored in long-term memory. What was observed among dementia of the Alzheimer's type subjects when they had to tell a tale based on a long-term memory storage is that the recall is impaired. Thus, the recall of events from long-term memory does not appear to be improved by the use of a schema. However, the recall of a tale without any visual cues does not allow one to distinguish between impairments in episodic (the events) versus semantic (the schema) memory. Another condition used in the study—the Car Accident story—was such that all the organized information was provided to build a story. The only thing subjects had to do was to verbalize the relations between pictured people and events. However, the performance of dementia of the Alzheimer's type subjects in the Car Accident story showed an impairment in the production of the story. Although all the information was provided visually, dementia of the Alzheimer's type subjects did not fully respect the schema in their efforts to organize the story. Thus, the results of this study have both neuropsychological and cognitive implications. From a neuropsychological standpoint, it can be suggested that the occurence of a dementia of the Alzheimer's type can result in a problem using narrative schema. However, from a cognitive point of view, it also appears that the presentation of visual cues does not seem to be sufficient to compensate for the efffects of the disease.

REFERENCES

Bayles, K. A., Kasniak, A. W., & Tomoeda, C. K. (1987). *Communication and cognition in normal aging and dementia*. Boston: Little, Brown.
Barsalou, L. W., & Sewell, D. R. (1985). Contrasting the representation of scripts and categories. *Journal of Memory and Language, 24,* 646–665.
Bartlett, F. C. (1932). *Remembering*. Cambridge, England: Cambridge University Press.
Bobrow, D., & Collins, A. (1975). *Representation and understanding*. New York: Academic Press.
Brewer, W. F. (1985). The story schema: Universal and cultural-specific properties. In D. R. Olson, N. Torrance, & A. Hildyard (Eds.), *Literacy, language and learning* (pp. 167–194). Cambridge, England: Cambridge University Press.
Butters, N., Grandholm, E., Salmon, D. P., & Grant, I. (1987). Episodic and semantic memory : A comparison of amnesic and demented patients. *Journal of Clinical and Experimental Neuropsychology, 9,* 479–497.
Cardebat, D., Démonet, J. F., Nespoulous, J.-L., Puel, M., & Rascol, A. (1991). Langage et démences. In M. Habib, Y. Joanette, & M. Puel (Eds.), *Démences et syndromes démentiels. Approche neuropsychologique* (pp.153–164). Paris: Masson.
Chang, T. M. (1986). Semantic memory: Facts and models. *Psychological Bulletin, 99,* 199–220.
Chertkow, H., & Bub, D. (1990). Semantic memory loss in dementia of Alzheimer's type. *Brain, 113,* 397–417.
Denhière, G. (1978–79). Compréhension et rappel d'un récit par des enfants de six à douze ans. In G. Oléron et M. Denis (Eds.), *La compréhension du langage. Bulletin de psychologie, 32,* 341, 803–819.
Fayol, M. (1985). *Le récit et sa construction*. Neuchâtel, Suisse: Dealchaux et Niestlé.
Garcia, L. (1991). *Conversational topic shifting styles in dementia of the Alzheimer Type: A multiple case study*. Doctoral dissertation, Université de Montréal.
Grafman, J., Thompson, K., Weingartner, H., Martinez, R., Lawlor, B. A., & Sunderland, T. (1991). Script generation as an indicator of knowledge representation in patients with Alzheimer's disease. *Brain and Language, 40,* 244–358.
Huff, F. J., Corkin, S., & Growdon, J. H. (1986). Semantic impairment and anomia in Alzheimer's disease. *Brain and Language, 28,* 235–249.
Joanette, Y., & Brownell, H. (1990). *Discourse ability and brain damage: Theoretical and empirical perspectives*. New York: Springer Verlag.
Kintsch, W. (1974). *The representation of meaning in memory*. Hillsdale, NJ: Lawrence Erlbaum.
Kintsch, W. (1985). Text processing : A psychological model. In T. A. van Dijk (Ed.), *Handbook of discourse analysis. Dimensions of discourse* (vol 2., pp. 231–243). New-York: Academic Press.
Kramer, J. H., Delis, D. C., Blusewicz, M. J., Brandt, J., Ober, B. A., & Strauss, M. (1988). Verbal memory errors in Alzheimer's and Huntington's dementias. *Developmental Neuropsychology, 4,* 1–15.

McKhann, G., Drachman, D., Folstein, M., Katzman, R., Price, D., & Stadlan, E. M. (1984). Clinical diagnosis of Alzheimer's disease: Report of the NINCDS-ADRDA Work Group under the auspices of the Department of Health and Human Services Task Force on Alzheimer's Disease. *Neurology, 34*, 939–944.

Mandler, J. M. (1984). Stories, scripts, and scenes: Aspects of schema theory. Hillsdale, NJ: Lawrence Erlbaum.

Martin, A., & Fedio, P. (1983). Word production and comprehension in Alzheimer's disease: The breakdown of semantic knowledge. *Brain and Language, 19*, 124–141.

Reisberg, B., Ferris, S.H., De Leon M.J., & Crook, T. (1982). The global deterioration scale for assessment of primary degenerative dementia. *American Journal of Psychiatry, 139*, 1136–1139.

Roman, M., Brownell, H. H., Potter, H. H., Seibold, M. S., & Gardner, H. (1987). Script knowledge in right hemisphere-damaged and in normal elderly adults. *Brain and Language, 31*, 151–170.

Stein, N. L., & Glenn, C. G. (1979). An analysis of story comprehension in elementary school children. In R. O. Freedle (Ed.), *New directions in discourse processing* (pp. 53–120). Norwood, NJ: Ablex.

Stein, N. L., & Glenn, C. G. (1982). Children's concept of time: The development of a story schema. In W. J. Friedman (Ed.), *The development of psychology of time* (pp. 255–282). New York: Academic Press.

Weingartner, H., Grafman, J., Boutelle, W., & Martin, P. (1983). Forms of memory failure. *Science, 221*, 380–382.

APPENDIX

List of Macropropositions

	Little Red Riding Hood	The Car Accident	The Bank Holdup
SETTING	LRRH* is a young girl who walks through the forest to bring food to her GM**.	A mother and her two children are in a car.	The robbery takes place in a bank situated on a street corner.
	4 ES***	3 ES	1 ES
INITIATING EVENT	LRRH meets the Wolf and talks with him.	The mother stops in front of the grocery store and leaves her children alone in the car.	The armed robbers enter the bank and demand that they be given money.
	2 ES	2 ES	3 ES
INTERNAL RESPONSE	The Wolf is tempted with the idea of eating LRRH and convinces LRRH into taking a long route to GM's house.	The children are left alone and want to play.	The staff and clients are frightened and raise their hands in the air. A passerby witnesses the events inside the bank.
	2 ES	1 ES	3 ES

INTERNAL PLAN	The Wolf arrives at GM's house and either eats her or gets rid of her. 2 ES	The boy decides to pretend that he is driving the car. 1 ES	a) An accomplice waits in a car. b) A bank employee hides under a desk. c) The passerby runs to get help. 3 ES
ATTEMPT	a) The Wolf disguises itself as GM, imitates GM and is asleep in bed when LRRH arrives. b) There is a dialogue between the disguised Wolf and LRRH. 5 ES	The boy heads towards the front seat of the car and releases the hand brake. 2 ES	a) The robbers seize the money. b) An employee phones the police. c) The passerby notifies a traffic cop. 3 ES
CONSEQUENCE	a) LRRH enters the house. b) The Wolf races towards LRRH and eats her. 3ES	The car, which is on a hill, rolls and crashes into a lamp-post. The car is damaged. 4ES	The police have been notified. Will they arrive in time? 1 ES
REACTION	A hunter passes close by to the house and kills the Wolf. GM is saved. LRRH is saved. 4 ES	The mother comes out of the grocery store furious and scolds the children. She then leaves with the car towards home. 4 ES	The police arrive and capture the criminals. 2 ES

* LRRH : Little Red Riding Hood
** GM : Grandmother
*** ES : Essential Information

CHAPTER 15

Narrative Discourse in Dementia

DOMINIQUE CARDEBAT, JEAN-FRANÇOIS DÉMONET, AND BERNARD DOYON

Since the pioneering work of Irigaray (1973), communication disorders, and more specifically language impairments, are identified as an integral part of the semiology of dementia of the Alzheimer's type (DAT).

During the last two decades, many studies aimed at specifying the linguistic disturbances observed in dementia patients by, most often, using methodological tools borrowed from aphasiology. The results of these studies, on the one hand, allowed labeling the different language patterns observed during the course of the disease according to the classical aphasiological terminology and, on the other hand, demonstrated the predominance of the lexical semantic deficits when the analysis is restricted to the lexical level.

The early stage of the disease is marked by word-finding difficulties in spontaneous speech, and the relatively isolated impairment in naming corresponds with that seen in anomic aphasia (Albert, 1980; Hier, Hagenlocker, & Shindler, 1985; Schwartz, Marin, & Saffran, 1979). At the mid and the mid-late stages of Alzheimer's disease, anomia appears important, and language becomes increasingly paraphasic with verbal and semantic paraphasias. Spontaneous speech is fluent but becomes progressively fragmented and sometimes incoherent. Auditory comprehension abilities are disturbed, whereas reading and repetition abilities seem to be relatively preserved. The dissociation between correct repetition and disturbed comprehension found in mid-stage dementia of the Alzheimer's type resembles the language pattern found in transcortical-sensory aphasia (Appel, Kertesz, & Fisman, 1982; Murdoch & Chenery, 1987).

In late-stage Alzheimer's disease, speech becomes nonfluent, partial or total mutism is not uncommon, and all the language levels are disturbed. The deficits reflect total language impairment, similar to that found in global aphasia.

The lexical semantic deficits that represent the major feature of the language semiology in dementia of the Alzheimer type have been explored specifically in many studies by using confrontation naming (Bayles & Tomoeda, 1983; Smith, Murdoch, & Chenery, 1989), word fluency (Bayles et al., 1989; Diesfeldt, 1989; Hart, Smith, & Swash, 1988) or word-association tests, but, here again, the studies, restricted to the lexical level, do not consider the discourse level.

However, some studies have focused on the analysis of the disourse of the dementia patients, and the results seem to evidence a discourse deficit independent of the disturbances observed at a strictly lexical level. The cause of this deficit can be memorial (see the study of Grafman et al., 1989, about the knowledge of the narrative scripts) as well as logical semantic (see Ulatowska et al., 1991, for analyses of narratives, and Blanken, Dittmann, Haas, & Wallesch, 1987, for analyses of spontaneous speech).

We report in this chapter the results of two multiple-case studies in which we adressed the issue of distinctive deficits of discourse production in patients presenting with DAT compared to elderly normal controls and to aphasic patients.

More specifically, the first study aimed at verifying whether the narrative deficits observed in dementia were qualitatively similar to those observed in normal aging, although quantitatively more important. If the results only pointed out quantitative differences between dementia patients and old normals, one could assume that, as far as narrative deficits were concerned, the pathologic processes involved in dementia of Alzheimer's type did not differ basically from the normal process of aging. So, we analyzed the narratives produced by dementia patients, by normal elderly subjects, and by very old normal subjects.

The second study aimed at identifying the narrative deficits of dementia patients in comparison with aphasic subjects without articulatory or phonemic disorders.

METHODS

SUBJECTS

The first study included three groups of subjects: a group of 25 normal old subjects (11 men, 14 women, ages 60 to 74 years), a group of 15 normal very old subjects (4 men, 11 women, ages 75 to 89 years) and a group of 19 DAT patients (7 men, 12 women, ages 75 to 89 years, Mini Mental Score [Folstein, Folstein, & McHugh, 1975] from 15 to 24).

In the second study, we analyzed the narrative production of 5 right-handed DAT patients (3 men and 2 women, ages 56 to 94, Global Deterioration Scale [Reisberg, Ferris, Mony, De Leon, Crook, 1982] score: 4) in comparison with 10 right-handed aphasic patients (6 men, 4 women, ages 31 to 72).

The aphasic subjects, seen 3 weeks after the stroke, included three Wernicke's aphasics, three transcortical sensory aphasics, one transcortical motor aphasic and three "subcortical" aphasics. This classification was based on the standard aphasiological terminology established by Lecours and Lhermitte (1977), except for the subcortical aphasia picture characterized by Puel et al. (1984). In all these aphasics, oral production was characterized by linguistic disturbances bearing exclusively on a lexical semantic level. These subjects did not show any anarthric disorders or phonemic and syntactic disturbances. Although their comprehension could be partly impaired, these patients were able to understand the instructions required by the test. The five patients with probable Alzheimer's disease (DAT) also showed lexical semantic disturbances in their discourse, but their comprehension, again, was sufficient to understand the instructions.

EXPERIMENTAL PROCEDURE

The experimental procedure was identical for both studies and consisted of a narrative sample referred to as the Dog Story, obtained from sequential pictures ($n = 7$) from the Leboeuf series presented to the subject in the correct order (see Figure 15–1).

The Dog Story can be summarized according to the basic components of a narrative structure (van Dijk, 1977). In the "setting," a little boy takes a stray dog home, and, because he is worried about his parents' reaction, he hides the dog in a wardobe; in the "complication," the mother finds the dog and asks the boy some explanations; finally, the "resolution" occurs in which the mother allows the boy to keep the dog.

To minimize memory effects, the pictures were left in front of the subject during the test. The subjects' productions (without time limit) were recorded and transcribed. The main elements of the story were named by the subject or the examiner before the test to eliminate major gnostic-type disturbances.

NARRATIVE ANALYSIS

Our methodology paid particular attention to the "surface features" which mark narrative deficits in our subjects' productions. These "sur-

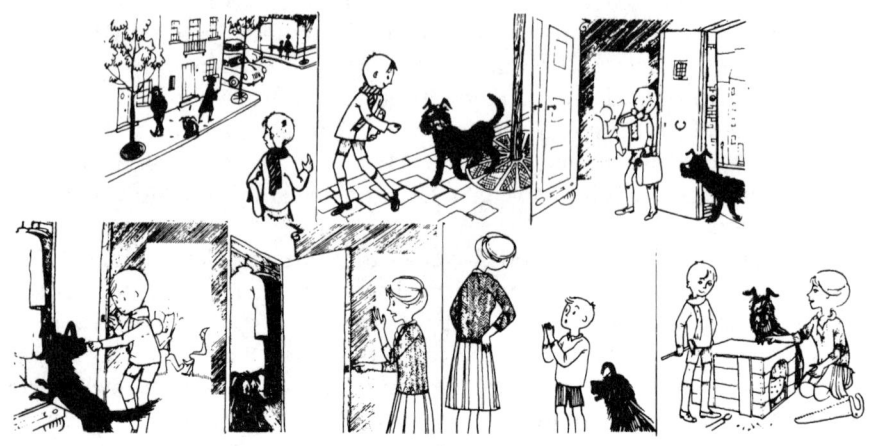

Figure 15-1. The narrative stimulus (the Dog Story) used in both studies.

face indices" can be grouped into two levels of analysis: (a) a surface level referring to the formal narrative organization, and (b) a macrostructural narrative level referring to the logical narrative organization.

In addition to the classical analyses concerning the surface level and the macrostructural level, we were interested in analyzing some narrative features pertaining to the pragmatic level of the particular situation of communication that is narrative, such as the strategy (descriptive or narrative) used by the subject and the position of the speaker in front of his or her narrative.

On the surface level, the analysis was twofold. The syntactic aspects were analyzed by:

- The number of words and clauses (characterized by the syntactic structure subject-predicate) in each narrative.
- The number of independent and subordinate clauses and the number of connectives.
- The number of anaphoric disturbances. In our productions, anaphora was generally represented by personnal pronouns (e.g., "he," "she," "it," and "they"). The disturbances related to an inappropriate use of anaphora covered three types of errors: anaphora without lexical referent, anaphora with ambigous lexical referent, and anaphora that was syntactically inappropriate.

The analysis of the content-word aspects concerned the anomic phenomena, the verbal deviations, and the gnostic deviations:

- The anomic phenomena referred to the absence of production of the target item indicated by a pause or the production of a vague generic term.
- Verbal deviations concerned both the morphological verbal deviations (formal resemblance between the target item and the one which is produced) and the verbal deviations of "close" and "distant" semantic type.
- The gnostic deviations concerned clear misidentification of the elements of the pictures during the narrative production.

On the macrostructural level, two phenomena were more closely studied: (a) the presence of one of the basic components of a narrative structure—the complication (van Dijk, 1977)—and (b) the presence of narrative paraphasias. The analysis of the "complication" of the story in terms of its presence or absence constitutes an indirect but essential indication of the level of comprehension of the story showed by the subjects.

"Narrative paraphasia" designate all the statements or partial statements, including at least one relation subject-predicate, that formed micro-narratives totally different from the target narrative. Using the classification worked out by Nespoulous (1980b), the narrative paraphasias can be called "non contextually determined narrative substitutions." In fact, these substitutions are not premature or misplaced actualization of actors, of actions, or circumstances of the narrative program, rather they reflect the introduction of narrative elements foreign to the target story which lead to a confusion affecting the narrative propositions rather than the "basic" lexical components. These elements can be borrowed from other stories, come from the speaker's personal life, or can be—apparently at least—invented by the speaker.

At the pragmatic level , two points were analyzed: the narrative strategy and the position of the speaker in relation to what he or she is saying. The narrative strategy of the subjects in front of the pictures was analyzed through the number of deictics that reflect a descriptive strategy more than a narrative one. They can appear in the test under different forms: definite articles in the beginning of the story, demonstrative adjectives and pronouns, and topographic adverbs and descriptive verbs.

The position of the speaker in relation to what he or she is saying was revealed by the enunciative modalizations (Nespoulous, 1980a). Indeed, the enunciative frame of the story, being highly constrained, assigns the speaker and the listener to a formal absence and to a maximum distanciation. Thus, the presence of enunciative modalizations in a story provokes the breaking up of the narrative macrostructure and may lead to enunciative incoherence (cf. the Meta-Rule of "enunciative non-contradiction" in Charolles, 1986).

RESULTS

The data hereunder reported are from the two studies described above, and results for each study are discussed according to the three different levels of analysis: the formal level, the macrostructural level, and the pragmatic level.

Although means and standard deviations of descriptive variables are presented, statistical comparisons between the narrative variables in the productions of our subjects were performed by non-parametric tests (Mann-Witney, Chi Square) because of the non-normal distribution of the data.

ANALYSIS I : NARRATIVE IN DEMENTIA AND IN THE ELDERLY

The major goal of this analysis has been to distinguish the narratives of dementia patients from those of both elderly and very old controls. Indeed, the narrative deficits exhibited by the dementia patients may also be found in the productions of very old subjects, although to a lesser extent. To do so, we analyzed and compared the narratives of an elderly group of controls (ages 60 to 74 years), a very old group of controls (ages 75 to 89 years), and a group of dementia patients.

As a general comment, our results did not show significant differences between our two groups of controls, although the very old group always occupies an intermediate position between the dementia group and the elderly group, whatever the narrative variable studied. Consequently, the analysis presented above will focus on the differences observed between the narratives of the dementia patients and the very old subjects.

FORMAL LEVEL

At the formal level, the narratives of the dementia patients presented disturbances (see Table 15–1) that were significantly more important that those observed in the very old subjects' narratives although no difference between dementia and very old subjects' productions was found with regard to the length of the narratives. However, the productions of the dementia patients were syntactically less complex than those of the very old group; such a syntactic simplification was showed by the significant differences observed for the number of independent clauses (more important in the productions of the dementia patients) and for the number of connectives (more important in the productions of the very old subjects). The poor syntactic ability of the patients was also marked by the significant inadequate use of anaphora. In the content-word analysis, no significant difference was found between dementia and very old subjects' narratives in terms of anomic phenomena. However, the dementia patients produced

Table 15–1. Comparison of dementia subjects' narratives and very old subjects' narratives—formal level

	Very Old Subjects (N = 15)	Dementia Subjects (N = 19)	
	Mean ± SD	Mean ± SD	
Number of words	116.3 ± 39.7	133.4 ± 73.1	NS*
Independent clauses	10.7 ± 3.7	14.7 ± 4.4	$p < .01$
Connectives	1.9 ± 1.2	0.3 ± 0.5	$p < .001$
Anaphoric disturbances	0.4 ± 0.8	1.9 ± 1.7	$p < .01$
Anomic phenomena	0.03 ± 0.15	0.4 ± 0.6	NS
Semantic paraphasias	0.1 ± 0.2	0.8 ± 0.8	$p < .01$
Gnostic deviations	0.6 ± 0.8	1.5 ± 1.2	$p < .05$

Note: Except for the number of words, the other variables are expressed in number of occurrence per 100 words produced.
* Mann-Witney test.

significantly more semantic paraphasias than the very old subjects. The same phenomenon was found for the gnostic deviations that were slightly, but significantly, more numerous in the productions of our patients.

MACROSTRUCTURAL LEVEL

The deficits observed in the narratives of the dementia patients at the formal level coexisted with important and specific deficits at the macrostructural level (see Table 15–2). Indeed, whereas almost all of the controls mentioned the complication of the story, none of the dementia subjects did.

Conversely, we never found narrative paraphasias in the productions of the very old subjects, whereas these paraphasias appeared in half of the narratives produced by the dementia patients. These "micro-narratives" could originate from the focusing of the subject on an element of one of the pictures that induced a parallel story but the target story could also disappear totally from the narrative replaced by the production of an episode belonging apparently to the life of the patient.

PRAGMATIC LEVEL

The incoherence provoked by the occurence of the narrative paraphasias was, moreover, strongly emphasized by the descriptive strategy used by the patients (see Table 15–3). We noted a significant difference concerning the distribution of the deictics, namely, the dementia subjects using significantly more deictics than the very old subjects. These deictics, the

Table 15–2. Comparison of dementia subjects' narratives and very old subjects' narratives—macrostructural level

	Very Old Subjects (N = 15)	Dementia Subjects (N = 19)	
Presence of "complication"	93%	0%	$p < .001$
Narrative paraphasias	0	53	$p < .001$

Table 15–3. Comparison of dementia subjects' narratives and very old subjects' narratives—pragmatic level

	Very Old Subjects (N = 15)	Dementia Subjects (N = 19)	
	Mean ± SD	Mean ± SD	
Number of deictics	2.4 ± 2.7	7.1 ± 3.4	$p < .001$*
Number of modalizations	2.2 ± 2.1	1.9 ± 1.7	NS

* Mann-Witney test

markers of the descriptive behaviour of the speaker, could sometimes be the precursor of a narrative paraphasia that totally diverged from the target story. Finally, the patients did not seem particularly aware of their deficits since modalizations were not more important in their narratives than in the narratives of the very old subjects.

RELATIONSHIPS BETWEEN THE NARRATIVE VARIABLES IN THE PRODUCTIONS OF DEMENTIA PATIENTS AND VERY OLD SUBJECTS

In addition to the analysis presented above, we studied the relationships between the narrative variables for our two groups of subjects. The study of pairwise correlations showed few significant relations in the dementia group (just 2 significant correlations), whereas we found 10 significant correlations in the very old group.

The lack of correlations in the dementia productions gave evidence of the incoherence of the narrative pattern of the dementia subjects. On the contrary, the correlations observed in the very old group, as it appears in Table 15–4, seemed to reflect an internal coherence. A first set of correlations con-

Table 15–4. Correlations between narrative variables in the very old group

	Independent Clauses	Subordinate Clauses	Anaphoric Disturbances	Anomia	Deictics
Subordinate Clauses	–.76 **				
Connectives	–.75 **	.79 ***			
Anomia			.55 *		
Semantic Paraphasias			.55 *	.99 ***	
Gnostic Deviations		–.54 *			
Deictics			.62 *		
Modalizations			.61 *		.77 **

Note: Only significant correlations are listed; negative correlations are indicated with a minus sign (–).
* $p < .05$, ** $p < .01$, *** $p < .001$ (Spearman r test).

cerned the syntactic level with significant positive and negative correlations between subordinate clauses, independent clauses, and connectives; these three variables reflected the syntactic style of the subjects and could not be considered as markers of a syntactic deficit. Two other sets of correlations concerned anaphoric deficits. The first one suggested a relationship between anaphoric deficits and lexical impairments (anomia and verbal paraphasias), a misuse of anaphora being coupled with lexical impairment in some very old subjects. These correlations between anaphoric deficits and anomia and verbal paraphasias would suggest that the anaphoric deficits in normal very old subjects' productions were, partly, the consequence of the lexical imprecision showed by the word-finding difficulties. The word-finding difficulties were also marked by the strong relationships between anomia and verbal paraphasias. Moreover, a second set of correlations (anaphoric × deictics and deictics × modalizations) suggested that anaphoric deficits could also point to difficulties in identification of the iconographic material. Problems of picture identification could induce anaphoric disturbances, because a correct use of anaphora required an accurate identification of the referent. It seemed that in some very old subjects, such a visual deficit has led subjects to resort to a descriptive, but inadequate, strategy producing deictics and to communicate their uncertainty through modalizations.

SUMMARY

When compared with the narratives of very old normal subjects, both the formal and the macrostructural aspects of the productions of the dementia patients are disturbed. From the visual analysis to the lexicalization, their productions include gnostic, semantic, and syntactic deviations. These formal deviations interact with macrostructural disturbances that support the hypothesis of a deficit of the cognitive narrative representation that places limits on production. Moreover, the dementia patient seems to have lost the necessary notion of distanciation (Irigaray, 1973) between speaker and narrative production. The object "story" has no clear frontier for the dementia speaker who gets into it through (often personal) anecdotes and, who, doing so, breaks up the enunciative neutrality of the narrative frame. Conversely, age does not seem to have a significant influence on the narrative production of the normal subject, even though the productions of the very elderly subjects may present some lexical semantic and gnostic deviations.

ANALYSIS II: NARRATIVE IN DEMENTIA AND IN APHASIA

The conclusions of our first analysis led us to compare the narratives produced by dementia patients with the narratives produced by moderately impaired aphasic patients whose deficits mainly affect the lexical semantic level. Indeed, the narratives of dementia subjects, when compared with those of control subjects, showed disturbances at the formal level as well as at the macrostructural and pragmatic levels. The current analysis was conducted to assess whether the narratives of dementia patients also differed from those of aphasic patients with respect to the amount and the nature of the narrative deviations.

FORMAL LEVEL

The comparison between narratives of dementia subjects and aphasic subjects at the syntactic level, as it appears in Table 15–5, led to few comments. Indeed, the length of the two populations' productions, in terms of number of clauses or number of words, did not evidence a significant difference. The narratives of the dementia patients, however, were more complex syntactically than those of the aphasic subjects since the dementia patients produced more subordinate clauses and used more temporal and causal connectives than the aphasics. The correct use of anaphora seemed to create more problems for the aphasics than for the dementia patients (although not in a significant way). Most of the disturbances for the aphasics came from the use of anaphora with ambiguous lexical referent, whereas the disturbances in dementia patients' productions concerned, as well, the use of anaphora with ambiguous lexical referent as the use of syntactically inadequate anaphora.

Table 15–5. Comparison of dementia subjects' narratives and aphasic subjects' narratives—formal level

	Dementia Subjects (N = 5)	Aphasic Subjects (N = 10)	
	Mean ± SD	Mean ± SD	
Number of words	163.2 ± 101.1	163.1 ± 121.2	NS*
Independent clauses	17.8 ± 11.1	20.2 ± 11.1	NS
Subordinate clauses	0.6 ± 0.5	0.4 ± 0.6	NS
Connectives	3.4 ± 2.3	2.5 ± 3.1	NS
Anaphoric disturbances	1 ± 0.7	2 ± 1.6	NS
Anomic phenomena	1.8 ± 1.9	3.2 ± 3.6	NS
Semantic paraphasias	0.6 ± 1.3	2.6 ± 1.2	$p < .05$

* Mann-Witney test

The distribution of the anomic phenomena was not different in our two groups. On the contrary, the verbal deviations were significantly more important in the aphasic narratives. One could add that, in the dementia patients' productions, the verbal deviations, whenever they existed, were of a "close" semantic type ("grandmother" instead of "mother") whereas in our aphasic group, several verbal deviations were of a "distant" semantic type ("soldier" instead of "dog").

MACROSTRUCTURAL LEVEL

At the macrostructural level, the presence or absence of the complication of the story did not seem to be distinctive, because our results did not show any significant difference between our pathological groups (see Table 15–6). Most of the narratives of our patients did not exhibit lexical indices corresponding to the complication of the story.

On the contrary, the narrative paraphasias seemed completely restricted to the dementia patients' productions, because these phenomena were never present in the productions of the aphasics. These micronarratives could be partial as shown by the intrusion of one or two elements that did not belong to the proposed narrative frame; for example, a dementia patient pointing to the picture representing the mother opening the wardrobe told us : "ça, c'est Bernadette qui va à la messe" ("that is Bernadette going to Mass"). But the disturbance could concern the whole production of the patient who, starting from a specific (and sometimes secondary) iconographic element of the story, built up a parallel story.

Table 15-6. Comparison of dementia subjects' narratives and aphasic subjects' narratives—macrostructural level

	Dementia Subjects (N = 5)	Aphasic Subjects (N = 10)	
Presence of "complication"	40%	60%	NS
Narrative paraphasias	60	0	$p < .001$

PRAGMATIC LEVEL

At the pragmatic level (see Table 15–7), although both aphasic and dementia patients had a deictic type of narrative behavior, the aphasics were generally more descriptive, their narratives being sometimes restricted to the production of an impoverished lexical storage studded with descriptive markers referring unceasingly to the iconographic material. Moreover, the narratives of the aphasics were, most of the time, interrupted by modalizations expressing the speaker's doubt about his or her production; these modalizations were never present in the productions of the dementia patients who seemed totally unaware of their narrative deficits.

SUMMARY

When considering each of the "surface indices" taken into consideration in this study (at the formal, the macrostructural, or the pragmatic level), the comparison between aphasic and dementia patients generally reveals more important deficits in the narratives of the aphasic patients than in the narratives of the dementia patients. These deficits seem to result from lexical and lexical syntaxic disturbances that exist also in the production of the aphasics when they are subjected to aphasia batteries.

Conversely, this type of deficit is not predominant in the narratives of the dementia patients. The major problem for these patients seems rather to concern the hierarchical selection of the main elements of the story, necessary to elaborate the narrative macrostructure; the dementia patients may focus on a secondary detail of a picture and, develop, from that detail, a narrative paraphasia. The same kind of disturbances applies to the apprehension of the content of the whole sequence of pictures. For the dementia patients, each picture constitutes a closed narrative world, and they find it difficult or even impossible to build hierarchical relations between pictures. These relations, nevertheless, are necessary to the building up of the story. However, in the way of handling icono-

Table 15–7. Comparison of dementia subject's narratives and aphasic subjects' narratives—pragmatic level

	Dementia Subjects (N = 5)	Aphasic Subjects (N = 10)	
	Mean ± SD	Mean ± SD	
Number of deictics	7 ± 7.6	9 ± 8.8	NS*
Number of modalizations	0.6 ± 1.5	0 ± 0	NS

* Mann-Witney test.

graphic support, the dementia patients show some dissociations that call for additional comments.

However, the iconographic support represents a crucial element for the dementia patient who turns out to be unable to go beyond a primary analysis of the discriminated elements. Conversely, the iconographic support and the requirements dictated by the narrative test seem to represent for the dementia narrators nothing but the starting point of a story that has little to do with the target story.

DISCUSSION

Our two analyses must be considered as exploratory and, perhaps, reductionist examinations of surface manifestations, namely disorders of the production of discourse in dementia patients, which may originate from a variety of causes. The number of such factors along with the intrinsic complexity of the set of psycholinguistic processes that come into play in discourse production probably account for the small number of studies in this topic.

The production of a narrative discourse implicates the combination of many processes and levels of representation pertaining to different cognitive spheres such as mnestic systems, gnostic functions, problem solving, and inferential processes. All these cognitive instances may be affected in dementia patients. Moreover, such cognitive impairments are far from homogenous and reproducible from one patient to another. The degree of overall cognitive impairments accounts for only a part of such variability, and various cognitive subtypes have been described (Celsis et al., 1990; Martin et al., 1986). Moreover, language deficits are heterogeneous even at the beginning of the disease (see Joanette, Ska, Poissant, & Béland, 1992), and it is also evident when looking at the reports on progressive aphasia that have been published in the past decade (see, for a review, Habib & Assal, 1991). Apart from the variations which are related to the severity of the disease or the cognitive subtypes, another source of variability arises from the well-known day-to-day variation of performances in dementia patients. In spite of these limitations, the pilot studies we have described point out some characteristic features of discourse deficits in dementia.

When compared to normal very old subjects, dementia patients are impaired in all aspects of language production: lexical, syntactic, and macrostructural levels. However, the comparison between the narrative discourses produced by dementia and severely impaired aphasic patients allows a more refined characterization of such disturbances. The most striking difference between the two groups of patients is the presence in dementia patients of those phenomena that have been called "narrative paraphasias." These kinds of narrative deficits, also mentioned by Ulatowska et al. (1991), seem to constitute the hallmark of narrative discourse in dementia. Indeed, narrative paraphasias were never observed in either aphasic patients or in the normals. These brief and deviant narrative elements are related to the iconogaphic material, but in a complex way. A picture element, irrelevant for the discourse structure, may play a trigger role to induce a narrative paraphasia whose content may originate from autobiographical sources. Although generated from the analysis of visual stimuli, these narrative paraphasias do not seem to correspond to impaired gnostic abilities, because the verbal production of patients reflects an accurate identification of picture elements. Narrative paraphasias seem to be generated because the dementia patients fail to establish hierarchy between various elements included in the pictures they were presented, according to their relevance in terms of narrative structure. For instance, we compared in the first sentences of the Dog Story the iconographic elements reported by the dementia patients and the very old controls. All the normals mentioned the main characters of the story, namely the dog and the boy, whereas they are mentioned by only 75% of the dementia patients. Even more interesting, those picture elements, which are secondary or even irrelevant as far as the story structure is concerned, are significantly more abundant in the productions of dementia patients than in the discourse of normal controls. As mentioned above in the context of narrative paraphasias, such a result seems to reflect a loss of the normal hierarchy between the main, secondary, and irrelevant picture elements of the story.

CONCLUSION

Impairments in the discourse of dementia patients may be related to various cognitive deficits that largely extend beyond the language domain.

Detailed studies of surface manifestations observed in "standardized" conditions, such as narrative productions with picture stimuli, seem to be a fruitful approach. Such studies would allow us to acquire descriptive data which might be interpreted according to the current, yet not comprehensive, models of discourse production like that built up by Frederiksen, Bracewell, Breuleux, and Renaud (1990). Then, specific experiments could be conducted to assess the first, inductive, interpretation. For instance, our hypothesis of loss of hierarchical function in discourse production could be assessed through an experiment in which variations of the number and the relevance of the picture elements in the proposed stimuli would induce changes in narrative performances of dementia patients.

REFERENCES

Albert, M. L. (1980). Language in normal and dementing elderly. In L. K. Obler & M. L. Albert (Eds.), *Language and communication in the elderly*. Boston, MA: D. C. Health.

Appell, J., Kertesz, A., & Fisman, M. (1982). A study of language functioning in Alzheimer patients. *Brain and Language, 17*, 3–91.

Bayles, K. A., & Tomoeda, C. K. (1983). Confrontation naming impairment in dementia. *Brain and Language, 19*, 98–114.

Bayles, K. A., Salmon, D. P., Tomoeda, C. K., Jacobs, D., Caffrey, J. T., Kazniak, A. W., & Troster, A. I. (1989). Semantic and letter category naming in Alzheimer's patients: A predictable difference. *Developmental Neuropsychology, 5*, 335–47.

Blanken, G., Dittmann, J., Haas, J. C., & Wallesch, C. W. (1987). Spontaneous speech in senile dementia and aphasia: Implications for a neurolinguistic model of language production. *Cognition, 27*, 247–274.

Celsis, P., Agniel, A., Puel, M., Le Tinnier, A., Viallard, G., Démonet, J. F., Rascol, A., & Marc-Vergnes, J. P. (1990). Lateral asymmetries in primary degenerative dementia of the Alzheimer type. A correlative study of cognitive, haemodynamic and EEG data, in relation with severity, age of onset and sex. *Cortex, 26*, 585–596.

Charolles, M. (1986). Grammaire de texte—Théorie du discours—Narrativité. *Pratiques,* 11/12, 133–154.

Diesfeldt, H. F. A. (1989). Semantic impairment in senile dementia of Alzheimer type. *Aphasiology, 3*(1), 41–54.

Folstein, M. F., Folstein, S. E., & McHugh, P. R. (1975). Mini mental test. A practical method for grading the cognitive state of patients for the clinician. *Journal of Psychiatric Research, 12*, 189–198.

Fredericksen, C. H., Bracewell, R. J., Breuleux, A., & Renaud, A. (1990). The cognitive representation and processing of discourse: Function and dysfunction. In Y. Joanette & H. H. Brownell (Eds.), *Discourse ability and brain damage. Theoretical and empirical perspectives*, (pp. 69–110), New York: Springer-Verlag.

Grafman, J., Thompson, K., Weingartner, H., Martinez, R., Lawlor, B.A., & Sunderland, T. (1989, July). *Script generation as an indicator of knowledge representation in patients with Alzheimer's disease*. Paper presented at the International Neuropsychology Society, Anvers, Belgium.

Habib, M., & Assal, G. (1991). Aphasie progressive primaire et syndromes apparentés. In M. Habib, Y. Joanette, & M. Puel (Eds.), *Démences et syndromes démentiels. Approche neuropsychologique*, (pp. 109–123). Paris: Masson.

Hart, S., Smith, C. M., & Swash, M. (1988). Word fluency in patients with early dementia of Alzheimer type. *British Journal of Clinical Psychology, 27*, 115–24.

Hier, D. B., Hagenlocker, K., & Shindler, A. G. (1985). Language disintegration in dementia: Effects of etiology and severity. *Brain and Language, 25*, 117–131.

Irigaray, L. (1973). *Le langage des déments*. The Hague: Mouton.

Joanette, Y., Ska, B., Poissant, A., & Béland, R. (1992). Neuropsychological aspects of Alzheimer's disease: Evidence for inter- and intra-function heterogeneity. In F. Boller, F. Forette, Z. Kachaturian, M. Poncet, & Y. Christen (Eds.), *Heterogeneity of Alzheimer's disease*. (pp. 33–42). Berlin: Springer-Verlag.

Lecours, A. R., & Lhermitte, F. (1977). *L'Aphasie*. Montréal: Flammarion Médecine-Sciences and Les Presses de l'Université de Montréal.

Martin, A., Brouwers, P., Lalorde, F., Cox, C., Teleska, P., & Fedio, P. (1986). Towards a behavioural typology of Alzheimer's patients. *Journal of Clinical and Experimental Neuropsychology, 8*, 594–610.

Murdoch, B.E., & Chenery, H.J. (1987). Language disorders in dementia of the Alzheimer type. *Brain and Language, 31*, 122–137.

Nespoulous, J. L. (1980a). De deux comportements verbaux de base: Référentiel vs. modalisateur. De leur dissociation dans le discours aphasique. *Cahiers de Psychologie, 23*, 195–210.

Nespoulous, J.L. (1980b). Du trait au discours: Les différents niveaux de structuration du langage et leur atteinte chez les aphasiques. *Grammatica, VII*, (1), 1–36.

Puel, M., Démonet, J. F., Cardebat, D., Bonafé, A., Gazounaud, J., Guiraud-Chaumeil, B., & Rascol, A. (1984). Aphasies sous-corticales. Etude neurolinguistique avec scanner X de 25 cas. *Revue Neurologique, 140*, 695–710.

Reisberg, B., Ferris, S. H., Mony, D., De Leon, J., & Crook, T. (1982). The global deterioration scale for assessment of primary degenerative dementia. *American Journal of Psychiatry, 139*, 1136–1139.

Schwartz, M. F., Marin, O. S. M., & Saffran, E. M. (1979). Dissociations of language function in dementia: A case study. *Brain and Language, 7*, 277–306.

Smith, R. S., Murdoch, B. E., & Chenery, H. J. (1989). Semantic abilities in dementia of the Alzheimer type. *Brain and Language, 36*, 314–324.

Ulatowska, H. K. , Allard, L., Donnell, A., Bristow, J., Haynes, S. M., Flower, A., & North, A. J. (1991). Discourse performance in subjects with dementia of the Alzheimer type. In H. A. Whitaker (Ed.), *Neuropsychological studies of non-focal brain damage: Trauma and dementia* (pp. 108–131). New York: Spinger-Verlag.

van Dijk, T. A. (1977). *Text and context. Explorations in the semantics and pragmatics of discourse*. London: Longman.

Index

Aesop's Fables, 171–189
Age-associated memory impairment (AAMI), 84
Alzheimer's disease (AD)
　assessment, 79, 84, 91, 94–97
　discourse, narrative, 317–331
　discourse patterns, 198–203
　formal level analysis, 322–323, 326
　macrolinguistic discourse, 204
　macrostructure, 321, 327
　memory, semantic, 300
　microlinguistic discourse, 204
　narrative schema, 299–313
　pragmatic analysis, 323–324, 328
　relevancy versus irrelevancy, 310-311, 304–305
　and script, 300–302, 308–310
　sequencing, 305, 308, 310
Aphasia, 151–168. *See also* Left hemisphere-damaged (LHD)
　assessment, 178–179
　attentional skills, 231–232
　Boston Diagnostic Aphasia Examination (BDAE), 178–179
　closed head injury (CHI), 199–203
　comprehension studies, early, 153
　directness, 160–165
　discourse patterns, 198–203
　fluent, 198–203
　formal level analysis, 326–327
　inference, 182, 232–234
　linguistic context, 156–158
　macrostructure, 222–224, 327
　Polish-speaking, 171–187
　pragmatic analysis, 328
　prediction, contextual, 215–216, 218
　redundancy, contextual, 218
　representation, mental, 158–160
　salience, 160–165
　semantic processing
　　context, 218–221

　speech rate and comprehension, 165–167
　stroke, 208
　Token Test, 154–155, 156
Assessment. *See also* Imaging
　Alzheimer's disease (AD), 79, 84, 91, 94–97
　Boston Diagnostic Aphasia Examination (BDAE), 166–167, 178–179, 198, 286
　cerebral infarct, 84
　computed tomography (CT), 255
　design, intraindividual, 85–90
　Dixon research stories (DHH), 94–97
　electroencephalogram (EEG), 255
　Huntington's disease, 79
　intraindividual, 79–86
　Mini Mental State, 255
　multiple sclerosis, 79
　Ravens Coloured Progressive Matrices Test, 179
　Reading Span Test, 106
　Token Test, 154–155, 156, 166
　variability, intraindividual, 82–85
　Wechsler Adult Intelligence Scale-Revised (WAIS-R)
　　Picture Arrangement subtest, 179
　Wechsler Memory Scale-Revised Logical Memory (LM), 79–80, 84, 85, 94–97
　Wisconsin Card Sorting Test, 111

Boston Diagnostic Aphasia Examination (BDAE), 198, 286
　aphasia, 166–167, 178–179
Broca's aphasia
　contextual prediction, 216

Centering theory, discourse, 36–43
Central nervous system (CNS)
  disorders. *See* Alzheimer's
  disease (AD); Closed head
  injury (CHI)
Closed head injury (CHI), 199–203
Comprehension. *See also* Salience
  and aging, 106–112
  causal networks, 9–11
  scene schemata, 8
  scripts, 8

Directness
  aphasia, 160–165
  right hemisphere-damaged (RHD),
    161–165
Discourse, 23–43. *See also* Narrative;
    Text
  and aging, 203–205
    comprehension, 106–112
    macrolinguistic, 203–205
    microlinguistic, 203–205
  Alzheimer's disease (AD), 198–203
    317–331
  aphasia, fluent, 198–203
  Centering theory, 36–43
  Churchland theory, 136, 137
  comprehension/aging, 106–112
  comprehension studies, 151–153
  co-reference, 34
  discourse purpose (DP), 29–30
  discourse segment purposes
    (DSPs), 29–30
  experimental tests, centering
    theory, 38–41
  French, longitudinal studies,
    120–121
  Given-New Strategy/language
    comprehension, 35
  global structure, 24–33
  Grosz and Sidner theory, 29–32,
    33
  inference, 34–35
  intentional structure, 29–31
  Kintsch and van Dijk model,
    28–29, 32–33, 34, 105, 136,
    137–139, 240–242

macrolinguistic ability, 199–200,
  202–203
macrostructure, 28, 138, 143–144, 241
memory, short-term, 34
and memory, working, 105–112
memory, working/aging, 106–112
microlinguistic ability, 199,
  202–203
microstructure, 28, 138
mind-brain puzzle, 137
monitoring, 246–267
Montreal Study, Syntactic
  complexity, 117–123
neuropsychology/aging, 135–145
patterns
  brain-damaged adults, 198–203
Philadelphia longitudinal study,
  116–117, 123–128
processing, 135–145, 240–242
production
  right hemisphere-damaged
    (RHD), 205–208
pronoun
  interpretation, 36
  memory/aging, 106–107
  reference, 35–36
right hemisphere-damaged (RHD),
  205–208, 239–270
schemata, 241–242
Single Photon Emission
  Tomography (SPECT), 135
speech rate and brain-damaged
  listener comprehension,
  165–167
structure, local, 34–43
structure and brain-damaged
  listener comprehension,
  160–165

Fable, 171–190
  inference, 182
  metis, 174, 184–186
  neurolinguistics, 171–172
  Old Woman and Doctor, 190
  Raven and Fox, 189
  Raven and Pigeons, 189
  semiotics, 171–172

structural features, 173–174
text transformation tasks,
  175–177
Two Donkeys, 189–190
French
  longitudinal studies, 130–131

Given-New Strategy/language
  comprehension, 35
Grammar, story, 1–8, 25–29
  encoding processes, 5–6
  memorization, 6
  schema, 4–5, 27

Huntington's disease
  assessment, 79

Imaging
  comprehension, language, 137
  memorization, 137
  positron emission tomography
    (PET), 137
  Single Photon Emission
    Tomography (SPECT), 135,
    137, 139–141
Inference
  discourse, 34–35
  narrative, 232–234
  right hemisphere-damaged (RHD),
    244–245, 259–265, 268–269, 286

Kintsch and van Dijk model, 11–15,
  17–18, 28–29, 32–33, 34, 105,
  136, 137–139, 240–242

Left hemisphere-damaged (LHD), 48
  208. *See also* Aphasia
  discourse patterns, 198–203
  narrative comprehension, 224–229
  narrative processing, 221–222
  neurosemiotics, 69–70
  text processing, 66–68
  thematic influence, 229–230
  Token Test, 154–155
  world knowledge modeling, 68
Lesions, cerebrovascular, 198–203
LINGQUEST analysis program, 128

Macrostructure
  discourse, 28, 241
  fable, 179
  narrative, 17–18
  right hemisphere-damaged (RHD)
    230–231, 284–288
Memory
  age-associated memory
    impairment (AAMI), 84
  intraindividual change, typical
    aging, 77–98
  qualitative differences/aging,
    103–112
  short-term. *See also* Memory,
    working
    discourse, 34
    narrative comprehension, 11–12
  working. *See also* Memory,
    short-term
    models, 103–105
Microstructure
  discourse, 28
  narrative, 17–18
Mini Mental State, 255
Modeling
  world knowledge
    left hemisphere-damaged
      (LHD), 68
    right hemisphere-damaged
      (RHD), 68
Multiple sclerosis
  assessment, 79

Narrative, 1–18. *See also* Discourse;
  Text
  Alzheimer's disease (AD), 317–331
  attentional skills, 231–232
  causal networks, 9–11
  comprehension, 213–234
    left hemisphere-damaged
      (LHD), 224–229
    right hemisphere-damaged
      (RHD), 224–229
  conceptual level, 16–17
  content, 8–11
  contextual influences, 214–221
  encoding processes, 5–6

Narrative *(continued)*
  expressive deficits, 279–293
  inference, 232–234
  Kintsch and van Dijk model,
    11–15, 17–18
  macroprocessing, 14, 15
  macrostructure, 17–18, 222–224
  memorization, 6
  memory, short-term, 11–12
  mental model, 11–15
  microprocessing, 12–14, 15
  microstructural, 17–18
  prediction, 215–217
  processes, 11–15
  redundancy, 217–218
  scene schemata, 8
  schema, 4–5
    Alzheimer's disease (AD),
      299–313
  scripts, 8
  semantic processing, 218–221
  story grammars, 1–8
  superstructural, 17
  thematic influence, 222–224
Neurolinguistics
  fables, 171–172
Neurosemiotics, 47–70, 69–70

Peirce, Charles S.
  semiotic theory, 70
Polish
  aphasics, 171–187
Psycholinguistics
  text processing, 55–58

Rate, speech
  and comprehension, aphasia,
    165–167
  and comprehension, right
    hemisphere-damaged
    (RHD), 166–167
Ravens Coloured Progressive
  Matrices Test, 179
Reading Span Test, 106
Right hemisphere-damaged (RHD),
  208
  attention, 232, 291–292

  conceptual processing, 239–270
  directness, 161–165
  discourse behavior, 242–246
  discourse production, 205–208
  expressive deficits, 279–293
  inference, 233, 244–245, 259–265,
    268–269, 286, 290–291
  integration, element, 288–290
  macrolinguistic processes,
    205–208
  macrostructure, 230–231, 243–244,
    260–265, 268–269, 284–288
  microlinguistic processes,
    205–208
  microstructure, 243, 259–260,
    268
  narrative comprehension, 224–229
  narrative processing, 221–222
  neurosemiotics, 69–70
  recall, 258–259
  reduced efficiency, 283–284
  representation, mental, 159–160
  salience, 161–165
  schema (frame) processing,
    245
  and speech rate, 165–167
  text processing, 48–50, 58–60,
    64–65, 66–68
  thematic influence, 229–230
  Token Test, 154–155
  world knowledge modeling, 68

Salience. *See also* Comprehension
  aphasia, 160–165
  right hemisphere-damaged (RHD)
    161–165
Schemata
  fable, 179
Semiotics. *See also* Neurosemiotics
  fables, 171–172
  neurosemiotics, 69–70
  Peirce, Charles S. theory, 70
  and verbal texts, 51
Single Photon Emission Tomograph
  (SPECT), 135, 137,
  139–141
Sociolinguistics, 115–129

Story
  grammar, 1–8, 25–29
    schema, 27
  schema, 4–5

Text. *See also* Discourse; Narrative
  definitions, 50–53
  linguistics, 53–55
  processing
    hemispheric influence, 66–68
    left hemisphere-damaged
      (LHD), 66–68
    neuropsychology, 58–60
    psycholinguistics, 55–58
    right hemisphere-damaged (RHD),
      48–50, 58–60, 64–65, 66–68
  recall. *See also* Memory

Token Test, 154–155
  aphasia, 166
  left hemisphere-damaged (LHD),
    154–155
  right hemisphere-damaged (RHD),
    154–155
  speech rate, 166
Token test
  aphasia, 156

Wechsler Adult Intelligence
    Scale-Revised (WAIS-R),
    179
Wechsler Memory Scale-Revised
    Logical Memory (LM),
    79–80, 84, 85, 94–97
Wisconsin Card Sorting Test, 111